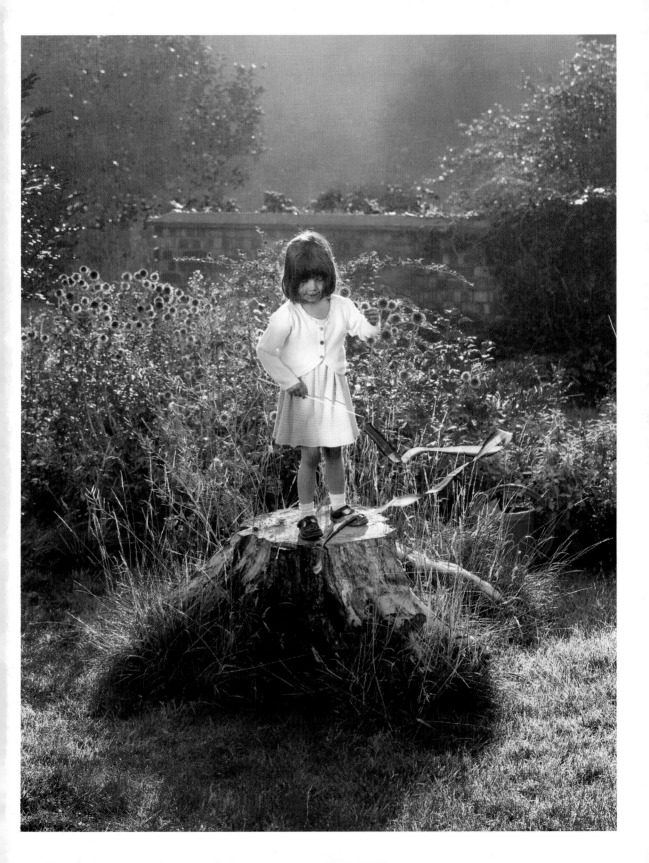

For P-J, Iris & Chula xxx

Text and photographs copyright © 2016, 2017 by Arabella Carter-Johnson
Illustrations copyright © 2016, 2017 by Alice Tait

First published in Great Britain in 2016 by Penguin Books Ltd.

Skyhorse Publishing books may be purchased in bulk at special discounts for sales promotion, corporate gifts, fund-raising, or educational purposes. Special editions can also be created to specifications. For details, contact the Special Sales Department, Skyhorse Publishing, 307 West 36th Street, 11th Floor, New York, NY 10018 or info@skyhorsepublishing.com.

Skyhorse® and Skyhorse Publishing® are registered trademarks of Skyhorse Publishing, Inc.®, a Delaware corporation.

Visit our website at www.skyhorsepublishing.com.
10 9 8 7 6 5 4 3 2 1

Library of Congress Cataloging-in-Publication Data is available on file.

Cover design by Rain Saukas

Print ISBN: 978-1-5107-1978-1
Ebook ISBN: 978-1-5107-1980-4

Printed in China

Iris Grace

*How Thula the Cat Saved
a Little Girl and Her Family*

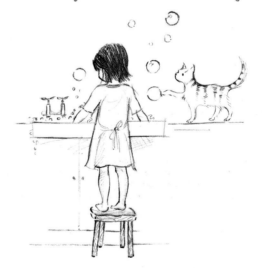

ARABELLA CARTER-JOHNSON

with illustrations by Alice Tait

Skyhorse Publishing

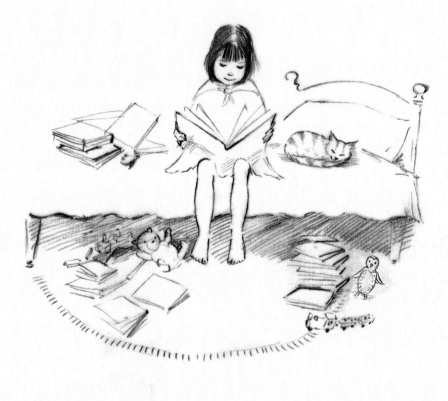

prologue

Iris's hand guided me back to the page of her book for the twentieth time. I repeated the words and she was content for a while. Her long dark eyelashes moved slowly down to rest upon her rosy cheeks . . . She was so close to falling asleep . . . but then she opened her eyes again, looking more awake than she had done for hours. My heart sank. It had been another long night of reading in bed. She didn't want me to leave her side or to stop reading and we were stuck in a cycle. Obsessions were friends and foes working with us and against us. Her desire to hear words, to read and to understand was a gift in her previously silent world. She still communicated mostly through body language but now she was becoming linked to these words. Powerful connections were forming that I didn't want to break. It was a driving force that needed to be balanced; her unique mind was busy, always busy and, while wonderful, that could be so destructive. As I stopped reading she was restless, fighting against her own tiredness and mine as I turned out the light once again. I hoped with everything I had that she would fall asleep. Days had merged into weeks then months and now years of sleep deprivation. How could we go on like this? Her beautiful face saddened me at times with those dark circles, and her behaviour was becoming more exaggerated and the intensity of her interests threatened to take over if she didn't get enough sleep. We would spiral down until we managed to have a good night, a break, until it started over again. My tiredness had become a part of me that I didn't like, slowing my mind as hers raced on and turning my thoughts to the darkness. I resented those who easily slipped into their dreams every night while we were still awake.

As Iris's frustrations mounted she started to cry, and her sobs filled the quiet room. I felt so hopeless as I held her close. Nothing seemed to comfort her apart from the book and I longed for some help, but she pushed away all who tried apart from me. The pressure of that was becoming too hard to bear. The highs and lows over the previous four years had been exhilarating but exhausting. Our minds were constantly trying to keep up and understand her world as she was learning to be in ours.

Downstairs, the credits at the end of the film were rolling and the fire in the wood-burning stove was almost out.

'What is it, Thula?'

My husband P-J looked at our new kitten who had suddenly got up off his lap. Her eyes focused towards the door and she had one foot raised, perfectly poised in the air. She was alert: something had grabbed her attention – cries that were undetectable to his ears were like sirens to hers. Then her legs were moving fast. Scooting round the corner, she flew up the stairs into Iris's bedroom and jumped on to the bed. She curled up next to Iris, ignored the crying and started grooming herself, licking her paws and rubbing them over her ears. Almost immediately, Iris's mood changed. She giggled at Thula's huge ears as they were folded down forward and then pinged back. The long tufts of black fur at the tips were backlit by the hallway, and her outline was adorable, with large ears set upon her tiny head. Fine longer hairs along her silhouette glowed in the darkness. The whiskers were next, and it was a performance like nothing I have seen before, combining comedy with beauty. Iris relaxed and put down her book. Seizing the opportunity, I slipped out of the room and waited at the bottom of the stairs, listening for the inevitable crying that would take me back to her side. There was silence: no bounces, no pages being turned, and no hums or cries.

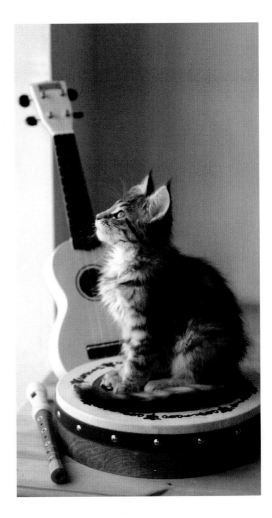

I waited till suspense got the better of me, then tiptoed to the door of her room and peeked in. Iris had fallen asleep with her kitten by her side and they were turned towards each other. Iris's hand rested on Thula's shoulders and I could hear a gentle purr. Their bodies mirrored one another with Thula's paws up against Iris's arm. Although still a tiny kitten and a new member of our family, Thula was already watching out for Iris, her faithful companion. She was a friend to me too, stepping in and helping when I needed it the most. I didn't even need to ask, she knew instinctively what to do and how to help. This magical kitten was changing our lives and this was just the beginning. She filled me with hope and made me smile as I thought about tomorrow.

•••

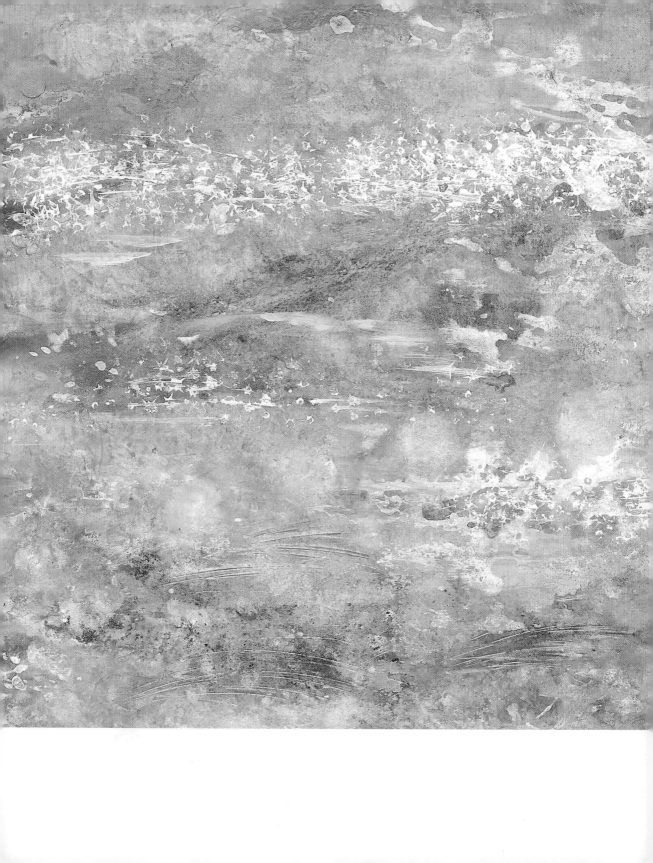

A-Where-Wa, watercolour, October 2013

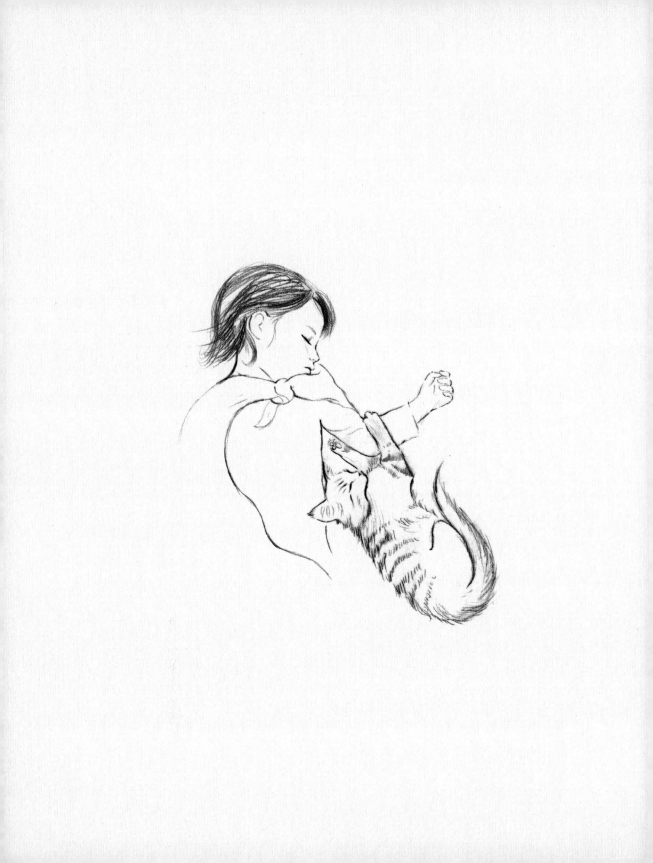

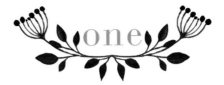

one

Outlined against the glass I saw a perfect cat shape through the clouds of dust: Meoska's silhouette. She was sitting neatly at the window with one paw up, trying to catch a butterfly on the other side. It was early summer in 2008 and my husband and I were making a start on our new project, restoring and redecorating a three-bedroomed house that we had bought in a village in the rolling hills of Leicestershire. Meoska and I had very different ideas about how to approach this project: like any Tonkinese she was letting me know what she thought of my DIY skills, regularly calling at me, nudging me and wrapping her small dark body and black tail round my legs to distract me. She abandoned the butterfly and pushed past my mug of half-drunk tea, almost knocking it over.

'Meoska, come here!' I whistled. She sat down and looked at me with her head on one side, her big blue eyes shining in the light and the cream fur on her chest puffed out and looking so beautiful. 'Why do you always go to P-J when he whistles and not me?'

She trotted over and brushed past my leg, making little meows. I could hear P-J laughing from the hallway. My mission was to rid our new home of brown. I never knew you could feel so strongly about a colour, but the floor-to-ceiling brown tiles in the kitchen were really starting to depress me. One by one I was knocking them off the walls. The brown wallpaper with swirls of green and the brown tiled carpet were like a heavy weight. I couldn't think properly in these dim surroundings and every surface was grubby with years of dirt and grime. Green was next on my list: the green bath, sink and loo, and the green-wallpapered room with the green door all had to go. I craved light and wondered if our decision to buy this house was a big mistake and that I was to blame.

'Look past all this,' I had said to P-J while he took his first look around the house a few months earlier. 'Imagine it once it's done – it will be beautiful, a brilliant family home. We could convert the barns, take down this tree, add an extension here . . .'

'Haven't we done enough of all that? I'm not sure if I want to go through it all again,' he had replied. He looked tired from his business trip and not in the right mood. He walked off around the garden, either to think alone or to shrug off his jet lag; I wasn't sure which.

We had returned that year from France, after a three-year adventure restoring an old farm in the Limousin, bringing back with us our cat who had arrived in a post van a year earlier. She was a beautiful cat, slender with a silky coat and dark points. We think she had hitchhiked her way to our farm, and unable to find her owner we took her in. She was a curious little character, almost dog-like, following us everywhere even when we went out on walks or rides on the horses. She came to P-J's whistle and entertained us as we worked on the farm. We would say she was our lucky mascot; whenever we felt low and tired by the physical work Meoska was there climbing up a tree or balancing on something with such a comical look on her face that it would make us laugh. She became a friend. It was at times a lonely life out in France. During the warmer months there was so much to do and we had visitors. But the winter was long and very hard: temperatures one year dropped to minus seventeen degrees Celsius and the snow was so deep that it made it almost impossible to work outside with the horses.

Meoska comforted me in those more isolating times and there was no way I would leave France without her.

While we were in France P-J was working in European sales for an American financial research company and so he was still busy with work when we returned to the UK. While I was hunting for a forever home he was taken up with business and had only just arrived back on a 'red-eye flight' from a trip to the US when I showed him the house. I had fallen in love with it and saw so much potential. Even the view, reminiscent of the Italian hills where we had once considered living, was hidden, waiting to be revealed. I felt at home and it was the first time I had felt that in a great many years.

•••

I couldn't really blame P-J for not being as enthusiastic as me about the new house: we had done so much work on our previous property and the thought of more was tiring to say the least. I could tell I was getting carried away but I didn't care; this was the one. When I had first walked around it on my own I had found a little nook behind the tall tree in the garden that gave me an idea of what the view could be like. There was so much to do within the house to make it a workable family home, but it was possible. It was totally rundown and pretty revolting in parts but that could all be remedied. We would have to complete the work over time and the prospect of that wasn't exactly appealing but with the prices so high this was the only option. I could visualize it all in my mind; it would be perfect.

From the moment I met P-J when I was just eighteen our travels abroad had begun. We'd been from Mexico to Venezuela, Italy and France, but now we were back, married and only a few miles from where I grew up. I knew this was where I wanted to start our family; we were home.

Tumpty Tum, watercolour, July 2014

I first met P-J at a twenty-first birthday party on Bastille Day. He had caught my attention as I drove up the tree-lined track to the party. Dressed as a musketeer, he had climbed over the post-and-rail fence and jumped off the other side. He looked confident as he brushed away his wavy dark brown hair from his face and placed a hat with a long feather on his head. My eyes followed him until he disappeared among the colourful crowd under the canvas marquee.

Inside, after chatting to the hosts I looked at the seating plan and made my way over to the table where I could leave my bag. There it was: the hat balancing on the corner of a wooden chair. Then the musketeer sat down beside where I stood.

'Hi, I'm P-J. I'm a good friend of Andy's sister. What's your name?' He shook my hand, looking at me with his bright blue eyes and I sat down next to him.

I wanted to know everything about this handsome musketeer and asked so many questions. He answered them all, looking at me intently with his kind eyes.

'I grew up on a farm in north Lincolnshire, but after university I went to work as an equity trader in London.'

'Is that what you do now?'

'Not any more. I left so that I could go travelling . . . Asia, Mexico . . .'

'My brother has been to Mexico. I would love to go.'

P-J and I had had similar childhoods in the countryside – he had a brother and a sister while I had a brother – but there was a striking difference of age, he was eleven years older than me, and I was so young, just starting my gap year.

'I'm meant to be doing a cookery course, but I'd love to travel afterwards,' I told him. 'I just don't know where to start.' He was so different from all the other men I had met: adventurous and exciting. We talked about the places I would like to see and my love of the arts, animals and cookery, and how I had wanted to be a sculptor but was also interested in photography. At first I didn't think of him romantically because of the age gap; I thought he was just being kind as I didn't know very many people at the party. But as we spent more time together that night I liked him more and wanted him to see me in that way. We danced together with a few interruptions from my protective brother. He spoke to P-J that night but I didn't need him to; I felt safe. When I think back to that evening I now realize how much it meant, what changes were on the horizon. At the time of course I was just enjoying myself and caught up in the moment. He kissed me by the fence where I had first seen him and he invited me to go travelling with him to Mexico. I have no answers as to why I didn't question it, why I was so calm about the idea of travelling with someone I had just met. My parents certainly weren't as happy.

'Darling, this isn't like you,' my mother said. 'I thought you wanted to do your cookery. You haven't mentioned wanting to go travelling before.'

'I'll still do the course and then go afterwards.'

'You'll be away for months. Can't you go with some of your girlfriends from school?'

I trust him; no we aren't going out; we're just friends . . . Even I could tell my answers weren't very convincing. They could tell how much I liked him and although he was a friend of a family friend there was a great deal of uncertainty about me leaving, but at eighteen years old and yearning to see the world they could see there wasn't much that would persuade me not to go.

So we went to Mexico in November 2000 and I got to see another world. I loved learning about another culture: the colours, landscapes, people and animals. Travelling with P-J was easy and we got on well as we drove around the country. We got into a flow: we seemed to want to move on from each place at the same time, having seen all we needed to and we had the same eagerness to see more further along our journey. He learnt about me – my eccentricities and my problems with low blood sugar and how I loved to plan, so he let me plot our adventures on the map and lead the way. He taught me to snorkel, how to use my lungs to stay down long enough to watch the colourful underwater world, to be suspended in the water and have perfect control through my own breath. He was patient with my sometimes overly ambitious ideas and swimming expeditions along the coast. I practised my photography and knew when we came back that I wanted to travel more. I had fallen in love with it all, and as my parents probably predicted, that included P-J.

In 2001 he was offered a job in Venezuela as a pensions and savings advisor to expats, so the year when I was just twenty years old we left on what was a much more challenging trip. A day after we arrived the country was on the brink of civil war and stayed unsettled for the entire year we were there. Our home was nestled into the foothills of the Andes, safely away from the unrest in Caracas. It was close to the university town of Merida and the countryside was breathtaking. We bought two stallions and rode them through the mountains, down into tropical valleys, through rivers, banana plantations and orange groves. We learnt so much out there, and had to do most things for ourselves; we even learnt how to shoe the horses. It showed me to be independent and strong, but like any incredible experience it didn't last for ever and our time in Venezuela came to an end. It was after my family came out to visit for my twenty-first birthday. We celebrated up high on Mount Bolivar and with a safari trip to Los Llanos, but immediately afterwards the embassy demanded that we all fly back on one of the last available flights home.

An idea had been forming in my mind for quite some time, inspired by my adventures in the Andes with our stallions; it was to run a horse-riding-holiday business in Europe. So in 2003 we went to France in our blue camper van and we found a farmhouse complete with two beautiful stone barns, a bread oven and an agricultural barn that we turned into an indoor riding school. Sixteen acres of grassland surrounded us, with oak woodlands in the distance and our very own stream. There was a network of bridleways that stretched out from the house through undulating countryside for miles on end, passing through woodlands, farms, fields and rivers. For three years we were really happy there. In between all of the work on the farm I practised my photography and started up a family-portrait business. It was in that house that P-J proposed and I said yes. But out on a ride one quiet Sunday everything changed.

'Isn't this just the best?' I said, turning round to speak to P-J. Tess, my thoroughbred mare, was striding ahead of Duo, a chestnut Arab gelding that P-J liked to ride.

'Couldn't be better!' P-J was looking to his right at the magnificent displays of blossom in the hedges and trees that lined the track.

We were deep in the countryside, miles away from anyone, when my horse, Tess, became spooked by something in the hedgeeow.

She leapt up in the air so fast, and with such power, that I was catapulted off and fell hard on my head. As my body hit the ground I lay unable to move or breathe, a sense of terror running through me. I was winded and my lungs wouldn't fill with the air I so badly needed and the pain in my chest was immense. My back felt like it was on fire and I could hardly move.

P-J was at my side: 'Can you get up?'

I shook my head. P-J looked worried but kept his voice calm for my sake. The reality of what was happening was sinking in for both of us. I couldn't move and we were in the middle of nowhere. It would take P-J hours to get help and I didn't know what I had done to myself. The pain was so bad I felt sure that I might have broken my back, and the winding made my chest unbearably painful.

'Whatever you do, don't move. I'll go and get help. I'll be back as soon as I can.'

Then he was out of sight. I could hear him running along the track but soon that faded and I was alone. Hours later I heard it: what sounded like a four-by-four vehicle coming my way. A team of French firefighters were soon surrounding me and lifted my body on to a stretcher. I couldn't have moved a millimetre even if I'd wanted to. We drove along the peaceful tracks back to the main road where I was transferred to an ambulance and given morphine, and after that it was like a dream: everyone trying to keep me awake and me struggling to make sense of the French voices.

The wait for an MRI was difficult: I was still in the stretcher and unable to feel if I could move my legs. They needed to establish if my fractured vertebra was stable and the thought of never walking again ran like fury in my mind. When the results came in, it was great news: the fracture was stable and I wouldn't need an operation, which was a massive relief. They predicted that by the end of the summer, after many months of recuperation and physiotherapy, I would be fine. However, the doctor said I would most probably never be able to ride again; the position of the fracture and the severe compression meant that the movement of the horse would cause me pain and I would probably get early arthritis. The news was a huge blow. I had loved horses and ridden since I was a child, and life without

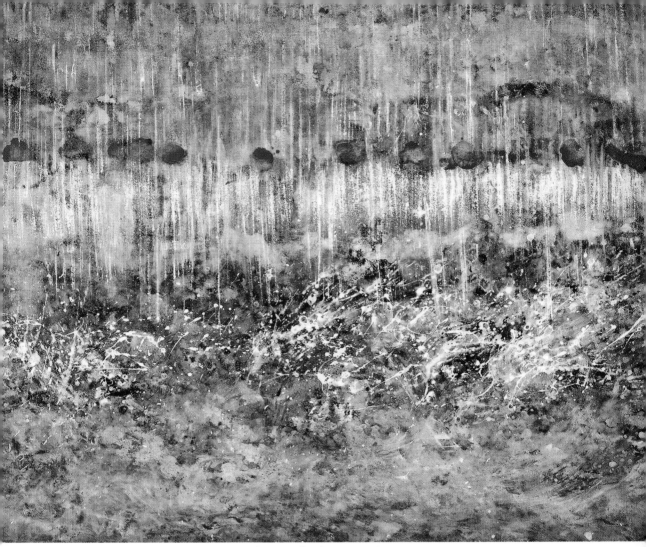

Anima, acrylic, August 2013

them seemed unbearable – all our plans and French dreams were based upon them. So many months later, with me still wearing an uncomfortable plastic body cast, we had to rethink our ideas for the horse-riding holidays. With the French doctors adamant I should never ride again and missing England and our families we decided to return to things that were familiar. By the autumn my cast was off and our property was on the market.

● ●

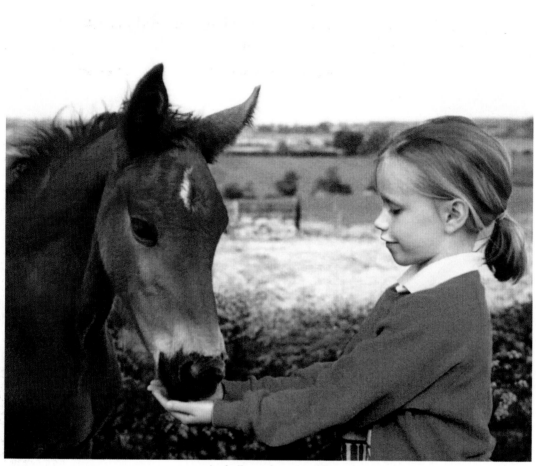

Arabella at six years old

We came back for our wedding in December. My mother had arranged it all as I was still recuperating. It was a dreamy English wedding in the evening by candlelight at an eighteenth-century house called Noseley Hall. My mother and I knew it well after many years of working there together creating floral displays for other people's weddings.

My parents were with me as I got ready in the bedrooms upstairs. 'The flares are lit!' my father said with a wide smile, slightly shaky after the ordeal of lighting over thirty flares that lined the pathway to the church in strong winds.

'That's great news. I thought you'd never be able to get them all done,' I said.

'You mean Arthur lit the flares with the blowtorch,' teased my mother. She knew my father would have needed the owner's help. 'Come on, you need to get ready. The photographer wants some photos of you both on the stairs.'

It was dark as I stepped outside arm in arm with my father and the cold air made me alive with excitement.

I think he was more nervous than I was. 'We are so proud of you,' he said, then he looked distracted.

Then I saw it: the noble thirteenth-century chapel glowing in the darkness.

It was pure romantic theatre; my mother had created the most enchanting scene. The chapel was filled with candles and flowers, the windowsills, pulpit, font and altar all bursting with beauty. Once we set foot inside I wasn't nervous at all: I felt at home and I adored every moment. Even when I forgot my left and right during the vows, to me it was perfect, and looking at P-J I knew he felt it too.

After the ceremony the evening reception seemed to fly by; before I knew it we were cutting the cake and the speeches were underway. My brother and father made a joint speech. James spoke of times in our childhood: 'Little Miss Doolittle, an independent spirit with her animals . . .' While laughter echoed around the room my father recounted how the wedding preparations began for him at my hen party. 'Picture seven gorgeous girls on a narrowboat covered in balloons and awash with champagne, with yours truly at the wheel. A shout from another boat: "How many birds have you got there, mate?" "Oh, just the seven today, thanks." Always the life and soul of a party, his charm and warmth created an atmosphere that was so joyous – the emotions always on the surface, immediate and true.

P-J carried the last bucket of broken brown tiles out of the kitchen through the front door and when he returned there was a great sense of satisfaction. We were getting there, slowly but surely.

'See, we'll get it done in no time. I always said this was the one,' P-J said with a huge teasing grin. He took off his dust-covered Panama hat and we both sat down at the kitchen table for a cup of tea with Meoska lying in front of the green Rayburn.

'So what's next on the list?'

'Steaming the wallpaper,' I replied, and went to the cupboard to bring out a rather peculiar-looking piece of kit: a mix between a kettle and an elephant.

'Right, unfortunately I have a very important conference call with somebody in America this afternoon and it might take a while . . .'

I knew what was going to happen: the steamer and I had become old friends in France. It's like when you first meet someone: you don't immediately get on and then you start to see their qualities. Well, I took the time to get to know this remarkably simple but oh-so-effective piece of DIY equipment, not sure P-J was ever going to.

As we talked about all the new plans for the house, possible changes, the garden and extension ideas, I realized how much I appreciated his positive outlook on life even though he did avoid some of the work. My arms gesticulated wildly as I tried to show P-J where the extension could go in our cramped little laundry at the back of the house. 'Sounds fantastic,' he said, 'let's go for it. Why don't you do some drawings of what it could be like?'

We didn't even have the money for it all yet but he never put me down or restricted my thoughts on what we could do. I was the planner, the worrier, always looking forward and rushing ahead, while he had a more relaxed approach, saying 'Let's deal with that if and when it happens' when I was leaping along thinking of all the potential problems.

In the following weeks our English village house slowly transformed room by room and P-J was busy making some alterations to the garden. The tall tree that had blocked so much light and covered our view was taken down branch by branch until all that was left was a tree stump that was the perfect seat to soak in the glorious view.

On our trips up and down the steep part of our garden we came up with another plan: sowing a wild-flower meadow in the orchard. We cleared strips of grass and prepared the soil, then sowed the seeds before the cold weather came. I couldn't wait to see the vibrant poppies in bloom, the chamomile, blue cornflowers, foxgloves and the cheerful ox-eye daisies. It would be a haven for birds, butterflies, dragonflies and bumblebees. Over by the hedge we would have red campion for a little pink among the grasses and corn marigold would add a touch of yellow. As I learnt about the grasses I started to love their names and their individual characters, which were adding a little fun into our orchard. Meadow foxtail with their tall flowering heads waving in the wind like cheeky foxes' brush tails and their light feathery seeds taking flight in the air as if by magic. Yorkshire fog, a tufted, grey-green downy grass with tightly packed flower heads that have a purple-red tinge to their tips.

Both the leaves and the flowers have a soft appearance that is so inviting to touch. What we didn't factor into our master plan was that it would take till mid-summer the following year for it all to cover over and bloom. Our orchard looked rather like a graveyard that winter and the following spring: not quite the idyll I had imagined. The impatient part of me couldn't help but feel disappointed, but nature has its own pace and will not be rushed, so with the saying 'all good things come to those who wait' in my mind I waited patiently.

The house was a continual work in progress but as soon as the old dining room was turned into a meeting and editing room for my wedding-photography business it was time for me to focus on my career. We had many more plans and ideas to improve our home, but for that to happen we needed the extra income. I wanted to update the profile photograph for my website, so I went into the local studio in town to get it done. It turned out that they had looked at my work before I came in and what I thought was going to be a portrait shoot turned into a job interview. A few weeks later I was the lead wedding photographer for a well-renowned portrait studio in town and wedding bookings were steadily coming in. The classic English countryside all around us is dotted with fine stately homes and private estates that very often open their doors for weddings and parties to help pay for their upkeep. So I captured couples' memorable days in these beautiful surroundings and, even better, with my mother already an established wedding florist, we were able to work together on many occasions.

It meant a great deal to both of us after so many years with oceans between us. I had worked alongside her before: when I was growing up I helped with the flower business and learnt how to arrange them. She would teach me along the way, saying the names of the flowers as we worked and telling me how to condition them. She would create arrangements for me to copy and step in if I was losing my way, but I never felt like she was telling me what to do. It felt more like suggestions: 'A little looser here, maybe more there. How does it look if you turn it this way?' She would talk about the flowers, their characters, what they needed, how best to use each one and when they were in season.

'Tulips,' she would say, carefully pulling the lower leaves from the stem, 'have soft stems.' She showed the bottom to me. 'At first glance they look strong and straight with an almost military feel but actually they respond better to gentle treatment. There's no point pushing them hard into the wet foam; they'll break. You need to create a small hole with a pencil, like this, see, and then slip them in.' She recut the bottom of another stem at an angle. 'This gives a better grip and also more surface area for them to drink.' Then slowly she pushed the tulip into the foam. 'In time they'll open but they do have a mind of their own, turning to find the sunshine, bending and curling as the petals open.' Without knowing it I learnt a great deal.

I loved how she adored horticulture. Flower magazines and books filled the bookshelves in our old playroom, and fresh flowers were always in vases on tables and windowsills. My childhood garden was at first glance a simple country garden, but each bed was beautifully thought out and the garden held many magical memories for all of us. It was opened once a year for charity and people would wander around its different 'rooms' and enjoy themselves immensely, as we did, in such colourful harmonious surroundings. I had my own part too, where I used to have a go at growing vegetables and I created a pond with my father. Really it was more like a puddle, but it was surprisingly full of wildlife. Even though it was filled in many years ago, frogs still return to the spot each year – the knowledge passed down through generations.

Meadow Foxtail, acrylic, June 2013

My mother's flower arrangements were always spectacular; she really understands proportion and never feels restricted by what others have done. Her displays were sometimes on a monumental scale and I would fill with pride as I saw the guests' reactions as I was photographing the weddings. People would gasp in delight as they came into the church or the marquee, and they were always a talking point. With her background as a set designer for the BBC, coupled with her love of flowers and English country gardens, it was a brilliant combination.

At first wedding photography was a nerve-racking job. I felt so much pressure, but the more I did the less intense that feeling became and I was able to enjoy it. It is, however, exhausting work being on your feet for a whole day and late into the night and running about, all the while trying to be discreet with an air of dignity and authority. Some of the weddings were unforgettable; the amount of time and thought that had gone into them astounded me and I made sure I captured every intricate detail. I liked to use natural light whenever I could and my favourite parts of the day were when I could just mingle, capturing those happy candid moments, all the laughter and joy that surrounds a couple's special day. I had to push myself to be confident for the large group photographs, with sometimes up to four hundred people staring at me while I got the shot of them all in front of a grand venue. It was a challenge for me, but adrenalin and my love of photography pulled me through.

Everything seemed to be slotting into place. It was a great deal of work and we would often take on too much but we both felt it was all coming together. We had talked about trying for a baby but with our move back to England the timing had never felt right. I was a nest-maker and needed to get everything prepared but I was feeling more settled and ready than I had before, so we decided that we were ready for the next chapter in our lives. I imagined us having a child together, a little boy or girl running through the meadow, learning to ride, enjoying the beautiful countryside that I had grown up in and loved. As we chatted in the kitchen about trying for a baby, with Meoska on my lap, we laughed about what she would think about the new addition, how much I wanted to see them playing together. P-J's thoughts were of adventures, travels in the future with his child, how much fun we would have exploring faraway places through new eyes. We were both very excited and it felt fantastic to be moving forward – a little scary of course but thrilling.

By the new year I was pregnant. We were delighted but tried to keep it a secret for as long as we could. But my sudden disinterest in a glass of wine at Sunday lunch with my parents gave us away in no time and my mother hugged me with such a big smile. Both our families were excited about the baby as it was their first grandchild. P-J was the first of three siblings to marry and it was the same for my side. I seemed to be swamped with hugs, all overjoyed at the thought of this new life coming into the family. My father is never one for holding in his emotions so I would suddenly be hugged or my hand squeezed as we took their dog for a walk up to an old farm where I used to ride as a child. He was so happy we were moving on to the next stage in our lives and excited to meet his first grandchild. Old clothes and toys from our childhoods were found and we started to prepare, buying all the things we needed. Our parents would chat about everything they would do with him or her as they grew up. My father wanted to go fishing, go on special holidays. My mother, who loved the mountains, wanted to go skiing, and P-J's mother wanted to go riding. All of them, of course, conveniently missing out the first five years and jumping to the fun bits. Even the topic of schools was discussed and researched. It was a busy time with my work too, with a full summer of weddings already booked in. Some were alarmingly close to my due date so I made plans, bringing in more help and putting back-up photographers on standby. As

I edited photographs during the week with Meoska purring on my lap I was very happy. My latest scan had showed that all was normal and fine with our baby girl and in between work I was getting her nursery ready.

Then one morning there was a knock at the door. The man on the doorstep was clearly upset and said that there was a cat out on the road: she had been hit, not by him but another driver who had driven off. Since we were the closest house he thought it might have been ours.

I looked out on to the road and saw her. Meoska was lying completely still. I ran over, took off my jumper and wrapped it round her, carrying her back towards the house. She was breathing, but only just. I grabbed my keys and put her on the front seat of the car and then ran back to the house, shouting upstairs to P-J who was in his office. I caught a glimpse of him at the door as I turned out on to the road, but there was no time to say anything else.

As I made my way to the vets I knew we were losing her. I could feel myself starting to lose control as tears ran down my cheeks. She died in my arms before we even got to the surgery.

I couldn't believe she had gone. I wanted her to get up and shake it off, to hear her meow and for her to nuzzle into me. I felt like my heart was breaking. This little soul had been there for me through the hardest of times, my best friend. I had never been lonely with her there and our house felt empty without her. We buried her in the orchard and for many weeks I sat in the garden under the apple trees thinking of her. All those pictures I held in my mind of Meoska playing with our child hurt terribly; the thought that they were no longer possible was like an ache.

I don't know if it was my hormones or the sudden loss of my friend, but I found it hard to recover from that day. Meoska had become so much a part of our family and I missed her dreadfully. I started to struggle with many aspects to do with my pregnancy, mainly an increasing fear about the birth.

The closer we got to my due date the more I feared hospitals. I had enquired about a home birth but was told they couldn't guarantee it. Then, when I visited the wards they were so chaotic and busy. The noise and constantly changing staff unnerved me and I was starting to lose my confidence. Everything that surrounded birth began to bring a sense of dread. My heart would beat hard and I would feel like I was suffocating every time I thought of the hospital.

So I researched. I wanted to find a private midwife who could help me regain my confidence and help make this a positive experience. Then I found Sue, the most kind-hearted and motherly midwife who did that and more; she became a friend and helped me in so many ways. Her experience and time with me certainly shaped what was to come. She taught me to be patient and to keep trying, and above all to trust my body and my instincts. After our sessions I would feel empowered and no longer scared. I began to feel what our baby was going to be like, getting a sense of her character. She would always move when music was played and she loved jazz the most. I felt calm in nature and spent a great deal of my spare time out on walks with P-J. We left from the back of our house, through the orchard, over the fence and along the footpaths to the gorse-covered hill. From this hill you can see for miles, to our local town and beyond. We talked about what we thought she was going to be like. I had a strong sense that our child would be unique in some way and wanted to find a special name for her. I know everyone probably thinks this, so maybe my feeling was completely normal, but sometimes I wonder if that feeling was a sign, that my body understood her better than any test ever could.

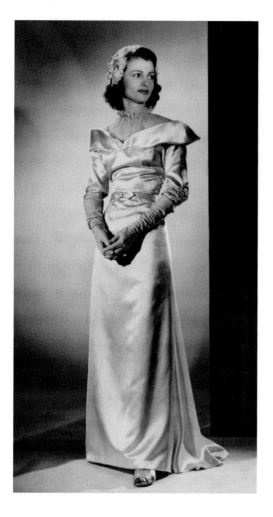

I never got to meet my maternal grandmother Iris; she had passed away while my mother was pregnant with me. My family would talk about her with such affection and no one could say her name without smiling. She became this ethereal figure in my childhood with her portrait at the top of the stairs and photographs of her around the house. To me she seemed beautiful inside and out. I was enchanted by her wide eyes, auburn hair and graceful pose. I got to know her through her belongings: china ornaments, jewellery, embroidery she had worked on, art she had created, and her clothes that I wore, which had come back into fashion. It's amazing how much you can sense from someone's belongings, seeing what they loved and enjoyed. It wasn't the same as knowing her, but these things meant a great deal to me. Her gentleness and love of art and nature was passed down to my mother and then to me. So when we were thinking about naming our baby girl, Iris was my first choice, and Grace was another favourite that both P-J and I loved, for no other reason than its elegance and beauty.

Can you hear me, Iris? I hope you know my voice by now. I can't wait to hear your voice and to know how you feel and what you think. I am waiting patiently to meet you, feeling more excited as each day passes. This evening I could feel you dancing to the music. You gave me energy when I needed it the most. I was photographing my last wedding of the summer and as the band played you kicked in time to the beat. How could I feel tired with you dancing inside me? You made me forget my aching body and the long hot day in the sun. Music is special to you, isn't it? I have a feeling it will give you so much comfort and joy.

You will need to be patient with me as I learn with you and we work all this out together. Let's stick together and keep your grandmother's words in our minds: 'It will pass. This is just one stage and it won't last for ever.' This will give us strength in those harder times. No matter what, I want you to know how much we love you and that you are not alone. So now we wait. We are ready and as prepared as we can be. You will know when it is time.

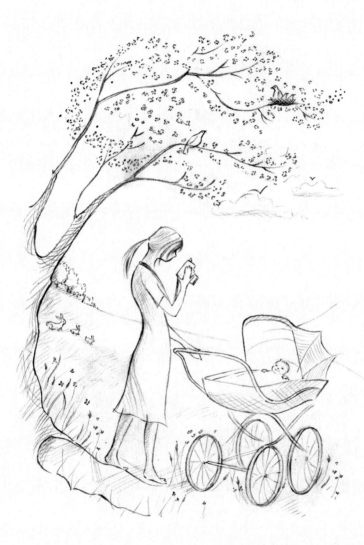

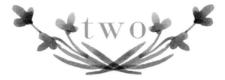

two

She tucked her little body against mine. Right away she seemed to fit, finding a position that suited and that was the one she was going to stick to, resting against my body upright with her head on my shoulder.

'You did it!' P-J said and then kissed me, smiling and holding on to Iris's tiny hand. She had lots of dark brown hair and I held her close for as long as I could in the kitchen. The day to meet our little Iris Grace had come sooner than expected. She was born a few weeks early in September 2009 at 7 pounds 3.5 ounces with brown hair and blue eyes. I will not pretend it was easy, but I never regretted the decision to have a home birth, not for one second. My midwife was incredible and I trusted her completely. I was never frightened or worried, but I did need space and quiet. I moved around the house, into the pool, out of the pool, up the stairs, down the stairs, lying quietly alone. I wanted the music on, then I needed it off. I followed how I felt and what my body was asking for and everybody tried their best to keep up with my wishes. I know it can't have been easy for my midwife, the second midwife and P-J who were up with me all through the night. There were moments when they were worried as I hadn't eaten for so long and I was exhausted, but I didn't want to eat – I couldn't. I just wanted to zone out at times and let my body rest with no interference, summoning the energy that I needed.

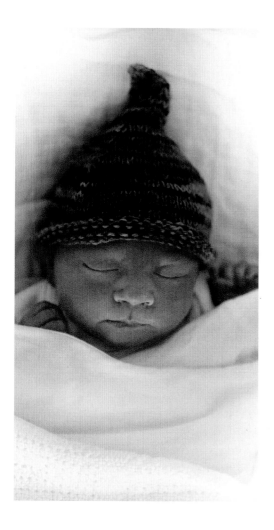

While I was with the midwife P-J had Iris in his arms and I shall never forget the look on his face: it was as though the two of them were in their own bubble. When I shut my eyes I could hear P-J whispering.

'Hello. How are you doing, Iris? How cool are you! You are simply wonderful and everything is going to be great. Your mummy is here; she will be fine soon. Don't you worry, little Iris, I'm going to keep you safe. Everything is going to be OK. We are going to have the most wonderful adventures in life – you just wait and see.'

I rested until I had the energy to move into the next room and on to the sofa. My comfortable nest, complete with blankets, tea, treacle cake and Iris in my arms, provided so much comfort. I laughed at the tiny hat that was a gift from the midwife. My little elf was content. She slept and I rested, then it was time for her first visitors, her delighted grandparents.

My father took Iris in his arms and it was clear that Iris made quite an impression on him immediately. He settled in an armchair with my mother kneeling at his side and they both looked at Iris adoringly and they couldn't stop smiling. 'Careful of her head; support her here,' my mother said as he passed Iris across for her to have a cuddle. It was a wonderful feeling looking at my parents holding their first grandchild. I knew that no matter what happened she would be loved by her family that surrounded her.

After Christmas, which was magical and totally exhausting all at the same time, we had Iris's christening to plan. But Iris's sleeping patterns were becoming less predictable and much harder to manage. As each week went by, that side of life gradually slipped out of control. Just getting her to sleep in the evenings was a mission; she would only settle with me and on my shoulder while I walked around listening to music, or rest on me in the rocking chair. Keeping her asleep also seemed impossible. She would wake after an hour or two and cry until she had the warmth of my shoulder again and the movement coupled with music. It was an exhausting process because by the time I got to sleep after settling her it seemed like I was being woken again. I couldn't believe my luck when Iris fell asleep in her christening gown as we walked with her to the church from my parents' house. She was tired from a restless night and for once that had worked in my favour: she slept peacefully for the whole ceremony until it was time for her part when she bravely let the vicar splash her forehead.

Afterwards close family and friends all came back to my parents' house opposite the church to have some lunch. Iris was uncomfortable so I changed her into some of her soft clothes but still she didn't like being held by anyone else apart from a few key members of the family. She loved the song 'She'll Be Coming 'Round the Mountain' – it was the only thing that seemed to keep her calm while she was downstairs with everyone around – so we all sang that to her, and then she needed to have some space away from the hubbub. The more I saw her act like this around others the more I would worry. She didn't enjoy company like other children and babies that I had photographed. She was very interactive at times with us and could hold eye contact – she laughed and smiled, even tried to copy – but these skills seemed so inconsistent, almost in waves of being social and then distant. At those times I felt like she was drifting away. Like in a daydream but more powerful, she would have a sad glazed look in her eyes and didn't seem to notice what was happening right in front of her. There were times when we would worry that she couldn't hear us properly because she didn't react to sudden noises or if we came into the room, but again that was so inconsistent that it really didn't give us anything concrete to go on. When I expressed my concerns to doctors I was told at six months it was far too early to be concerned and that she was a happy, healthy baby. I was just tired from the lack of sleep that all parents experience and there was no need to worry. My anxieties eased with these words and I felt a little embarrassed for even bringing it up. With so little sleep you start to doubt every move you make and the assurance put my mind at rest for a while.

By around seven months all her dark brown hair had fallen out and was replaced with a much lighter blondish brown. By eight months she had said 'dada' and was using various sounds. She was hitting all the various milestones, maybe a little off on some, but nothing that would cause alarm. However, the sleep issues continued.

'Tomorrow will be better,' I whispered to Iris, her body clinging to mine as we rocked in the chair. We had been through a succession of long nights and difficult days for weeks. The sleep deprivation was really starting to take its toll and many times out in the car I had to stop because my eyes hurt so badly from the light. I had even resorted to having both sun visors down and wearing two pairs of sunglasses. It attracted strange looks but I was beyond caring. I would open the window for fresh air,

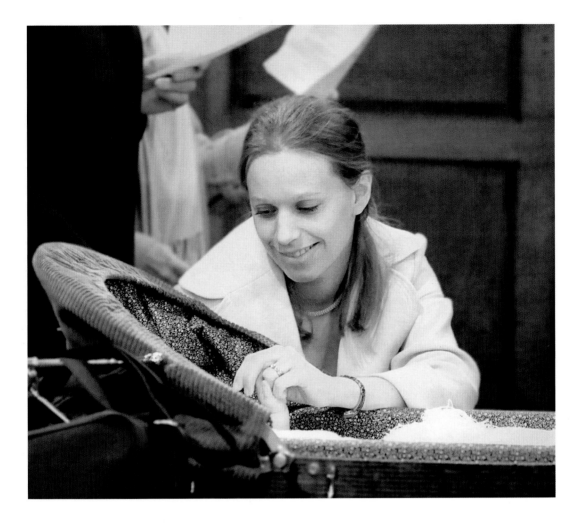

paranoid that I was going to fall asleep at the wheel.

Hour after hour passed and Iris fought sleep like a night warrior, determined with every part of her body to stay awake as I willed my body to stay awake for her. During the day I had become used to the dizzy spells and the nausea brought on by what felt like a permanent and extreme state of no sleep. But as I rocked Iris to her favourite piano music I realized that this could not go on for ever. Something had to change because all our methods

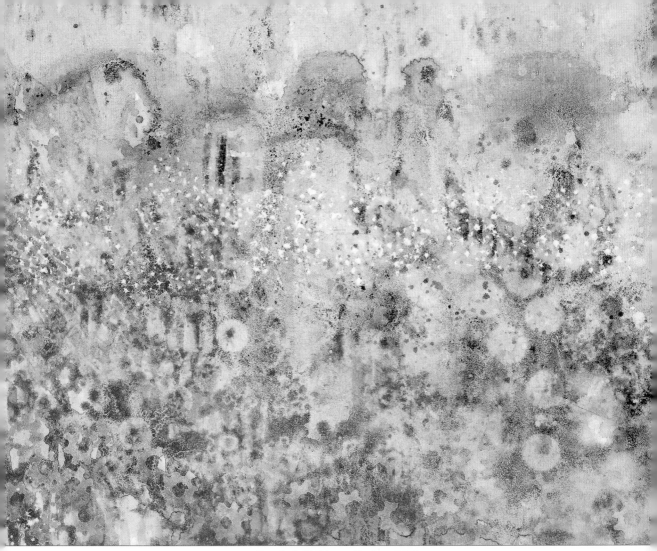

Tuesday's Child, acrylic, June 2013

were failing. I was only surviving because of my support network: my wonderful mother dropped off cooked meals and sandwiches almost daily and P-J did trips to the shops while I edited wedding photographs and sent out quotes, trying to get some work done in the few precious hours while Iris was asleep during the day.

Iris's body slumped across to one side and I felt her breathing becoming more even; she was finally drifting off to sleep. Now the transfer: a delicate operation. First, rising from the comfort of the rocking chair without the dreaded squeak; moving her body in a smooth motion over to the French bed; and then rolling her over on to her side – all the while keeping her blanket over her. I waited for a little while longer, putting off this defining moment. I kissed her and then started to cry, trying not to but unable to control it. Why was this so hard? Why couldn't she sleep? I knew this wasn't normal. This wasn't what everyone else was going through with their children. I knew something was wrong, and the desperate hopelessness of the unknown hurt from the inside out. It ached. We were spiralling downwards. While everyone else seemed to be rising from the newborn sleep-deprived days, we were sinking. I could hear my mother's voice in my head: 'It will pass. This is just a phase – one stage and before you know it things will have moved on.' Then my own voice screaming in my mind: 'It isn't passing! What am I doing wrong?'

•••

After Iris's first birthday her behaviour seemed to become more exaggerated and her sleep problems were increasingly noticeable. Her interest in books was intense. Before she could even turn the pages properly with her fingers she was using her feet lying on her back. She would spend hours looking at her books in this way and then once she had full control of her fingers she was fully immersed. If she was looking at her books, a whole funfair could be going on and she wouldn't even look up. It was as if she was linked, connected in some way that was so powerful that it created an impenetrable orb around her.

One morning I was editing photographs with Iris playing in my office. The clock on my computer told me it was time for Iris to have a feed. It made me think. Iris had been content playing with books on my office floor for hours with unbroken focus, looking at each page, turning them with her feet and hands. My first feeling was incredible pride that my baby had such amazing concentration skills that would rival a six-year-old, but then the realization came that this wasn't a six-year-old, it was my baby girl.

Suddenly it felt like I could hear everything: the hum from the computer, Iris turning the pages, my own heart. It was beating fast and I felt strangely cold: something wasn't right here. Iris hadn't wanted my attention all morning. I had been singing nursery rhymes while I worked and she had been so happy looking at the books that it hadn't occurred to me that she didn't seem to mind if I was there or not. She was in her own world, a different world, consumed by the books and the colourful pages. She hardly ever made an attempt to talk any more. After her 'dada' at eight months old she had made a few other sounds, but since then she had been gradually more and more silent as the months passed. The lack of speech was frustrating as we knew she was capable of making the sounds; it was as if she had a complete lack of interest in doing so. I became very good at understanding Iris through her body language and by watching her eyes, which alleviated some of the frustrations. Well-meaning advice from others made me feel that it was my fault for doing too much for her, for anticipating her needs and wishes. When she wanted something she would try to get it herself but if it was out of reach I would help. But perhaps these were chances to try to get her to communicate verbally. What everyone else didn't see is that I had tried many times, but it would cause Iris so much distress that I was unable to handle in my sleep-deprived state. It's all too easy for others to see fragments of time and make judgements, but really it's

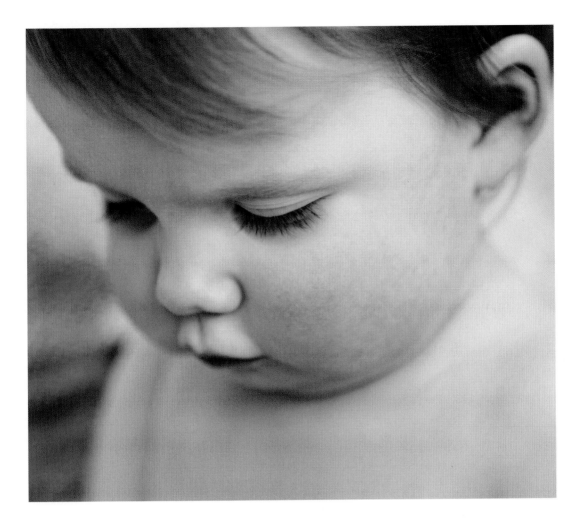

the parents who know. That uneasy feeling that I had all those months ago returned in a quick and powerful surge. What was happening to her?

From the age of four months Iris had had another pastime that she dearly loved as much as her books and that was Tom and Jerry. She would watch these cartoons for as long as she could. By the time she was over a year old we had the complete set of old Tom and Jerry cartoons. They gave her so much pleasure that

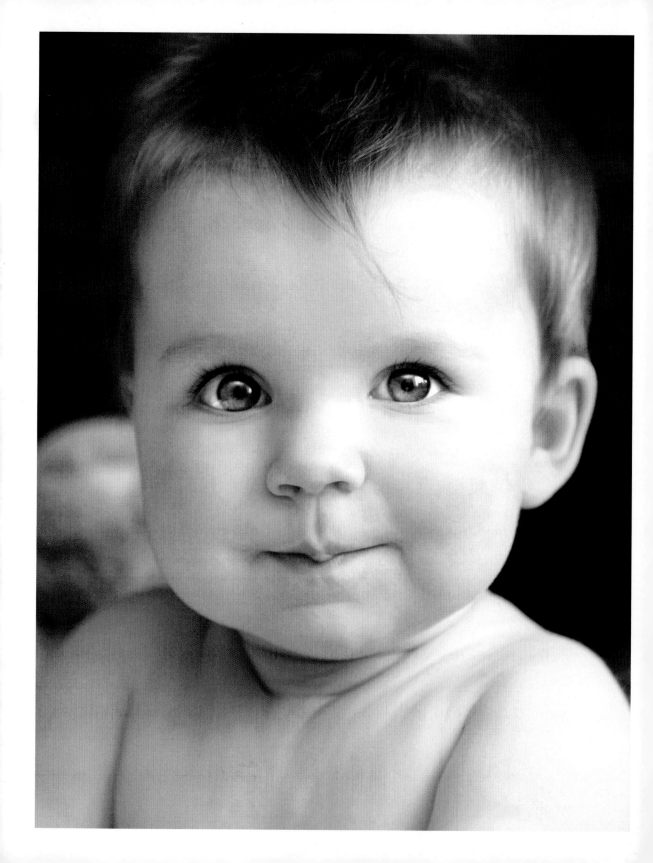

I didn't see any harm in it. I knew her gentle nature well enough to know that she wasn't going to take the cartoons literally, but many found her deep interest in something so specific worrying. She would laugh hysterically at the jokes and her legs and hands had a life of their own, completely connected to the action on the screen. It was almost as if the excitement was on a different level than we feel.

Music had a similar effect. While she listened to music her hands would be out in the air, her little fingers twitching, moving and feeling the music. It was as if her senses were heightened, so acutely at times that it was an electric state of euphoria. She was able to concentrate for hours at a time with unbroken focus and we saw the same reactions when she watched the wind in the trees, or other movements in water and nature. Watching her while she was like this was bewitching: a child so young connected in a way that we could only imagine. I had no idea what it meant or why it was happening, but we could see and feel that she was experiencing life on a different plane to us. Sometimes the profound way that she experienced the world was like a destructive force. In social situations, with all the chat and movement, she became either distant or distressed, crying uncontrollably, and if she wasn't removed from the situation she would quickly get very agitated and angry. Her attention to detail and her ability to see a vast amount in a short space of time was also troublesome at times. As soon as she came into a room she was able to take it all in and if I had moved a book or a toy from where she had last left it she would notice and became anxious. She looked to the place where the item once was and would make her way over to it, then putting her hand to the spot she would start to cry until it was back in its place. If she couldn't reach the item it would become even more confusing as she cried and got more wound up until I eventually figured out what had been moved. Certain items had to be left in their exact position on the floor; if you moved them even a centimetre, she would know and move them back. These distinct wishes weren't only limited to her toys and books; she was insistent on what clothing she could tolerate – soft cotton bodysuits, T-shirts and baggy comfortable bottoms were fine, anything with complicated buttons, zips, too much detail or labels were not. Tights, socks and shoes were like torture, and you could forget dresses. Most of the time when we were out people would mistake her for a boy, but that was the least of my worries.

The customary weeks for mothers filled with play dates and toddler groups came with heartbreak for us. I would bundle Iris's favourite toys and books into a bag, shutting my eyes and wishing that today, for once, our outing would go well, that Iris would enjoy herself like the other children could, and that she wouldn't hide away behind the piano lining up crayons in order. I would wish that I would be able to take my eyes off her and turn round and see her smiling. Oh how I would wish that, but no amount of wishing, crossing fingers or hope would change the outcome.

Instead, once again, I would find myself back in the car after another disastrous attempt at enjoying ourselves. Iris would get desperately distressed when a child came close to her and then spend her time hidden away under the piano, obsessing about a tiny mark on the carpet. I would have to take her home. How many times could I do this to her? She was only a year and a half old. One day, after a typically gruelling session, I made a decision. She obviously hated it and the experience was making me feel terrible. I promised her that I would stop; I would not make her feel like that again and that somehow we would figure this out. I thought about all the outings we had tried, how I had somehow in my sleep-deprived state been persuaded to sign up to a whole term of a baby gym, and how Iris was fixated upon anything but the fun equipment that was in front of her, how she would find minuscule imperfections in the play mats and with her face centimetres away from them inspecting them in great detail while the rest of the group circulated the room, having fun on the balance beams, slides and trampolines. When she wasn't obsessing over such minor details she was over by the tennis-court net, figuring out the intricate way the net was formed. She would do anything but be engaged in the group's activities. Circle time was a particularly tortuous affair that always ended in us leaving early, with Iris screaming down the corridor and out of the front doors of the building. Yet as soon as we were outside she would stop crying and peace resumed. She couldn't wait to return to the safety of our car and make her escape, and I was starting to feel the same way.

I couldn't bear the looks from the other parents – at first pitying glances and then frustration that we were disturbing the group. It was like being an outcast for something that I couldn't even name and didn't understand. All I knew was that we didn't fit. We didn't seem to fit in anywhere that was your typical toddler experience. Even the playground parks were arduous affairs. While other children happily slid down slides, were pushed on swings by their mothers, played in the sandpit or spun on the roundabout, Iris would be inspecting the nuts and bolts that held the playground equipment together. She had very little interest in being on the different apparatus: she was in pursuit of knowledge, wanting to find out how it all worked. Each time we visited the same routine would commence: she would return to the exact same pieces in the same order and work systematically around the park, gesturing to me where she would like to go to next. I did have some success with the swings but it had to be one particular swing and other mothers just didn't understand why it was so important for them to move their child on to the next one so Iris could use her favourite. There was a reason her attention was so fixed on that swing and it was a simple detail: the joins in the chain loops were smooth, whereas on the other swings they were rough, and Iris liked the smooth ones better

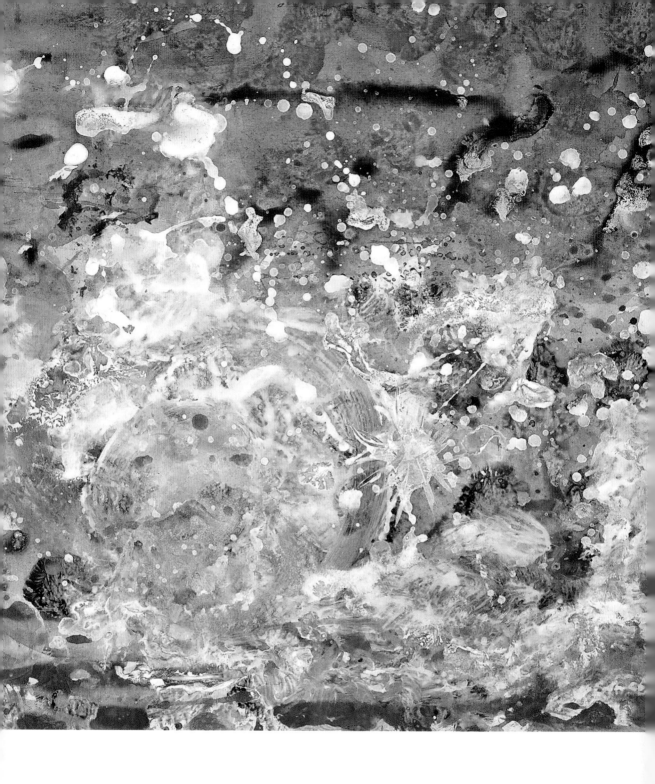

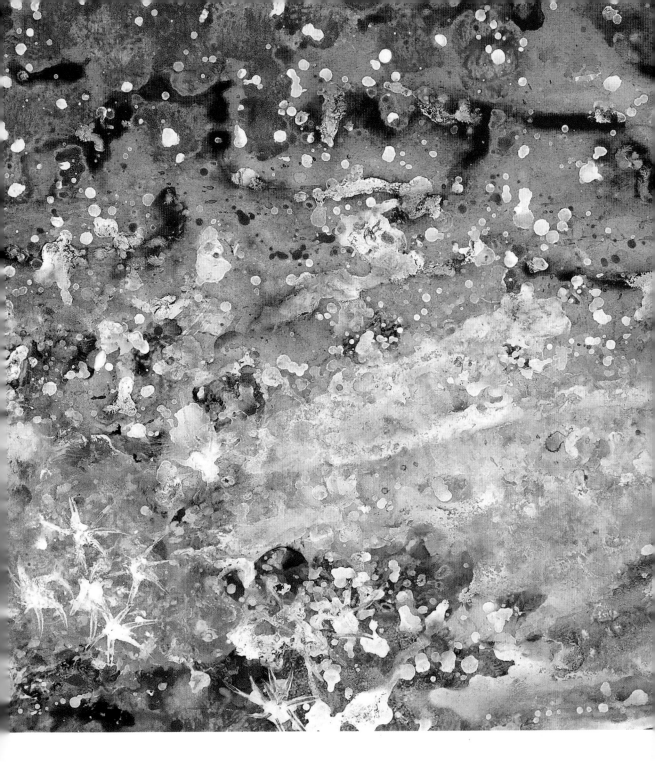

Music at Sunrise, acrylic, March 2013

against her skin. I began to take her to the park in less busy times to secure her swing and I found that she was more relaxed with fewer people around, so we did many early-morning visits to the park. Our only adversary at that time of day was the street cleaner that made its way through the park, but its presence was short-lived and Iris could see that it would be leaving soon. She would bury her head into my jacket and I would protect her ears from the unwanted noise.

It was the unpredictability of being out and about that proved so taxing for Iris: children would suddenly squeal or scream, cars beeped, alarms were triggered, people chatted and shouted across the park to their friends or their child that was straying too far, and mobile phones rang with different ringtones all over the place. When we went into cafés the coffee machines hissed and clunked, the cutlery clinked and chairs scraped against the floors. Iris would recoil and cry at the intrusive clatter that seemed to reverberate around her. After lunch at my parents' on a Sunday, if the Formula One racing was on my father would have the television volume up and Iris would either be hyperactive or get upset by the noise. In these tricky situations I couldn't help but feel the urge to scoop her up and take her home, where I could at least control her environment to a certain extent to reduce the triggers. This feeling led to many weeks spent avoiding most public places. I could feel myself becoming more detached from the outside world. I was still working hard with my wedding photography so spent most weekends in meetings or at weddings; my life was at polar extremes: super social to the point of being relentless and exhausting at work, then isolation at home during the week.

Iris was most happy at home, or when we were out and about checking venues for weddings, locations for photo shoots, or exploring churches and gardens. It soon became clear how much Iris enjoyed spending time in the garden; it was the one place

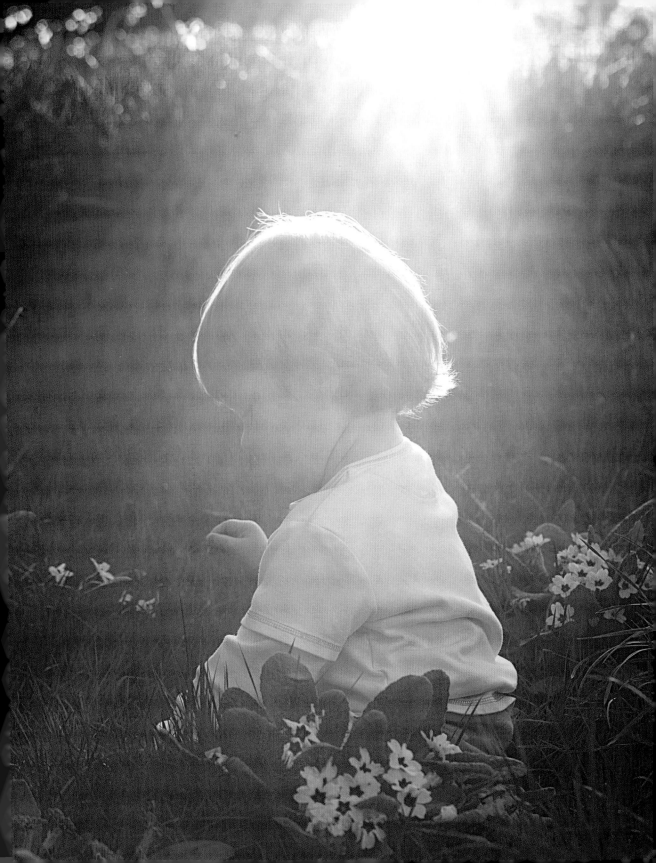

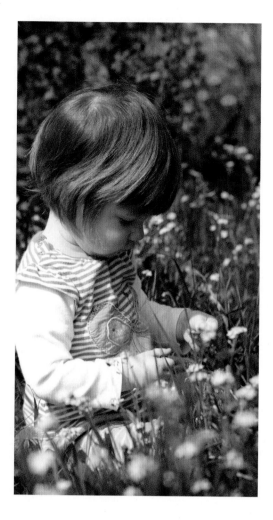

where she didn't retreat with her books. She was happy there and I found I was too. We would look at the flowers and I would talk about everything we saw. Walks were also a comfort: daily outings pushing Iris's stroller along the country roads, with her watching the canopy above, but even they came with an added sting. Iris would not under any circumstances wear anything on her feet – not socks or shoes. When the weather was cold the disapproving looks from others hurt. I could tell what they were thinking as I tried once again to cover up her feet with a blanket but out they came like a spring in a jack-in-the-box, her tiny pink feet determined to feel the cold air.

In the summer of 2010 when Iris was ten months old we tried all sorts of different activities and outings with her, but the same issues arouse again and again. The problem appeared to be rooted in being around other people, especially ones her own age. She found their random actions and chaotic nature deeply disturbing. I began to research, to try to find some answers to why life was more challenging for Iris. P-J started to see what I was observing too and was convinced it wasn't her hearing after doing some of his own ad hoc tests at home. Then in June his family went through the darkest of times with the loss of his father. His death came as a massive shock and P-J was, of course, grieving. He threw himself into organizing everything: the funeral and then the probate of the estate, managing all the affairs. I didn't want to burden him with more turmoil so for a while my search went on alone.

I was lucky to have my mother as a support. Once I turned up at her door after a play date in tears as the differences in Iris were too hard to deny. I felt like I had been clobbered with the reality that something was seriously wrong; I had been concerned before but hoped she just needed time to develop. Iris was slipping further behind her peers and the more we pretended all was well to others the worse I felt. It was like I was living this double life in so many ways, saying what people wanted me to say, that everything was fine and that we were well. My smile was hiding how I really felt, and I couldn't smile any more. It used to be easy: Iris was such a pretty girl, everybody warmed to her as soon as they saw her and there was always a plausible excuse for her behaviour around others: 'She had a bad night', 'teething', 'tummy ache', 'I've forgotten her favourite toy . . .', but I was on the edge. I couldn't go on pretending.

Although we thought she could hear us we couldn't ignore the fact that there might still be a problem with her hearing because it would explain so much about her behaviour and her speech delay. She still wasn't saying anything more than those initial first attempts at 'dada' and 'mama'. In fact, she had regressed and we weren't hearing any more sounds. She was communicating physically with a few gestures and was very independent, unlike her peers who by now were learning many words and starting to put together short sentences. She hardly wanted our attention at all; most of the time, if we tried, she would cry or move away, and that became even more intense with everyone else apart from me. At times when we were alone and the house was quiet I would see a glimpse of how she could be but I was seeing that less and less. I always had to feed her from the left side with no one else around. It had started with breastfeeding and now it was the same with anything we tried to give her, like her water bottle. She had become sensitive on many levels. Her reluctance to socialize and her fear of busy places also couldn't be overlooked any more.

We began the process of getting her hearing tested. But after many frustrating meetings and assessments without any definite conclusions, P-J found a charity in Cambridgeshire that could see Iris right away, so that we could have her hearing tested extensively. With these results we had enough information to fast-track Iris through the system, justifying an auditory brainstem response test in the local hospital to prove once and for all if she had any hearing problems. She was sedated and they placed electrodes on her scalp to pick up the signals that were generated in the inner ear. These signals travel along the nerve to the brainstem then into her brain.

As we waited for Iris to wake after the test the doctors were analysing the data. I couldn't help but think of all the information I had already read about, and what we would do if she was deaf. I had started learning some sign language already but the reality of what we were potentially facing really worried me. This wasn't just research on the internet; this could be our lives from now on – Iris's life from now on. It broke my heart to think that maybe all this time she hadn't been able to hear my voice. I didn't know how to reach her when she was in her own world and without my voice I felt helpless. I also felt confused. Why did music have such an effect upon her? Was she just feeling the vibrations? Was that why she was so sensitive, almost feeling the music with her fingers? The waiting room felt like it was closing in on me so I paced up and down the hallway. I couldn't wait to leave but we needed to face this: I needed to be strong for Iris and when she woke I stroked her forehead and told her that I loved her and everything would be fine, but without knowing if she could hear me or not I felt like crying. A doctor came down the hall with Iris's file in her hand and talked us through the results. It was what we had been hoping for; her hearing was, in fact, better than normal. She could hear everything just perfectly.

With that question answered, for a while life seemed to settle. There wasn't any kind of follow-up from the professionals and there was such a sense of relief within the family that Iris's hearing was fine that it felt like respite from the worry and uncertainty. It was a brief indulgence that only made what came next even more difficult to handle.

We had decided to take our first holiday. Iris was still so young, not yet two years old, and preferred being in nature, so we thought Cornwall would be perfect. In May 2011, before the busy holiday season, we drove the 310 miles down to a very pretty area of the coast. The car was packed full. I seemed to have fitted a whole children's library and playroom into the boot, along with buckets and spades. I had been thinking of my first holidays in the Isle of Wight, nostalgic thoughts of my brother and me happy on the beach, making sandcastles, paddling, exploring and looking at rock pools. We made the last turn down a road that became a single-lane country track and caught our first glimpse of the coast. The sea was turquoise and the rugged landscape exhilarating.

We drove along, trying to find our rented cottage. Iris had been very well behaved on the journey but we had all had enough and couldn't wait to stretch our legs and have a cup of tea looking at the view. However, the directions to the cottage weren't clear and we ended up driving to the owner's house so then had to back our way out to find the right turn. As P-J reversed down the steep curved drive the car slid down the bank and we found ourselves in a precarious position with the car's passenger-side back wheel a metre and a half in the air above the steep slope and the cliff not too far away.

'Oh, well, this is just fantastic!' I said sarcastically, angry and upset. 'Now what?'

'I think you two should get out now. Carefully,' replied P-J, shocked.

I twisted back and got Iris out of her seat, gave her to P-J and slowly opened my door. I climbed out, then carried Iris to safety. P-J gently got out of the car and we sat looking at the stupid scene before us – my car with all its underbelly showing and the stunning view beyond in the late-afternoon sun. I felt upset with P-J for ruining the start of our first holiday. Of course I was relieved everyone was fine but I felt agitated: we had been looking forward to this and it was a much needed change from the cycle of sleeplessness at home. I needed some relief from dramas and this was meant to be it; instead it felt like we were facing another enormous problem. We discussed the idea of finding a local farmer with a tractor but soon came to the conclusion that we had better just use the AA; it might take a while but we didn't want to start our holiday by annoying the neighbours. I needed to keep calm for Iris, so we went off to the cottage while P-J rang the AA to come and salvage the situation. Hours later, with the car back on all four wheels and finally all unpacked our holiday began.

To make up for the disastrous arrival, P-J suggested an evening walk down to the sea and with Iris on his back we made our way down the pretty coastal paths to the beach. The sun was low, there was a golden mist above the crashing waves and we walked along the beach for a while. Iris was tired but content on her father's

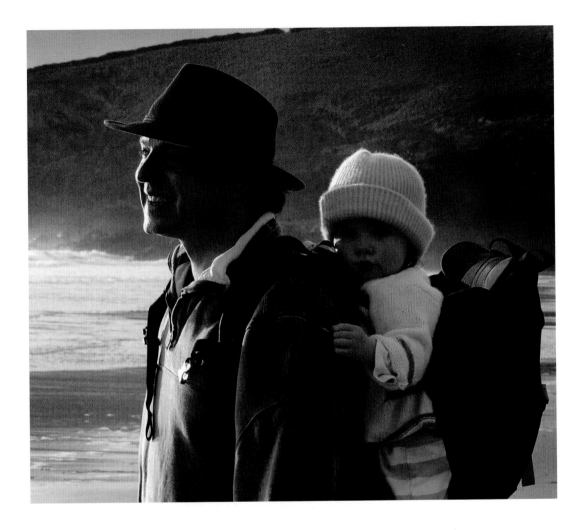

back. The sea's majestic beauty made me forget everything and with peace restored we made our way back to the cottage.

Our week was filled with highs and lows. Iris walked for the first time freely with no help and it was like lift-off in that department. We had been hoping for a while that she would walk as it was another milestone that was of concern, so we couldn't have been more delighted when we watched her make her way across the cottage kitchen all on her own. The blissful

Sunflakes, acrylic, January 2014

moment was short and sweet as the realization about where we were and our total lack of preparation for this event crashed in on us. I hadn't brought any gadgets with me – no stair gates – and we had rented a cottage at the edge of a cliff because when we had booked Iris couldn't walk unaided.

The nights were even harder than at home. I can't recall her sleeping for more than an hour at a time for the whole holiday. Our routine had changed and that wasn't a good move in Iris's book. I would hear her during the night and find her sitting bolt upright staring into space, a distant glazed look in her eyes, unresponsive when I talked to her. She would only fall asleep again lying next to me. She became more controlling over what toys she played with and what she watched. She would need the same cartoons playing over and over and she would become anxious if she didn't have a crayon in her hand. It was the latest in a succession of items that Iris needed to hold on to; they were like a security blanket to her.

One day P-J went on a diving trip to see basking sharks. We managed with Iris in the diving shop as he rented his wetsuit, but only because there was hardly anyone else in there. Once we had left to go on our own little adventure the story wasn't so great. Iris and I went to visit a local town filled with quaint shops. Well, I am assuming they were quaint – I couldn't get through the door of most of them. As I held Iris to go into the shops she would turn herself into some sort of starfish. Her legs and arms would shoot outwards and catch hold of the door frame. She had become surprisingly strong and would scream if I pushed forward. If it hadn't been so comical, I would have broken down in tears. We ended up returning to the boot of the car, which was like a makeshift playroom complete with a library and duvet. I parked up in one of the clifftop car parks and it was there that I realized how isolating her behaviour was when I wasn't at home. I didn't have the support of my mother bringing meals and the safe retreat of our garden. We needed to go into shops and restaurants, but they were impossible places for Iris: she would cry every time someone came close to her or when there was too much noise. I wondered why we had made this trip: was it to run away from it all? Was it more pretending: living the life we thought we should? Of course what had happened was that we were confronted with it head-on. But the worst thing was that I didn't even know what 'it' was. No one could give me any answers. All I had got was advice, tonnes of parenting advice, most of which had been proved useless.

Later I parked the car, waiting for P-J to return from his diving trip. I wasn't sure if it was the adrenalin from the unbelievably steep track down to the sea or the concerns over Iris but I was starting to feel very tired. I just wanted to go to sleep and forget it all, to wake and find my life as I had planned it. Well, maybe not quite as planned – I realize not everything can go to plan – but I wished that sometimes we could enjoy the things that others did with ease. I hadn't slept properly for what seemed like an eternity and I could barely think straight any more. But underneath this I knew something was happening with Iris and that we needed to find out what it was.

P-J arrived and slung all his kit in the back and kissed Iris, then swapped places with me to drive.

'So how was it?' I asked, trying to keep my voice upbeat and enthusiastic.

'Amazing! We went out on the boat for about thirty minutes. The captain warned us we might not see any sharks and then we saw three! One was so interested in the boat and when it was safe to get in I saw the biggest one swim towards me. Its huge mouth was wide open and then it went right under where I was, so I got to see all of it from the top too.'

'How big were they?'

'About eight metres long . . . How was your day?'

'Not great.' I looked back at Iris, who was completely absorbed in her alphabet book. 'Tell me more about the trip: was the water cold?'

'Freezing. It gave me a headache after a while so I could only do short stints with my head down but it was so worth it.'

I listened to P-J as he enthusiastically talked about his incredible adventure and tried my best to share his excitement – after all, it was giant basking sharks, a once-in-a-lifetime experience, and by the sounds of it he had had a mind-blowing encounter, but I was struggling.

We had tried our best and yet most things we did seemed to upset Iris. I felt she was becoming more distant from us at times, pushing us away to play alone and not wanting to look at us, avoiding any contact. But then she could be so affectionate and loved to snuggle in and hug me, although that wasn't the case with P-J. It was very hard for him to connect with her apart from when he served a purpose, like when she rode on his back in the baby carrier. Whenever she pushed him away at home there was always the distraction of something else to be getting on with, but in that small cottage with just the three of us and no work to do these issues were highlighted.

As P-J sat down beside her she waved her arm around and then shot it out sideways to push him out of her space.

'What's wrong, Iris?' He tried to hug her but she pushed him away again and started to cry.

I gestured for him to move away from us. 'She doesn't want you to sit there.'

'Well, where am I meant to sit then?' He walked off to the kitchen, clearly agitated.

With only one sofa and a rather uncomfortable chair as seating options I could see his point. I understood how painful it was to be pushed out but I hated seeing Iris upset. My first reaction was always to sort the problem and so often that meant P-J being sent away, and I worried that it was moving us further apart too. It was like a double rejection from both of us, but I was too exhausted to do anything but keep the peace.

In more difficult times P-J would remark that it wouldn't matter if he was there or not, but I didn't believe that – I could see she loved him. It was hard to hold on to this, though, when so often our efforts would backfire. When we tried to involve ourselves in her play it would more than likely end in tears, sometimes on both sides. She detested the feeling of sand on her feet and would scream wildly if I tried to put her down on the beach. I felt like chucking the brightly coloured bucket and spade off the cliff. They were a constant reminder of yet another childhood experience that she was missing out on, another aspect of our lives that I was failing miserably at. The only time she seemed happy was on P-J's back supported by the baby carrier. Then she would put her arms and feet out, spreading her fingers wide to feel the coastal wind.

I had to admit defeat and we returned home a few days early to try to regain some energy and to refocus. I needed answers.

Many of the quirks and behaviours we could shrug off and laugh about, but others were impossible to deny. P-J believed that she was a slow developer in certain areas like her speech, but he had heard from family that it wasn't an unusual trait, so at first he wasn't as concerned as I was. His happy-go-lucky nature believed that she would get there soon enough, and he always looked at her so fondly while she was absorbed in her books. He generally spent time with Iris when I was at work and that meant there was always a plausible reason for her behaviour – she didn't like change and wanted me home – but I knew none of these excuses were getting to the heart of the problem. She was fading into a world with her books and I was scared that soon, if we didn't do something, it would be too late.

She was losing many of the social skills that she had had in the early days. There were times when she would giggle hysterically at P-J as he did something silly like balancing something on his head or tickling her, and she would occasionally smile and look straight at me through the lens of my camera. That had all gone.

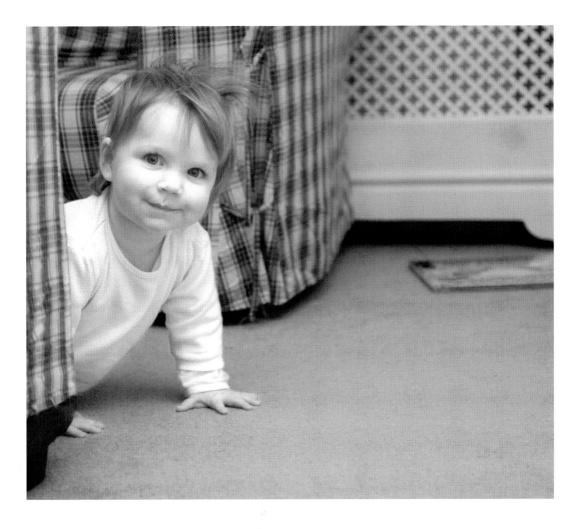

She now ignored me when I tried to photograph her. I was finding it harder to reach her than ever before. Even our hugs seemed brief, mostly just when she was exhausted and needed to sleep. When I tried to get her to look at me she would always turn away or look down at her books. I wondered if that was why she loved them so much; they gave her an out, and opened a door into a place where no one made demands upon her and where she was free to explore without pressures. Everyone seemed so pleased and accepting if she had a book in her lap and it enabled her to have some space and

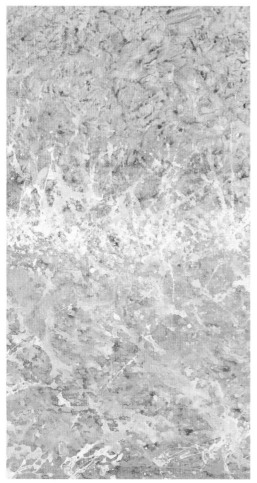

Kupros, acrylic, September 2013

to avoid face-to-face contact. I couldn't even remember the last time I had heard her say anything or even attempt a word.

Then one night I found the answer. The house was quiet, Iris was finally asleep and I prepared myself for what had turned into my nightly ritual, climbing into bed with P-J's iPhone where I could get access to the internet along with the comfort of a soft duvet. I was searching for answers, knowing in my heart that something about Iris was profoundly different from other children.

Constant questions and frustrations ran through my mind, driving me on trying to find a clue. It was about 2.30 a.m. and I felt hopeless and alone. I read about a child on a parent forum who sounded remarkably like Iris. The post was about another two-year-old. I read on, leaping through posts from other mothers until I saw a list of signs referred to as 'red flags'. My eyes filled with tears – if I could have physically ticked the items on this list, I would have ticked nearly all of them – until, unable to see properly through my watery eyes, I reached the word 'autism'. I didn't understand the full meaning of it but I knew enough to realize that this would change all our lives. The future I had in mind for our daughter vanished and was replaced by fear and uncertainty. I woke P-J up immediately.

'What's wrong?' P-J put his arm on my shoulder and looked at me. My eyes were swollen from crying and I wiped away my tears and gave him the phone. 'What's this all about?'

'Just read it.'

As he read, he sat up on the bed, then got up and started to pace around the room. 'But I don't even know what it means. What's autism?'

'I know. It's OK. I didn't either. Well, I thought I sort of knew what it was, but I had to look it up.' I burst into tears again. 'Most websites say there's no cure; it's a lifelong condition. Nothing we can do. But there must be something. There's got to be something.'

'Look, we don't even know for sure yet. We might be wrong. Iris could just be slow at developing in certain areas.'

'Look at the list. This is the answer we've been trying to find. I know it is. She doesn't respond to her name, avoids eye contact, doesn't speak and gets upset with minor changes. She's obsessive, flaps her hands when she is excited, gets upset by sounds and other senses, plays alone, has no interest in others. There's no "pretend" play. She's hyperactive, she has sleep issues . . .'

To my relief he didn't brush it off with a positive spin. He listened and I could tell how serious he was. 'Right,' he said, 'I'm ringing the doctor tomorrow. We can try to get a specialist to see her. There must be someone who can help us with this.'

It was as clear as day what I had been observing all this time, and now he could see it too. I finally fell asleep with the assurance that in the morning we would follow this up and make an appointment for Iris to be assessed.

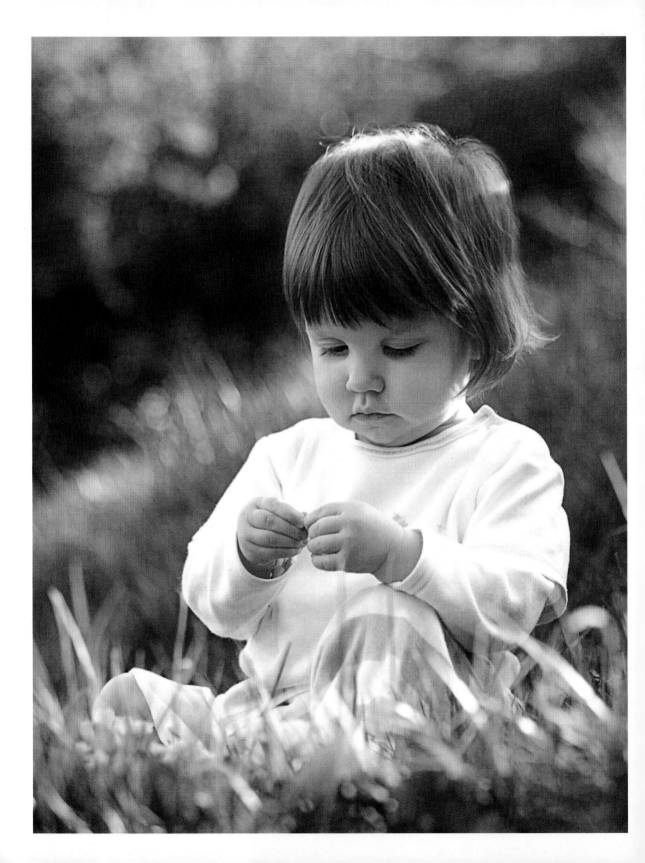

A sense of certainty and hope is with me this morning that I haven't felt in a while. Last night I felt fear from my discovery, but now there is an overriding feeling of power running through me. Finally I have the answer and now I can act on it. For so long I have felt hopeless and questioned everything I've been doing. Now I can focus and we can make a difference. I know what I read last night comes with depressing predictions for the future but there is hope and I will hold on to that.

Iris was up in the night only an hour after I fell asleep so she is lying next to me and to my delight sleeping peacefully. Her rosy cheek rests against my arm and her lips slightly open. I can feel her breath against my skin; it's like a comfort blanket, the regular warm puffs of air reassuring and calm. She stirs and links her arm through mine. I want to hold on to this moment before life moves on. Iris's long eyelashes start to open and she looks up at me with her gorgeous eyes. I want to explain to her that everything is going to be OK, that we will keep her safe and find out how to help her, but I know if I talk I will lose her. She will look and move away so I cherish every second of her eyes meeting mine and as her eyes close and she drifts off to sleep again I hold her close.

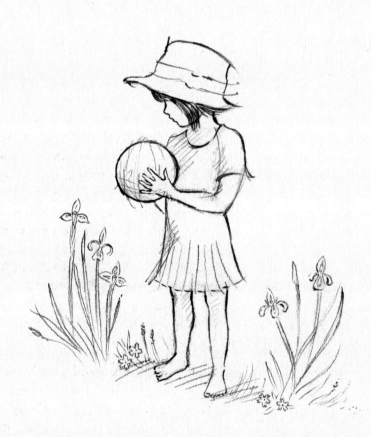

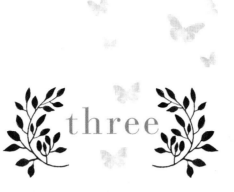

three

Having a plan in our minds and following through with everything that needed to be done to get Iris diagnosed was one thing, but what we hadn't anticipated was 'the system' – the frustrating pace and the amount of chasing we would have to do to secure appointments and assessments to get her diagnosis. There was talk about getting Iris a 'statement' for school so she could get the support she needed, and for us to have the formal diagnosis so we could access the speech therapists and occupational therapists that were available. I felt like we were being swamped as I waded my way through all the acronyms: ASC, PDD, HFA, PECS, ABA, TEACCH, DIR, SLT, OT, SI, PT, AIT . . . It was exhausting just reading the information when it was all so new to me, constantly figuring out what everything meant. It was as if Iris and I were struggling together in a world filled with information that was hard to decipher.

I researched extensively on the internet and bought many books on autism, watched films, went to talks and became immersed in the topic. Piles of books lay by my bed with little torn-off pieces of paper sticking out at various pages, makeshift Post-it notes to mark vital information for me to remember. From what I could tell at that point, autism was a really hard condition to describe because it varied so much from person to person. Some would describe it as a grouping of three closely related developmental disabilities: impaired social interaction, impaired communication and restrictive, repetitive behaviour, interests and activities. In the books there would be a diagram of a triangle around the three groups and in the middle, where all these overlapped, was the word 'autism'. It affects how a person perceives the world and how they relate to it. When someone like Iris walks into a room their senses are sometimes overwhelmed with the visuals. They notice tiny details, see it as a whole and everything in between, meaning that with added extras like people talking or sudden movements from other children they get upset and want to be alone. I was learning that Iris's reactions to her senses were not uncommon and that much of her behaviour was a reaction to her environment. For example, the way she flapped her hands quickly when she got excited by something or when she felt happy. There was a term for that; it was called 'stimming', a release of energy with repetitive movements, allowing her to regulate her own system.

I struggled with the idea of Iris always needing support and the possibility that she might never talk or be able to live an independent life. Every adult on the spectrum lived a completely different life, with abilities that varied as much as anyone else, ranging from having a fantastic career and a family of their own to being in supported living at a residential home, unable to look after themselves or communicate with others. I couldn't figure any of that out then, how it would all work. Every time I thought of it I felt like bursting into tears. I couldn't understand why this was happening and needed answers. But the more I learnt the more I realized that there weren't any concrete answers. Every week there seemed to be new research out contradicting the last and with every new theory, a new potential cure. The emphasis always seemed to be about causes and a cure, which was also a difficult concept. If Iris was autistic, what part of her was that? What would she be like without her autism? When do you say this is an autistic behaviour, symptom or trait, and this is not? Did this come from me? I too struggle in noisy environments and P-J has some tendencies too. His mind easily fixates on a thought or certain way of doing things and he also stays away from crowded spaces. After all, we both worked from home running our own businesses. Was this inherited? If we had more children, would they be autistic too? So many questions.

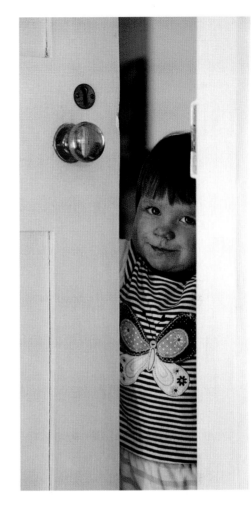

I read about what it might feel like if she was diagnosed. Parents described themselves going through a period of mourning, of saying goodbye to the child they thought they would have. This made me so angry. I couldn't even contemplate the idea of mourning for Iris, as if we had given up on her. She was here. My incredibly perceptive, funny, beautiful, curious little girl was right here with us, and she needed us to believe in her. The very idea of it made me stay up into the early hours every night, learning and researching. It wasn't that I didn't accept the situation; quite the opposite, I was seeing things clearly and seeing the difficult road we had ahead. But I knew I needed to stay positive. I didn't want Iris to miss out on any of the dreams we had all had for her

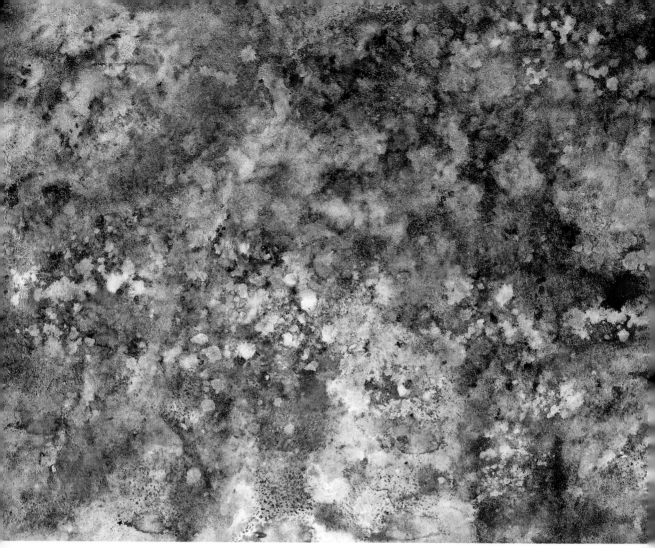

Hiatus, acrylic, April 2014

and I was going to do everything in my power to make sure we gave her every opportunity possible. We would never give up, no matter how hard it got.

P-J came to my rescue many times and when I was too tired to manage all the paperwork involved he took over. The waiting lists were long for assessments and we quickly realized that if we were to help Iris we needed to act fast and on our own while we waited. We were told it could easily be six months before we got to see a specialist doctor, and that was relatively quick: some cases could take up to a year or more. This was frightening news since everything I was reading was confirming my thoughts on how critical early intervention was, and that the faster we moved on this the better.

I found out about various techniques and therapies that could do no harm. Every night I would spend hours reading up on what I could do to reach Iris with a type of play therapy called Floortime and another called Son-Rise. They were therapies that resonated with me and sounded similar to how I had learnt to communicate with horses. The idea is that you use the individual's 'language' on their level, building a bond by achieving a non-verbal conversation involving smiles, looks, pointing, gestures and pure joy over sharing a moment of interest together. These beautiful social communication moments can be missing or less obvious in children with autism. As with horse whispering, a technique I had learnt and used with my own horses, the principles are all about observing body language carefully. All a person's actions are considered to be purposeful and shouldn't be ignored. At first you follow the child's lead, finding out what interests them, so I watched Iris and made notes about the nature, toys, textures, colours and items she spent longer inspecting or which made her bounce with excitement. I would fully absorb myself in the activity, gaining a deeper understanding of why it was motivating to her. I learnt about the simple pleasures of feeling texture, sitting beside her we would run our fingers gently over the surface of a copper-relief sculpture my grandmother had made out in Africa. I felt the cool metal, how smooth and pleasurable the sensation was, and the intriguing formations felt delightful under my fingertips. I enjoyed the perfect round surface of the balls in the ball pool and felt the weight of play-dough just resting in my palms or how sand felt as it poured on to my hand. Then I would move away and think about how I could use this information, how I could create an activity based on my findings that allowed Iris to enjoy spending time with me, playing alongside me using her interests. It was all about focusing on her strengths instead of her weaknesses and expanding on them. It's a framework for understanding a child and creating a comprehensive programme tailored to their needs. Some aspects of the Son-Rise programme made so much sense to me: for example, the belief that children engage in what appear to be exclusive or repetitive activities for a reason. It could be that the child has a different sensory-perceptual system and needs to reorganize stimuli in a way that they can better deal with. These activities are seen as useful to the child rather than something to be stopped or redirected. With this in mind I made sure that Iris had plenty of places to jump and bounce. She seemed to need to do that and I knew that there must be a reason for it even if I didn't know what it was yet. So we put a mattress on the floor in her playroom and a small trampoline in my office.

My aim was broken down into parts. At first it was to reconnect: I needed Iris to accept me playing alongside her. She had become more accustomed to pushing everyone out of her space and even out of the room she was in. Pretty much the only time she would hold someone's hand was to take them to the door and then she would run off back into the room. It was an amusing trick the first time but now it was becoming a routine. So that was first on my to-do list. Then I wanted us to do something together, focusing on the same thing and achieving 'joint attention'. To begin with I would ask Iris to respond to me, asking for joint attention and to be involved, then the hope was that she would gradually initiate activity. It was crucial for Iris in starting to be comfortable looking at me and most importantly at my face. I could see that Iris's verbal skills were never going to improve unless she was able to look at me and watch my mouth moving while I spoke. Her lack of speech, to my mind, was directly linked to her antisocial behaviour: her avoidance of interactions with others and that she found it so hard to look at their faces. She wasn't picking up on all those language skills that babies and toddlers are constantly immersing themselves in when they require all of your attention. The long-term goal was to open up as many opportunities as I could for Iris and to encourage communication, but I knew I was a long way off all that. So for now I decided I would just learn about Iris in a way that I hadn't tried before. I would follow her and try to understand her world instead of always trying to make her fit into ours.

For many nights I had similar dreams: memories from when I was working with our horses in France. Our Arab pony Duo was an old hand at endurance riding, and his heavenly floating trot and easy-going nature meant he was a joy to ride and perfect for our horse-riding-holiday business. But when I fractured and compacted my vertebra I couldn't ride him or the other horses. Being able to run the business, all the duties and work involved, were now impossible. I needed to start to think about selling some of the horses and that meant getting them all in top condition.

To keep them fit I worked with them in the round pen: no equipment, just the horse and me. I was still in my plastic body cast and fragile, so didn't want to risk any further injuries through one of the horses pulling on the rope or reins. Natural horsemanship was a great interest of mine and I read many books on the topic. Years earlier I had attended a Monty Roberts horse-whispering workshop in the UK. From him I learnt 'Equus', a silent language that is conveyed through the body and gestures. I had already been using the techniques in more subtle ways, so I decided I would make use of the rather grim situation and practise and learn more. If these were to be my last months with my equine friends, I wanted them to be great and for us all to get something out of it.

Using 'Equus' is a combination of gestures and body language. Every move you make is observed by the horse as sound doesn't play a central role in the horse's communication system. Horses' eyes can magnify five times more than a human eye and are highly sensitive to movement; they are very much visual thinkers, which is something as a photographer I could totally relate to. They constantly react to the image they see before them in a particular moment. It's an essential part of their survival to be acutely aware of their surroundings, their entire environment, and to be distractible. It is why my accident happened: Tess had suddenly been scared of the bags in the bushes. This wasn't her being naughty; it was an inbuilt response – to her those bags could have been a predator waiting to pounce.

My dreams would fill with moments from those days and the connections I formed with our horses. Duo was my favourite to work with in the pen. I found him easy to understand and I learnt how to read his body language and to communicate with him through mine. After a while I didn't even use my voice. I could request for a change in pace by looking at certain parts of his body, slightly changing the angle of my body to his and ask him to turn with just a slight movement of mine the other way. It was like dancing and he loved being understood and enjoyed the sessions. As each day went by, the easier it got, until I didn't even have to think about it any more and it was as simple as having a chat with a friend on the phone. At first I would send him away to canter or trot around the pen and I would look for his gestures, beginning with his ears, which told me so much. Once he was listening to me in the pen, the inside ear, the closest one to me, would be locked on me. Then he would make his circle smaller around me, feeling safer. I would still keep up the eye contact and he would start to chew a little and lastly he would drop his head, almost touching the ground. This was what I was waiting for and as I took my eyes off his and

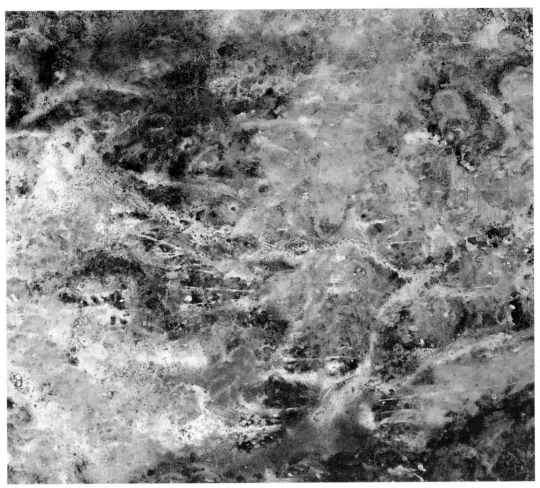

Arien, acrylic, April 2014

lowered my arms, curving my body inwards, looking down at the ground, he would come over to me and stand quietly behind me, waiting. Without looking at him I would turn towards him and stroke his shoulder and neck and then his forehead. This is known as 'join up'. From here I could move in any direction and he would follow. I could ask him to go and exercise around the pen with ease. From that point I had his trust and working with him wasn't work any more; it was a joy.

There are many ways to train horses. The most popular method seems to be to 'tell' them to do something, rewarding the behaviour you desire and punishing the unwanted response. No relationship is formed on this basis but it does generally produce the desired result quickly. There is another way and that is to 'ask' using their language. There is great delight in working together and respecting one another. I wanted that same feeling again, but with Iris. I know it may seem like a strange comparison, a horse and a child, but Iris had a similar flight response; she was reacting and responding rather than initiating. She had a phenomenal memory, was a visual thinker and her trust was easily lost. She was highly sensitive to her surroundings and like a horse extremely distractible in some environments due to her ability to see everything all at once and notice changes instantly. For a horse this is a survival technique, but for Iris it had drawbacks: she would easily become overwhelmed by her senses and upset by small changes. Also, like a horse, she was using body language and gestures to communicate. Using similar methods to interact with Iris would take time and rely heavily on my observation and understanding of how Iris perceived the world but I wanted to try my best and to see what was possible.

Our at-home therapy sessions began with me finding my way carefully, following Iris's lead. I would sit next to her on the floor and copy what she was doing. At first I would get pushed away and then slowly I was accepted. She even found it amusing and appreciated my presence. I was always careful about my eye contact as I knew this was difficult for her and I kept as quiet as possible. I started to learn when I could join her and how long for. I would be interested in and smile at the pictures she liked in her books, feel the textures on objects, bringing them up to my face like she did. I mimicked and followed her until I sensed that she had had enough. At first it was only playing together for a few minutes, but over time that increased.

With the information I learnt about what she liked and what was motivating her I was able to fill her life with those things. She loved books so we bought more every week on topics that she was interested in. Animals were a firm favourite and she also loved books with textured surfaces. As our library expanded so did the array of sensory toys and other homemade things like tubs of coloured rice, sand and play-dough. They were like little precious keys into her world, allowing me to get closer and form a stronger relationship with her. It felt great to be doing something positive and for it to be working. Her eye contact was improving and although there was still no improvement at all in her speech and her relationships with others I could tell we were making vital steps in the right direction. She welcomed me beside her and enjoyed our time together; she even started to initiate some joint attention with the use of a water pen on an aqua pad. This was a rather addictive addition to our kit: a pen filled with water and a white pad that turned dark blue as the pen touched its surface. As the water dries the marks disappear and you have a fresh pad to work on. Simple but effective. An everlasting doodle pad with no mess. Iris would prompt my hand to make a mark, then she would take the pen and have a go, passing the pen back to me when she had finished. We were working together, and although they were small things probably undetectable by most or which would be taken for granted, to me they felt huge and I celebrated them. Each time I was accepted and she played alongside me or wanted me to be involved I felt like I had won a fantastic prize, a funfair and celebrations happening in my mind. I wanted to do a lap of honour running around the room, but settled for smiling and giving Iris some praise.

Iris was intrigued by pencils, pens and crayons, playing with them for many hours a day. Most of the time it seemed the walls were being covered in some sort of toddler mural and I had lost count of the amount of times I had repainted. With my perceptions altered, I saw that this was clearly an interest and a strength that I could encourage. I just had to figure out how I could redirect the interest from our walls. I found large rolls of wallpaper liner in the local DIY shop and cut pieces to the same length as the wooden coffee table and then taped down both ends. Iris thought this arrangement was perfect and she scribbled away for hours. She would cover the paper completely with multicoloured swirls and circles, all interlocking and overlapping each other. She bounced on her tiptoes, humming sometimes. She would even use both hands, both busily working away, spreading the colours blissfully, free and so happy. The table covered in paper had been a marvellous success and the walls stayed spotless for many weeks, but it didn't last for ever.

My eyes followed a blue crayon line along the wall, zigzagging all the way to the door frame and then making a gentle loop-the-loop back to me. Iris must have been here not that long ago – only moments before this wall had been untouched. Just as I was thinking about how once again I could explain to her that 'we do not draw on walls!' I noticed the change from the angry craggy mountain range to smooth, petal-shaped loops. It hinted at a delightful shift in her mood. Always drawing information from anywhere I could to understand and help her, I recognized this as another opportunity to connect. So I took it. The basket of washing was shunted to one side and replaced with paper and pens. Together we peered over the paper. I started with a smiley face and passed the pen over to her. She giggled and, her eyes meeting mine, she looked down, drew a straight line, then passed the pen back to my hand, guiding me to the paper. I drew a stick man and added the ground, a tree, a bird in the sky and a sun with triangular rays, telling a story as I went. We took turns adding details to the picture, Iris happy with this arrangement for a while. We were working well together, understanding each other, and then a car pulled up, the heavy sound of the gate, and the disturbance and intrusion into our world closed the window of opportunity and she moved away. The washing basket was back in my arms again but my thoughts were with the stick man and the next story I could tell. I wanted to use this latest interest to interact with her so I drew. I drew stories, and masses of them. They were just with stick men and funny animals, but they proved to be vital in moving Iris's attention on to what I was doing and allowing me into her space even more. All these little steps gave me the hope and the energy I needed as I did my best to manage my business, life at home, Iris and this new project that I hoped would have an immensely positive impact on all of our lives.

● ●

We knew how much nature and the garden already meant to Iris and we were on a mission to bring some more happiness back into our lives. The previous months, with P-J's father passing away and the discovery of Iris's condition, had been hard for all of us and this project was something new and positive to focus on. The plan was to knock down the ugly laundry that hogged the beautiful view at the back of the house and in its place build a barn-like structure out from the kitchen that would become known as the garden room. We knew a build like this would be very difficult for Iris in the short term but the long-term benefits would make it worthwhile. It was to be a living space, occasional dining room, playroom, music room – one of those spaces that I hoped could be anything we wanted it to be. I needed more light and the feeling of freedom you get from looking out on to nature. Iris was responding well to my methods of interaction but it would have been much easier if we had a bigger space to work in. I had also been noticing how Iris was easily distracted from our activities by the road. If a car parked up, it would destroy any connection we had made. She would be nervous about the gate opening and shutting, and I couldn't wait to work with her in a space away from all that on the other side of the house. Also, because Iris got so distressed while we were out and about meant that for many weeks we hadn't ventured out very much, apart from to my parents' house and walks out in the countryside. It wasn't that I was embarrassed by her outbursts; it was more the way they took their toll on all of us later on. If she had been upset by something, I could say goodbye to getting any sleep that night, as she would be restless, which would affect the following day. It was a domino effect and I tried everything I could to keep all the pieces upright, but that in itself was destructive in its own way. At times the isolation was hard to handle. It was like life was happening, thriving to a constant beat beyond the walls of our home, but we were standing still, alone.

Over the summer Iris spent more and more time out in the garden, inspecting the wild flowers that were in full bloom. She was so interested and intrigued by all the sounds and sensations that surrounded her. It was as though she was in a jungle of petals and butterflies; in patches they towered above her. She made her way through, taking flowers by their stems and bending them down to her height to take a closer look. Her little index finger on her right hand pointed outward gently, feeling the surface of the petals and she would hum excitedly when she found one she loved. A single object was always in her left hand, like a solid comfort blanket she kept with her at all times.

The latest permanent fixture was a pink ball, a plastic pink ball from the ball pool, but it had to be one in particular and she would know right away if I had lost it and replaced it with another. I couldn't tell the difference between 'the one' and all the others, but there was obviously something very special about this

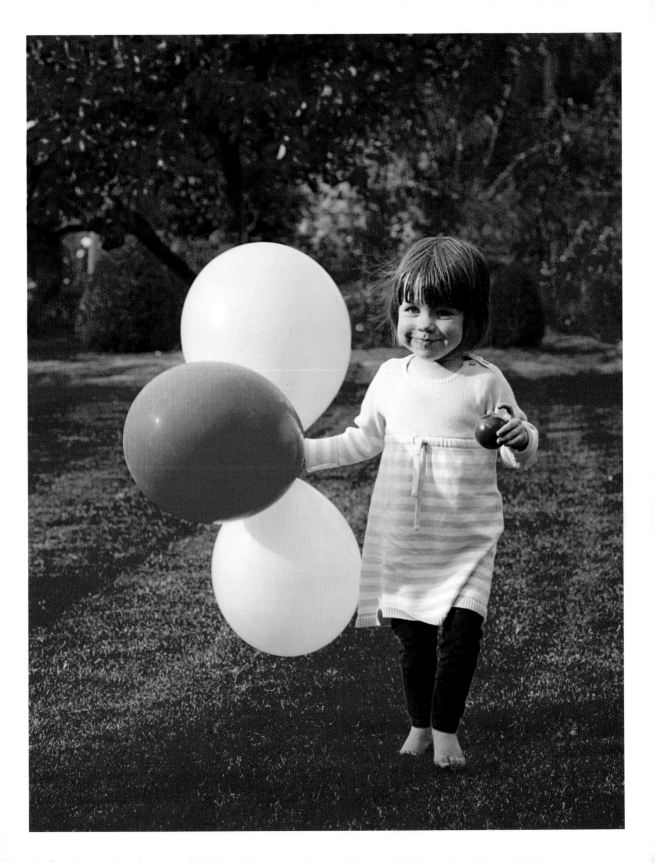

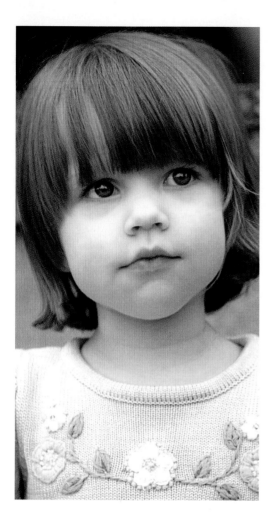

particular one that Iris liked. She would take it everywhere with her and I had to stretch all the cuffs on her clothes so I could change her tops without causing her distress while she kept it in her hand.

As time went on and I was able to connect with Iris more through her interests and love of nature I began to feel that maybe P-J was right: she was just developing at a different rate from other children. Then there were occasions where I felt like her potential diagnosis was as clear as day. However, even with all our best efforts, Iris found it difficult to enjoy her second birthday. It was, of course, a social occasion, with many family members, and she avoided everyone as best she could. Even the chocolate Tom and Jerry birthday cake didn't improve the situation. She ignored most of her presents and was willing everyone to leave her alone. Once they had all left she ran freely around her grandparents' garden with her balloons, giggling, content, totally at ease in nature and away from the social interactions. We watched her from the kitchen, smiling and laughing at her running so happily across the grass, but I could tell both P-J and I were thinking the same thing. Our thoughts were about what this meant, how we could help her and why this was happening.

By the autumn the build had started and as we predicted it was a difficult time for Iris. She found the noise of the digger and all the various deliveries distressing and we shut ourselves in the far corner of the house while P-J managed the builders. So, to avoid the noise, we spent more time over at my parents'. My parents had bought a new black Labrador puppy called Indigo, Indy for short. She was adorable and she loved Iris. Yet the connection wasn't quite there on both sides: Iris didn't like to be licked, but she was amused by the puppy and tolerated her bouncy play. It was wonderful to watch Indy try to interact with Iris; it wasn't always successfully but I appreciated her efforts. As soon as we came in through the front door she was there

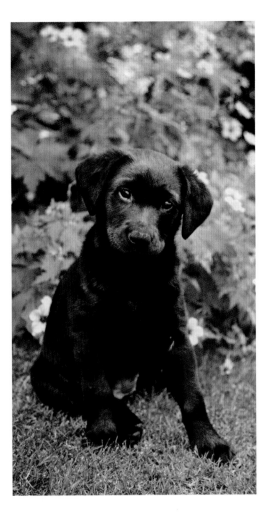

to welcome Iris and she would bring her toys, reaching out to her whenever possible and never appearing to feel hurt if Iris rejected her. I couldn't help but envy the dog's resilience about being dismissed. It was so unlike the rest of us who would feel sad about being pushed away. Yet she didn't show it, not once; she just tried again later with the same buoyant nature.

I decided to take on that attitude. I knew that Iris loved us dearly but just couldn't show it in the way that other children so easily could. Instead we would have to be patient and keep trying to reach out to her however we could. This concept wasn't easy for everyone to take on board. My father couldn't help but feel disheartened every time he was pushed away. No amount of explaining would help; he needed time. One week she would tolerate and even enjoy being more tactile with him, allowing his hugs and kisses or wheelbarrow rides around the garden, then other weeks she just couldn't handle it. My mother was incredibly patient, more than all of us, and waited — she knew that Iris would come to her when she was ready. And the more I worked with Iris, the more I saw improvements with her relationship with P-J. They were only hints at first, but they gave him hope. If I was away photographing a wedding, Iris would transfer many of the skills she used with me to him. Unfortunately, when I arrived back her loyalties would switch straight back to me. For the majority of the time I was Iris's rock, her translator. I understood her more than I had ever done before, and I began to hear her like I used to listen to the horses. I could read her body language and started to get better at seeing when I needed to take a step back, reducing the likelihood of a meltdown. I could see that for now Iris could only manage to interact with one person at a time in this way and I understood that these skills were new and still very difficult.

The inspiration for the type of extension to our home came from the time we had spent in Venezuela. Our house there had provided safety for us. The high ceilings, strong beams and the views of the Andes through its huge triangular windows had given me courage in uncertain times. Now I wanted that same feeling of protection for Iris. So we went for it: the whole gable end was glass; there was even glass between the king post truss. We found a builder and a carpenter to work on the project with P-J and he managed the build himself. The whole experience from start to finish was packed with highs and lows. P-J broke his finger, and there were moments when we just wanted to pack it all in, but then we would figure out the problem and see everything coming together again. In between calls to suppliers P-J battled on with chasing the doctor to try to get Iris's assessment brought forward, and one day we received a letter giving us a start date for the three-day assessment.

It was December and the weather had been unusually good so the build was going well; we actually had a shot at being in there for Christmas. The plan was for P-J to carry on managing the build and I would take Iris to the assessment and stay with her. It was at a Child Development Centre in a city close by and over the three days we saw many different professionals in the field. The assessment was difficult for both of us. Iris was unnerved by many aspects of the main room. It was too hot and the fans blew balloons from the ceiling. There was constant movement to deal with. Once they were removed she settled, and at first it was about observing her play in the different areas set out, before moving on to different sessions with the different departments. All her endearing traits were noted, analysed and catalogued. The process was difficult to watch. Every time Iris picked up an object, she wouldn't play with it like the toy was designed to be played with. She would inspect it in great detail – how it was put together, the texture, how it felt across her cheek, how it fitted into her hand, how it looked in different light, how it fitted in my hand, which hand she preferred it in. She was always silent; there was not a word or sound until something excited her and then she would flap her hands and hum. The doctor was making notes and I was willing her to put the plastic broccoli on to the plate or to pick up the tiny cup for a sip of tea – anything that would be more typical for a child of her age. They watched me feed her and made notes. It was a very strange experience, as if we were both being judged, and I couldn't help but feel awkward. All the doctors and nurses were kind and understanding, which helped, but then it was time for more formal assessments where she was asked to do different activities, all of which she had no interest in, and the doctors found it impossible to engage with her. It was as if the doctors weren't there or, as she made her feelings clear with wild screams and by running to the door, that they were an annoyance that needed to be dealt with.

I knew I should feel happy that they were seeing what I had observed, that they were taking her behaviour seriously, and that the most likely outcome was that they would agree that she was on the autistic spectrum, but all of a sudden it didn't feel that way. I wanted her to 'pass' with flying colours. I wanted to be proud and for them to say 'Nothing to worry about here. All is well, my dear, off you go home now.' Of course that wasn't the case and I left each day feeling more and more certain of what the outcome would be. We didn't have to wait long for the diagnosis – the doctor had said that he didn't want us waiting over the Christmas holidays – so on 20 December 2011 we went in for a final meeting to discuss their findings and to receive Iris's diagnosis.

P-J and I were sitting close to one another on low uncomfortable chairs. The heating was on full, and it was unbearably hot in the hospital consultation room of the Child Development Centre and I could feel my cheeks flushing red. As the doctor talked to us, describing his findings from the three-day assessment before finally getting to the diagnosis, I tried to keep my breathing slow and regular, constantly fighting the urge to cry. I didn't want to cry in front of this man. I respected him as a doctor; but although he was obviously knowledgeable, I didn't like his cold manner, his depressing outlook on life. If I let him see how I felt it would spread like wildfire within me. I couldn't open myself up to that, so I stayed calm and took some notes on the file of papers we had been given. I knew P-J and I both needed answers, but now that we had them it didn't feel any better. In time that would change, but at that moment it felt as though I was being suffocated by information. Our daughter was autistic: a lifelong condition with little known about its cause and no known cure.

'There are an abundance of therapies you can try,' the doctor said, 'and you can try any that are safe for her, but in my opinion very few work.'

With those words I felt like I was being crushed. Over the past couple of months, while we waited for this assessment, I had worked with Iris and had seen real improvements, and had truly believed that we were making progress and that our methods were working to a degree; but his words seemed to belittle everything I had worked so hard on. The doctor read out some of his conclusions: 'Iris demonstrated early-learning and language skills of a nine- to twelve-month-old baby at two years old. She has difficulties with social interaction, social communication and repetitive play. All these behaviours confirm a diagnosis of Autistic Spectrum Disorder.'

He then drew a line on a piece of paper, telling us this was the spectrum. At one end he wrote the words 'severely autistic' and at the other 'Asperger's'. He made a mark close to the severe end and said, 'She has a significant impairment in speech development, language and early-learning skills.' He repeated that as I stared at him and the look in his eyes hurt. I could tell he needed me to take this on board properly, to believe and accept it. What he didn't realize was that I had already come to terms with the likely diagnosis. What I needed was hope, not to be told that she may never speak. I needed him to see the light in Iris that I saw when I was interacting with her at home, while I was drawing or watching the way she reacted to nature, her unbelievable concentration span and her interest in books. These were all strengths, yet it was as though they counted for nothing. Even worse than that, they were used as cons and I couldn't bear it. I hated that piece of paper. I wanted to screw it up, to burn it and to never think of it again. I realized it was irrational. We were there for one purpose:

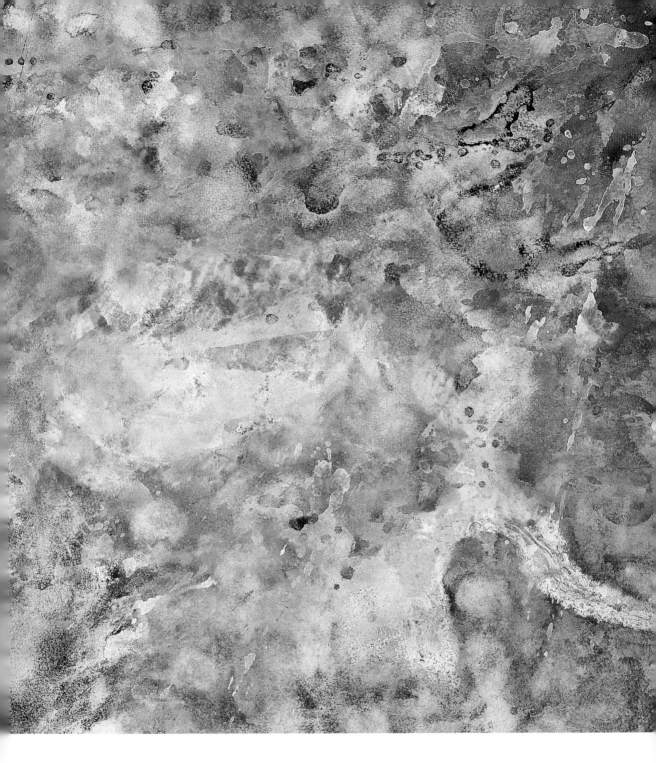

Fable, acrylic, July 2013

for Iris to be diagnosed so we could get her the help and support she needed, but no amount of rational thinking would mend the sadness sweeping through me. As I looked at the doctor I felt angry: angry at him for being negative, angry at all the doctors for not finding any answers for us other than a name, for what we were facing and for instilling the belief that nothing could be done, that all hope was lost.

All I wanted to do was hold my little girl but she was with my parents at home. As P-J and I drove back we were both quiet. It was sinking in and we needed time to think: for P-J to come to terms with what he had just been told and for me to focus on the positive and to believe that we could really make a difference and help Iris. We had known for months that this diagnosis was a very high possibility, but I think we had both been secretly hoping that it was just developmental delays and that everything would be fine, especially since I had been seeing some improvements. P-J was normally so positive but this news felt firm, almost concrete, and it seemed to squash all hope, making his usually happy face look cold and withdrawn. As I opened the door my mother was there. I didn't need to say anything. She held me and then I hugged Iris. I heard her say, 'We're here for you. We'll get through this.'

Our plans for Christmas were a welcome distraction. We had invited both families; it was to be a party of twelve. I'm not sure how the idea came about, but I was thrilled about having something to look forward to and to finally be in the new part of our home. There was just one hitch in the plan: the extension wasn't anywhere near ready yet. With only a week to go it was action stations to make it all happen. We were both more determined than ever to have a wonderful holiday. But the more we tried, the more things fell apart.

'It will be amazing!' said P-J. Then the delivery van arrived with our long-awaited oak floorboards and they were awful: terribly stained and with knots all over the place. They were not what we had ordered and all of them had to go back. The next delivery wasn't going to be until the second week in January.

'Don't worry, who needs smart flooring? We can just use rugs or something. The concrete will be fine if it's swept.'

'Not quite the romantic Christmassy look I was going for, P-J,' I replied.

Then we received a call about the special spotlights I had ordered – they weren't going to be shipped in time. Massive delays there too. P-J grinned at me, his Panama hat, ski jacket and work gloves on in our cold, slightly damp, extension. 'Candles?'

I couldn't help but laugh at the room. 'For heaven's sake, this is getting ridiculous.' The doors had only just been fitted during a very heavy rainfall, which didn't exactly improve the mood of our cantankerous carpenter, and the plaster wasn't dry enough to paint due to the delays in putting the glass and doors in. Ladders, buckets, paint pots and rubbish were dotted about the room and there was a rather unappetizing smell.

P-J started sweeping the floor: huge clouds of grey concrete dust totally obscured my view of him and all I could hear was a muffled voice.

'What?' I said, then saw him looking even more ridiculous with a bandana over his mouth to stop him breathing in the dust.

'Don't worry!' he shouted out to me. 'It'll be fine!'

Undeterred by the various problems, we marched on. I pulled in a favour with one of our local wedding venues and borrowed a huge roll of old marquee carpet. We lined the floor with giant tarpaulins, which in the end wasn't the greatest plan, since even with the carpet over the top they gave a sort of squeaky crunch underfoot.

'It sounds terrible. Do you think we should just take the tarpaulins away?'

P-J was beginning to bring in some of the furniture we needed: extra chairs and another table to extend our dining-room table. 'No way! There's no time. This will have to work as it is.'

I adorned the beams with foliage from the garden and Christmas decorations: little robins and red berries among the greenery. We set up side tables and lamps, candles for more lighting and I decorated an enormous three-metre-tall Christmas tree late on Christmas Eve. The effect was very festive, with fairy lights and greenery framing the view of the gable end. It was romantic and pretty – if you squinted your eyes and ignored the rumpled carpet and drying plaster. With ivy draping from the trusses and the fire roaring, champagne in the fridge, and all the food bought and ready to be cooked we were in fine spirits on Christmas Day morning. And then the oil-fired Rayburn cooker went out. I couldn't cook anything on it or in it or even heat water.

You would think that we would take notice of the signs, but oh no. On we went.

'You can't be serious! Why don't you all just come over here?' said my mother on the phone. 'Darling, you've done your best, but the room just isn't ready yet – and now the cooker. Blooming thing. Do you remember when ours went out? It's always at the worst time. Did you try to turn it up? Change the settings? Anyway, I'm worried. You're taking on too much. I know you must be tired.'

I almost burst into tears. My mother could tell what I was thinking. I needed the distraction, I needed not to think about the future and I needed to enjoy a magical Christmas. Ever since I could remember my mother had turned their country house into

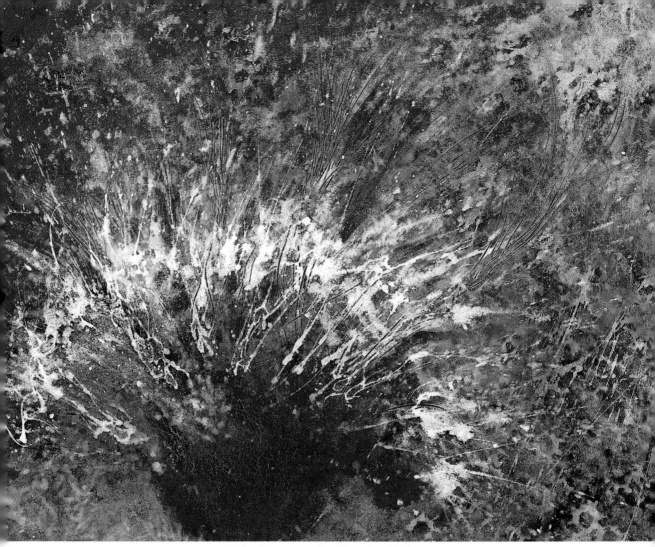

Tale of Green, acrylic, November 2014

an enchanted wonderland at Christmas. We would decorate the tree and beams together and listen to carols, going completely overboard on the decorations, and there would be flowers, log fires, candles and a party on Christmas Eve. I adored it all and it was always a very special time of year for me. I hated the idea that everything was going to be ruined because of a stupid old cooker. And yes, we had tried to turn it up. It was as if it had said, 'You have to be kidding me,' and gone to sleep, not to be woken until the new year when we would be able to get it serviced.

'I've got an idea,' my mother said. 'I'll cook everything here. I can bring over the hot plate and do the last parts with you but I'll get the turkey done and all the roasted vegetables and gravy . . . and I'll bring it all over in the car.'

The logical thing to have done would be for everyone to be over at my parents'. Their house was just ten minutes away, but I was way past logic. We were on a mission and needed to see this through. So my poor mother brought a whole Christmas lunch for twelve in her car, spilling some into the boot as she raced over to ours to try to keep it all warm.

The idea of Christmas at ours was, of course, different in reality. Factors beyond my control meant that things went from bad to worse. Some of the family were really late to arrive after getting lost on their journey, which meant after all that effort the food was past its best and everyone was very hungry, ate too many canapés and had too many drinks before lunch. Iris found the whole situation hard to handle and instead of having fun and it being a break from our worries it only compounded them. Apart from my parents, we hadn't told anybody else about Iris's diagnosis so it was hard to explain her behaviour. I couldn't talk about it yet; I just wasn't ready, and it certainly wasn't the right day to start. P-J and I took it in turns to check on Iris in her playroom and I sat with her for a while after lunch while everyone was having their coffee. She was completely absorbed in her favourite book, hardly even noticing me or what day it was, apart from the fact that she wanted to stay as far away from all that noise as possible and ignore everybody, and that included me. I tried to hug her and she pushed me away, and then the guilt set in: all the progress we had made over the past months and I went and did this. Was I mad? It had been a more testing day than I had ever imagined in so many ways. I now wanted Christmas to be over. I was failing at what I had set out to do all those months ago and I wished for it to be a new day and a fresh start so we could try again.

My heart is heavy with a sadness that I can't shake off. It's Christmas Day and our darling girl is alone in her playroom. She has tried to be with us, a quick dip in and out, but cannot cope. Too many people, too much noise, the furniture has been moved and she hasn't had any time to get used to the extension. There is wrapping paper everywhere, the tearing and unwrapping noise rips through her. Every time she goes close to anyone they call out her name and she runs for safety away from it all. I follow her to see if I can be of some comfort but she pushes me away, her eyes are filled with tears and now so are mine. How could I have been so thoughtless? It is as though I have lost my way, in all our efforts to enjoy a perfect Christmas and to move on from that diagnosis day in the hospital I have forgotten everything I have learnt from Iris.

I make a vow to myself, never again. I did not consider the consequences of this tradition for her. She is my Christmas and now she sits alone. I feel empty without her.

A Christmas Promise
I will take more care, smaller steps and make adjustments.
I will modify our traditions so we can all be together for Christmas Day.
Dear Iris, I promise next year will be different.

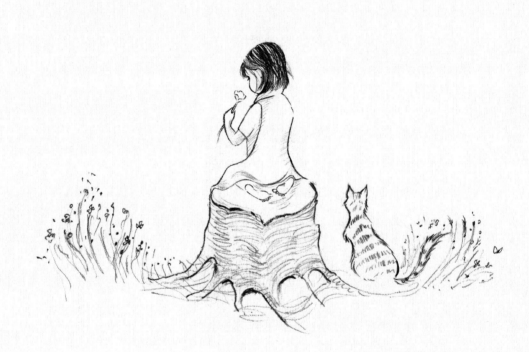

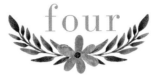

four

Everyone was asleep and the outside world had gone quiet. I tiptoed over to the window – even though it was early, it seemed brighter than usual. The snow covered everything: no one wanted to brave the hill and not one car had passed our home. The new year had brought so much hope. Hope for all the help we would finally access. We would no longer be doing this alone. I was looking forward to learning more and working with professionals who could guide us.

But as the weeks wore on, and more difficulties arose at home with Iris's behaviour, I realized there we didn't have the great support team I had been hoping for after the diagnosis. Instead there was just a file containing basic information about autism and contact details for charities and groups that might offer support. Most of them turned out to be out of date. Some numbers did work, but as the tired voices at the other end explained how with a lack of funding they had been closed for a while the reality of what I was facing began to sink in. I would need to pick myself up after the disappointments at Christmas and carry on as planned. I had to follow Iris, to understand her behaviour and the difficulties she experienced. To move forward we needed to build on her strengths.

Her more repetitive behaviour, like ripping up pieces of tissue paper, appeared at first to be irritating habits that caused mess, but I began to look at life in another way and to use behaviour like this to our advantage. They were an opportunity for us to interact, to do some speech therapy with her by counting as she dropped the ribbons of tissue that gracefully fell to the ground. I realized that Iris liked to watch things fall, so I bought a bulk load of large colourful buttons that she could drop into water and after their success many more items followed, providing times where we could interact easily. Sometimes I didn't know if feeding her interests in this way was the right choice. Although she was only two years old she would get easily stuck in a repetitive loop, wanting to see the same action again and again. She could be very persuasive in getting what she wanted, taking my hand or P-J's back to the items, and we were so happy to be included in her play that mostly we went with it. But at times her obsessive nature would escalate and if the activity was taken away she would become inconsolable like any child her age. As these tensions and anxieties mounted, my most reliable solution would be to take her outside into the garden where she immediately relaxed. It seemed to work almost every time but when the weather was bad that wasn't possible. I would then see her plummet out of control and I felt helpless as I tried to avoid the inevitable meltdown. It wouldn't take much if she was on the edge; it could just be the sound of newspaper being crumpled up to light the fire. They were like tantrums that were beyond Iris's control. She cried and shook with frustration, and all I could do was to try to minimize what seemed to be upsetting her. If I tried to hug her, she would lash out. At times wrapping her duvet round her would help, as it seemed to calm her, but at other times this would aggravate her to a whole other level. It was as though when she felt like things were out of control — externally from a noisy or confusing environment, or internally from her own compulsive behaviour — it triggered anguish inside her. She threw herself to the ground, hitting the floor with her fists and even hitting her own tummy or biting her wrist. She didn't seem to care about her safety and it was frightening to watch. She would bite into her toys with her face turning red and shaking, not looking at me or even caring if her actions were getting a reaction from us. It wasn't attention-seeking or a cry for help; it was like she didn't have any control any more and that her feelings had to come out somehow. Sometimes these episodes would last for hours, while other times we would have days that seemed to be one meltdown after another.

I started to hate the winter and the grey days with curtains of rain trapping us all inside. Some meltdowns would seem like they were over until the pressures started to build and once again Iris's fury would return. P-J and I would take it in turns to help her through them. Then there would be nothing for weeks and there was a sense of relief – maybe it had just been a phase – but then something would happen to trigger another. Generally they came after she had been managing well in a social situation but we had pushed it too far and stayed too long. Quite often it happened when we got home. All it took was a noise like the dishwasher being unpacked, and the clattering of plates and cutlery would overload her mind and she would fill with uncontrollable emotion. Some people describe meltdowns as if the child is shutting down, but for Iris it seemed more like everything was going at full speed and I needed to find a way to slow it down, to help her before she got to that moment of chaos. I dreaded it happening when we were out. People would try to help by waving a toy and trying their best to distract her. But these movements and noises and the intense face-to-face contact were agony to Iris, intensifying the turbulent world surrounding her, and I felt it too. Dealing with her meltdowns was the most exhausting process. I felt like I had been hit by a truck. They affected me emotionally for days. The sadness I felt from seeing our darling girl like that was heart-wrenching; it was as though I was being tortured in the worst possible way. I

Thistledown, acrylic, September 2013

wanted so much for her to talk to me, for her to tell me what was happening so I could try to somehow prevent them. The frustration and hopelessness of her mostly silent world was as relentless as the sleep deprivation.

P-J and I discussed the problems at length. Knowing what was causing the meltdowns and how best we could stop them from happening was a good place to start. Meltdowns seemed to be a part of autism that the doctors expected at one time or another and they looked on them as commonplace, but I couldn't understand why they were so accepting. Up until Christmas she hadn't had that many meltdowns but the gloomy weather in the new year brought many more and I could not accept the doctors' view on this. I wanted to do everything in my power to understand Iris on a deeper level, using observation and taking her lead. I needed to be more vigilant and watch for the signs, to forget about what friends thought if I left early or wasn't at the table for lunch, to forget about social pressures and to focus on Iris.

The snow made me feel like it was a fresh start, I wanted to wake Iris and P-J and go sledging, to replace the difficult memories with happy ones. Iris had not been out in the snow yet and I couldn't wait to see what she thought of it, intrigued to see our little nature lover in her magical garden cloaked in white. Of course there was the issue of her not liking anything on her feet; I would need Iris to be OK with her boots and gloves on. Another problematic hurdle to overcome, but first I needed a cup of tea.

I went downstairs to prepare myself for another day. While the kettle boiled I sorted Iris's books that were scattered over all the surfaces. There were forms on the kitchen table that I had filled in for various courses for Iris. January had gone by without any particular change. We were on a waiting list for a speech therapist and had enrolled in a class to teach us all about autism and how we could help Iris. Some of the information we gleaned there was very useful, but as each week went on I found their attitude and approach unsettling. I just couldn't understand how their techniques were going to work with Iris. It all seemed so rigid and some of it out of date compared to the latest research I was reading. The system they were suggesting was called PECS, Picture Exchange Communication System. With this system, a child is taught to communicate with an adult by giving them a card with a picture on it. The trouble was Iris wasn't responding to this method at all; in fact, it was having the reverse effect. It was causing upset and frustrations, causing Iris to move away from us and wanting to spend even more time alone. It didn't seem to matter how many beautiful cards I made. They never conveyed the concept, item or wish she desired. It was as if we were on a conveyor belt of parents with diagnosed children. This was the standard information that they gave out to everybody; it hadn't changed for quite some time and there were no alternative options or therapies that they recommended. It was their set routine to follow, packed full of visual schedules all neatly laminated, their generic formula or nothing at all – and that was something I didn't trust. This was definitely not a one-size-fits-all situation. After all, the definition of autism itself describes it as a 'spectrum condition'. The information we had wasn't tailored to Iris, her age group or our needs; it was just a guide to what has worked for schools and families in the past. Another massive file of notes with more contact details.

I found a pen in the kitchen and went through my notes, highlighting the points that I believed in and the suggestions that I could see working. I spread them across the table, and began to write down more: plans, ideas, items I needed to buy, things that I knew Iris liked. Every note sparked off more and more ideas. Before I knew it I had months' worth of activities all plotted out in front of me and I hadn't even had breakfast yet. I was going to take play therapy to a new level. Our house would become a fun house, a sensory wonderland. I would learn from Iris what calmed her, what excited her, what intrigued her, and create spaces that facilitated and encouraged learning and communication as well as helping her with her sensory needs.

I had highlighted one note that I kept coming back to. It was about the positioning of furniture in a room and how it had an impact on behaviour. I began to think about our home and what I had already experienced. How if a table was placed in the middle of a room, surrounded by open space, it enticed Iris to circle it in an almost uncontrollable movement, around and around. However, with the table banked on one side, her focus was clear. By taking the time to understand her behaviour and the reasons behind it, and seeing the world through her eyes, I would be able to connect with her more effectively. Such minor, seemingly insignificant details can make the difference between chaos and harmony. With that in mind I noted what furniture I wanted to move, seeing how I could mould our house to help Iris.

'What's all this?' P-J said, still in his dressing gown and looking at me with his scruffy mad-professor morning hair. 'More lists I see! What are you up to, Bean?' Bean was my nickname and it had morphed into Iris's too. She was known affectionately as 'Beanie Deux', but mostly we would drop the 'deux' and just call her Beanie.

'Well, you know we haven't actually seen the speech therapist yet, and I don't know how many sessions we will get. They are talking about five or six a year; it doesn't seem right! So, we need a plan. I think we were making progress before Christmas, don't you?'

'Yes, definitely,' he replied a little too quickly. I wasn't sure if that was a man's answer, filling in the blank with what he thought I wanted to hear, but he had only just woken up so I went with it.

'So, my thoughts are that I need to carry on with what I was doing but make it even more fun. I have a good idea now about what she loves, how she interacts with her toys and I want to expand upon that. Here is a list of the things we need to get.'

P-J looked at the list. 'But we already have plastic balls for the ball pool.'

'We need loads more, masses of them, as many bags as you can carry from the shop back to the car. I want to fill a large paddling pool with them; we can create our own at-home sensory room for her. Ball pool, sensory lights, chill-out area, slide made from a mattress . . .' The lights were expensive, but I was sure they would be worth it. Iris loved colour and I was convinced they would really help her calm down when she was upset or let her focus on something beautiful if she was anxious.

'Right. I'll be in charge of this list. I can get all of this. A big trampoline, great. Let's get a huge one.'

'Don't get too carried away – I want it to fit inside in the garden room. I think we will have to move the dining-room table out, but we hardly eat in there as it is.'

P-J was already on his iPhone, looking up trampoline options. He looked at the list once again: 'This last note here: MUSIC. What do you want me to get?'

'I've been thinking how about my parents' piano. We can put it along the side of the wall.' I moved into the garden room to show him the position just between the two main beams, in the middle of the room against the side wall. I felt really strongly about this last item. I could see how much it would mean to Iris. She loved music so much and lately the only music she would fall asleep to was a CD of piano music. I wanted to be able to play it to her myself. P-J had also played a bit as a child and we resolved to start learning properly again. I had been reading about music therapy for children with autism and how much it helps them . . . It felt like a good option for the future. I started to make more notes of all the things that I needed to research: music therapists, music teachers, piano tuners, restorers . . .

'Right, I will get all the rest of the things on this list today then.'

'But we can't go out today, look.'

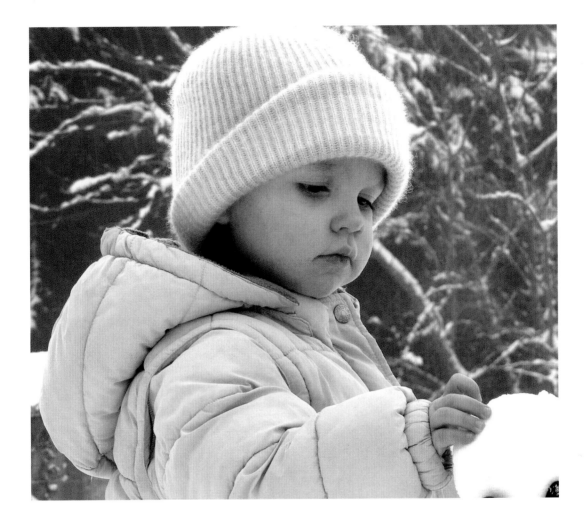

P-J looked out of the window and took in the snow for the first time. 'Good point! Let's go sledging!' he said excitedly like a small boy. 'Where's Beanie?'

I had been a little ambitious thinking I could get Iris to happily wear the gloves; they turned out to be an absolute no-go area. I couldn't get them to stay on for more than one second, so I abandoned them and went on to her boots. It took hours for me to persuade her they were a good idea, pairing them up with music and her favourite toys. She wanted to feel every part of them, to understand how they were made and that she could get them off easily if she wanted to. With them finally on we stepped out into the snow. The crunch unnerved her, so they went out into the garden together, Iris in P-J's arms. She gently touched a ball of snow in his hand with her index finger. The cold sensation was enough for her to decide this was interesting but not for her. No amount of encouragement would get her into the sled. This was going to take some getting used to – to forget our agenda and to follow Iris. To leave all those expectations behind, to try not to just replicate all our happy childhood memories and instead to focus on what Iris liked to do. Then when she was ready for new experiences to take them slowly and allow her to understand the whole process. So I sat in the snow with Iris on my lap and I let her shake off her boots. She watched the snow fall from heavily laden branches. With joyful hums, her hands occasionally flapped at the movement before her as if the forces of nature were transmitting their energy and then quickly being dispersed through her fingers. Listening to the gentle crackling sound of the snow as it melted and the dripping water from the slate roof, she was in a state of elated calm.

In the late-afternoon golden light a long strip of tissue paper floated gently to the ground to join its friends. Ribbons of white created an effect like a giant piece of modern art on the floor. 'Beanie has been busy!' P-J said to me as he came into her playroom. A ritual that had once filled our days was luckily today just a jaunty journey down memory lane inspired by the snow. Iris's interests could turn into addictive fascinations that seemed to rule the land. From water to bubbles, rice to sand, and tissue to feathers, the connection between them all was movement and gravity: to watch them fall, to see them spread. The motion always totally captivated her, so before interrupting I tried to think twice, suppressing my urge to tidy. What to us might seem a repetitive obsession could be important to the workings of Iris's mind, helping her figure out the world and the delightful effects she had upon it. I viewed it as an invitation into her world and joined in. Always carefully observing her, always watching for signs to see if the activity was being taken too far: was she getting frustrated by her own actions or enjoying them? If she was starting to feel pressure from herself, her body would be tense and her movements would become more repetitive and her hands would flap but at a much higher speed with quick movements right close to her chest, her hums becoming more intense. I would have my 'Mary Poppins' bag at hand, which was filled with intriguing sensory toys – squishy, stretchy and tactile objects that were so alluring they would take Iris's mind away from what she had become fixated upon so she could relax.

Our home gradually changed. Every room came to serve a purpose in Iris's therapy. At times even the corridors were obstacle courses designed to encourage interaction and speech. My mother would arrive at the door with a cooked meal for us all and barely be able to get to the kitchen. There were sand tables and water tables, and even my photography equipment played its part. The massive silver reflectors created fantastic circular bases for me to put plastic balls to encourage Iris to play. With every sofa and chair in the house stripped of its cushions, I made ramps, walls and ball pools. I dotted Iris's favourite books at strategic points along the way to inspire her to move on to the next activity. She would reach out to me, needing my help climbing over the cushions all piled up or for another go down the mattress slide into the ball pool. Before I helped her use the slide I would say, 'One, two, three,' and then pause, waiting for her to look up at my face. As soon as she did I would say 'Go!' and get her going down the slide. After a while she began to even mouth the 'g' for 'go' and I knew we were on to something. By keeping it fun and rewarding for Iris and using what she loved she was responding and many more sounds reached our ears. She was beginning to use language to communicate. While we played whenever she looked at me

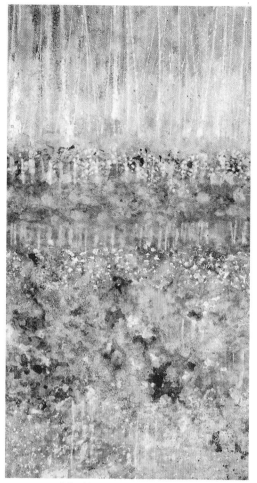

Tip-Toe, acrylic, June 2013

I would say 'good looking', always praising her for these achievements no matter how tiny they seemed to us, then letting her rest afterwards. She found it tiring and I knew if I pushed too hard she would retreat, moving away from us and taking a book on to the sofa where it became difficult to get eye contact.

With all this sensory play we began to see improvements in other areas. For instance, she started to tolerate socks and shoes and wear a few accessories like hats when we were out. We also made some progress with her speech. Using some basic techniques from the speech therapist and highly motivating activities like bubbles or her favourite toys, we would encourage her to say some sounds. Iris practised simple actions like blowing and became more lively – giggling and joining in with all the fun, using more gestures and sounds to show me what she wanted. It was slow but we were moving forward. The coffee table was always prepped with paper and crayons for us to use. I would feel her warm grasp on my hand pulling me over to the paper where I had been drawing stars, guiding my hand to the crayon and placing it on the paper: she wanted more. The paper was already full: a celestial heaven. Again and again she watched in delight at the two triangles overlapping each other. She was safe and secure in the comfort of repetition, the superhero cloak of knowledge providing confidence and peace. Our little Beanie was a creature of habit and quickly organized objects and even people into their place. There was order to her kingdom and veering off was not on the agenda. We encouraged change softly, little by little, by being there for her when all became overwhelming – a balancing act of challenges and allowances.

The garden room was proving so valuable, the light that shone in through the floor-to-ceiling windows inspiring us. I was still working hard photographing weddings at weekends. Iris's sleeping had improved a little, largely due to a visit from my aunty Sally-Anne, my father's sister, a mother of five. She wanted to see Iris's room and when I showed her she suggested that I made some changes. She didn't believe in keeping children's bedrooms plain so they could sleep better. Quite the opposite: she wanted to see more pillows, rugs, teddies, books, paintings, drawings, cosy areas, fairy lights – anything that would make Iris think this was a wonderful place to be and for her to want to go to bed, to want to relax up there and for it to be a magical place. Her plan worked well and the more additions I made, the more enchanting the room became and the better Iris settled in the evenings. It wasn't a complete cure; she would still only need about five or six hours before she woke up but at least we were heading in the right direction. Almost weekly there would be a blip and old habits returned. It was still difficult to manage. My exhaustion was a continual battle, but the garden room gave me so much strength.

But I worried that P-J and I were drifting apart. I spent so much time with Iris; it was all-consuming from the moment I woke till I went to bed. Some days I didn't know if I could give any more. How could one person be split so many ways? I was pulled in every direction – between Iris, work and my relationship with P-J. When I was around Iris just wanted me. She would take P-J to the door and quite literally push him out at times. And when she was upset I would do the same to him. I knew what I was doing was horrible and must be hurting him but when tiredness set in it was a reflex. Iris's behaviour towards him was painful to watch. When she didn't want him around, her hand would shoot out with her palm facing him like a stop sign. She would turn her body away and there was no doubt what it meant.

For so long P-J had to be brave and love her from afar. Iris saw him in a more functional role, taking my place when I was gone. He desperately wanted to play, to laugh with her and to create happy childhood memories, to be the father he wanted to be: fun, loving and the adventurer. He waited patiently for those moments of laughter and giggles, all the while watching me get closer to her. He didn't yet understand her like I could, even when I explained how I was achieving it. When he tried, it didn't seem to work in the same way – she reacted differently towards him and to others who tried.

'As long as it's working for one of us. Whatever works. Look how much better she is with you these days,' he would say with a smile, but I could see he was struggling to hold that smile.

He wanted it to be him for a while and sometimes I did too. I wanted for someone else to take some of the load, for me to have a break. I also wanted to comfort him, to make time for us as a couple, to mend what was breaking, but there never seemed to be enough time. But in the darkest moments the glass gable gave me light, filling every part of me with hope. We spent happy times as a family under those beams and they were mending our somewhat fractured lives.

One great new addition was the piano. Iris loved it from the start and right away went to sit on the red-velvet-covered piano stool. It was as if she already knew this old piano from years ago and they were old friends reuniting. The lid was always to be

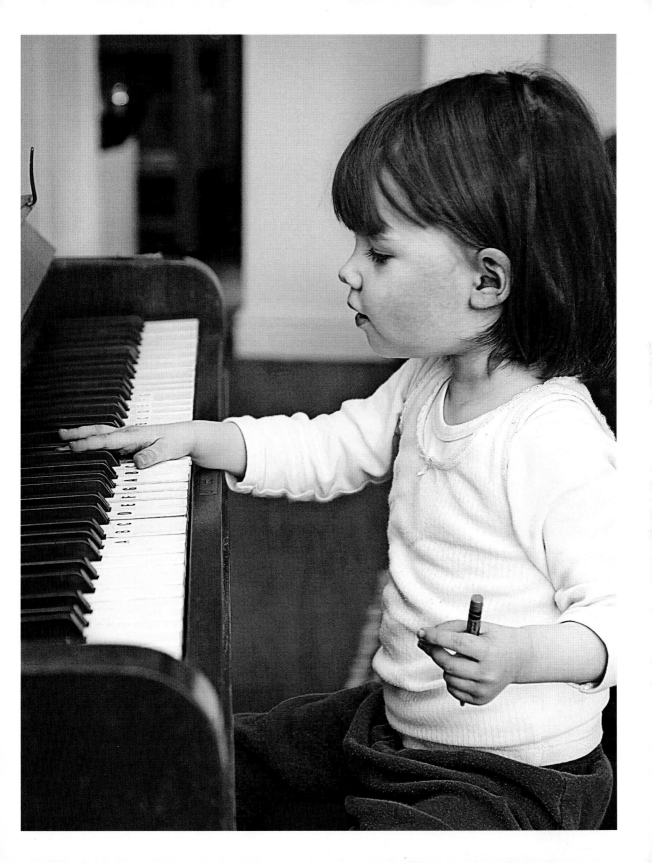

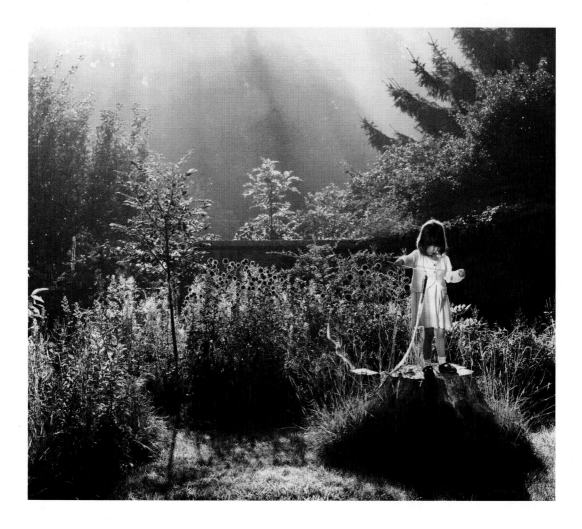

kept open, inviting a conversation and time to play. Once the piano had been tuned it sounded fantastic and gave a warmth to the room that could only come from music.

Then, as the seasons changed so did our view, and the garden beckoned Iris to explore. I began to see the garden as another space for us to work in and the decking area was perfect for all the sand and water play. We bought a swing chair for Iris and every day when the weather was good enough I would spend an hour or so in the morning setting up play areas: a cosy comfortable area with cushions to read books and an array of activities spread throughout the garden to encourage her to move on and to interact with me and the nature around us. When she needed space she would sit alone in the swing chair looking out at the trees. Watching leaves in the wind, she was so peaceful, almost serene, looking far older than her years and a whole world away from the anxious little girl I would see when we were surrounded by other people. Her repetitive and often obsessive behaviour would disappear and was replaced by a child filled with curiosity. She was no longer distant or disconnected. As the leaves moved, her hands reached out, her fingers gently moving with them, almost conducting, dancing and connected. I came to realize that the garden was doing more for her than I first thought. Her frustrations calmed and she could relax out there among the grass, flowers and trees, but they were offering her more than relaxation; they were helping her make sense of the world around her – soothing and nurturing at the same time.

There was one spot in the garden that Iris would return to again and again: the tree stump. So much had happened since we had cut down that tree in the garden, which had hidden our house in the shadows. I loved the stump as much as Iris did. It was a solid reminder of all the energy and dreams I had had back then and I didn't want to lose that. From a distance time seemed to have had no effect on it, but if you looked closer there were changes. Life thrived within the bark. It was home to all sorts of creatures and Iris loved inspecting their habitat. It was well positioned in the garden for many activities. The ground around it was flatter than other parts, perfect for laying a rug out with cushions. It was also more elevated, providing a great lookout tower. In the early summer P-J and I watched Iris as we ate our breakfast. Her calf muscles tensed and ankles flexed, and her heels rose up high, little toes curled from the pressure of standing perfectly still in the breeze as she surveyed her garden from on top of the tree stump. Everything was in order. She did an appreciative nod, then climbed down on to the grass and danced on tiptoes over to the flower bed, springing to the sky effortlessly like a ballerina on her unusually long legs. This was a sight that has become a signature quirk of her condition. The common link between autism and walking on toes isn't yet clear, but we could see that Iris gained comfort and a release through the sensation. She would bounce from the balls of her feet when she was happy, exhilarated or surprised, but they lay flat on the ground when she was calm – a striking indicator of her mood. Later that morning she placed her hands on top of the stump, feeling the grain, running her index finger along the many growth rings. She hummed contentedly and stood completely still with her feet flat on the ground. Then her attention turned to the bark and all its varied textures and colours. She climbed on top of it, feeling every part with her feet too, placing both feet and palms against the wood at the same time, as if she was drawing energy from the stump. Once again I saw a child so composed – not in a world of her own, but linked with the nature that surrounded her. As I watched her from the decking it was as though she cast a spell over everything. The world felt more alive and interesting to me too; it was enchanting. Her interest in the elements and attention to detail was inspiring and I started to see the world through her eyes, noticing intricate details, listening more intently and appreciating the beauty. My own senses were heightened, giving me a deeper understanding.

On another day 'monsoon' rain fell heavily on the garden-room roof. From the kitchen doorway I could see Iris's silhouette at the window, looking out on to the decking at the huge raindrops bouncing up high. A sheet patterned with concentric rings. She was mesmerized, her slim figure rigid and still, then suddenly, with an excited spring, she started to bounce, imitating the drops on the other side of the glass. As I approached she turned and smiled at me. Running over she

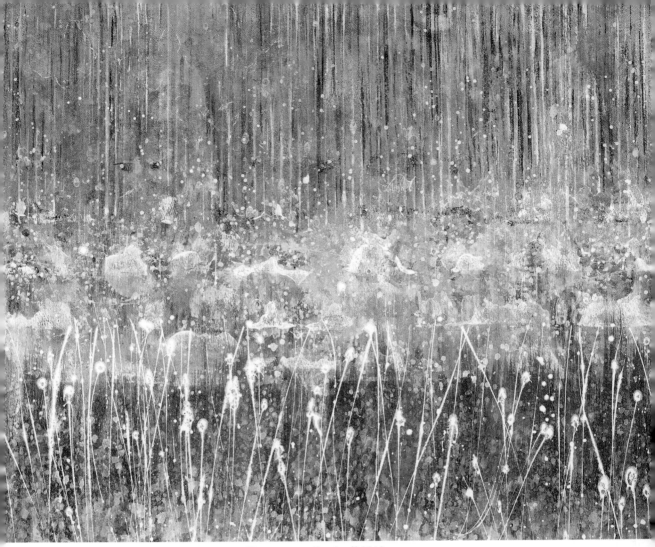

Monsoon, acrylic, April 2013

grabbed me by the hand and took me to the door, wrapping my fingers round the door handle. No words were needed to understand that she wanted to experience every part of this and that meant going outside. So we ventured out – pitter-pat, pitter-pat – her bare feet and the rain in harmony together. She darted in and out of the door, coming in when it all got too much. Sitting down just in from the rain, she watched it fall at ground level. I wrapped a warm towel round her and we sat together watching the raindrops. My mind was as busy as the patterns we watched, bursts of thought, ideas forming and then leaving, my tiredness catching up with me.

•••

With all these improvements in Iris's second year I had begun to look forward, to the future and the next stage of Iris's life: the preparation for her to go to school. This wouldn't be a quick or easy process; she would need to attend a preschool first for a few days a week when she was three years old and then build from there until she was going five days a week when she was four. The goal: Iris happily attending preschool, interacting with her peers and teachers. Then, at four to five years old, attending school. I knew we still had much to overcome, as we certainly had our fair share of challenging days when no matter how hard I tried things just didn't work, but they were being outweighed by better days, and I started to imagine Iris happy in a preschool setting and myself regaining some balance in my own life.

Iris was enjoying our activities and becoming so much more confident. By the time she was two and half she was interacting more with P-J and the rest of the family. She would raise her hands up for P-J to pick her up, and she wanted to be comforted by him and wanted his attention even when I was around. He would play her music on his iPhone, and they shared this appreciation and it became a way for him to connect with her. She was also more confident with other people around, and we had many happy Sunday lunches with friends and family at my parents' house.

I sat on the sofa beside my father one Sunday afternoon. He was ecstatic. 'She came up to me and kissed me! Did you see it? Just here, three little kisses on my cheek. Oh, Iris!' We had all seen it and knew how much it meant. Then he tickled her and she moved away: a step too far that made me laugh.

Our lunches were traditional in one way, mostly roasts, but they were different in another. My parents had learnt not to pressure Iris to sit at the table, and I fed her at home before we arrived. A little routine would commence. We would arrive always at the same time, about twelve thirty.

'Hello, darling,' my mother would call out from the kitchen. 'I've put some things out for Iris, taken the wool blanket off and her water is there.'

I would then lay out Iris's books and encourage her to explore the toys her grandmother had put out for her, grateful that the wool blanket wasn't on the back of the sofa. Iris's skin was sensitive and materials like that might cause an upset. While we ate our lunch in the dining room Iris would stay in the playroom with Indy, who was probably eating her snacks. Then she would dart in and out of the dining room, inspecting the ornaments on the table. There would be moments of interaction with each family member and then off she would go to the playroom again. No matter how much we tried no one could take their eyes off her while she carefully rotated the china or silver in her hands. There was something intriguing about the way she handled objects. The way she appreciated and looked after things was so alluring; you wanted to touch it too to appreciate what had caught her attention. When Iris needed space and went to sit on the sofa my mother would remind my father 'Just leave her for now. She is busy looking at her books' or 'Turn the volume down' as he watched sport on television next to her in the playroom. If my parents had friends for lunch or more of the extended family were there, we would make sure we arrived beforehand so Iris could settle and it was always a balancing act with Iris dipping in and out of the party so she could manage the additional people in the house. Having a quiet space just for her was essential on these occasions. But it didn't always work. Sometimes she would get distressed about the noise and movement of others and I

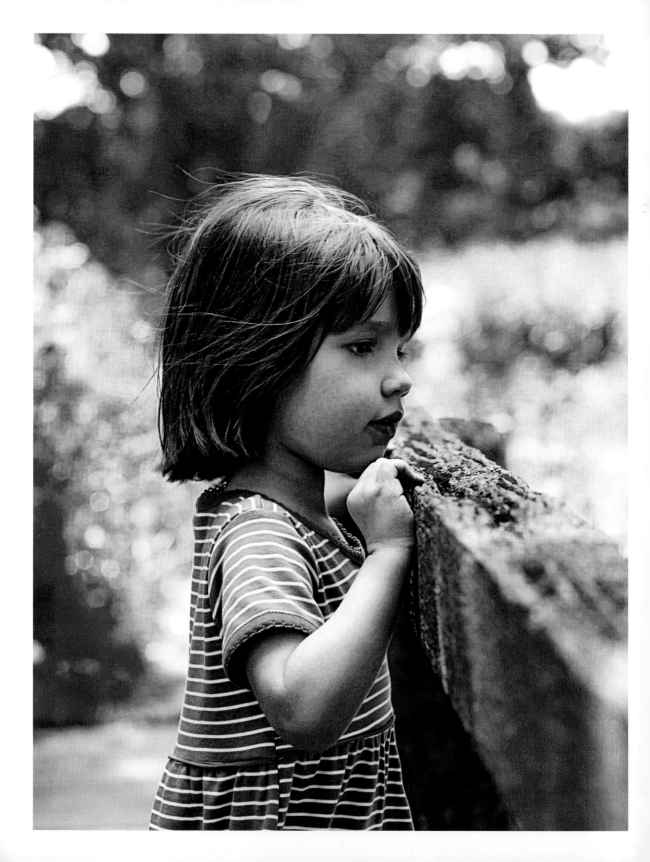

would take her for a drive in the car, which always helped: some time out and peace, looking out on to the countryside from her seat in the back of the car.

Although she was still not saying anything verbally beyond a few sounds, she was able to make herself understood by guiding us to what she wanted and showing us. Best of all, she was now able to do that not just with me, but with everyone in our family, so I had high hopes that it would eventually extend to teachers at the preschool.

In June, with only a summer to go until Iris turned three, I was starting to feel the pressure of what was to come. Her time at preschool would be the perfect way to prepare Iris for school, but I also wanted her to be prepared for preschool itself, which would be a massive change for Iris as her social skills were still so basic. She didn't follow verbal instructions, still found other children very confusing, and really her only way of communicating was through body language. Was there something I was missing, something I hadn't thought of to help Iris, another type of therapy perhaps?

I revisited an idea that I had looked into in the past, but to make this one work I would need to persuade P-J. Since Iris had been diagnosed I had made enquiries for her to be on the waiting list for an assistance dog. I had read how they had helped children in many situations and after the loss of Meoska I was missing having an animal in the house. I believed wholeheartedly that only good could come from having a pet and wanted Iris to experience the pleasures of having a faithful friend. The idea that a dog could be trained to help Iris, that it could provide support for her and help with her social skills was so special. Unfortunately my research and enquiries were not going well. Most of the waiting lists had been closed due to high demand. A lovely lady from one charity suggested I contacted a friend of hers who ran courses about how to train your own dog to be an assistance dog. A plan formed in my mind, to find a dog for Iris that we could train with some help from a professional. To my surprise P-J wasn't averse to the idea. He didn't want to walk the dog, but I loved going for walks so that was easy enough to negotiate. The obvious choice was to find a golden retriever and there happened to be one that was a year old being advertised for sale locally. A gamekeeper was cutting down on the amount of dogs he had on his farm and wanted to sell his youngest, Willow. I was so excited about meeting her; she sounded perfect for us. I kept in mind all those times I had seen Indy be kind to Iris and I began to visualize all the ways in which Willow might be able to help Iris when she was anxious or upset: giving her confidence and helping with her social skills, perhaps even coming in the car as we took Iris for her first day at preschool and all the other firsts that were yet to come.

'She's the one, I can feel it,' P-J said, as he came back to the car on our first visit to see her. I was waiting with Iris just in case the dogs were too noisy. As I approached Willow I could see what he meant: she was gentle, loving and very attentive. Her lovely face was so graceful and she had long blonde eyelashes and beautiful brown eyes. We took her back home that day with the agreement that we could have her on a two-week trial but we were both thinking this would be her forever home. I adored her already and hoped Iris would too.

But the trial didn't go well. As I heard P-J's voice through Iris's cries I knew that this hadn't been my greatest plan.

'Look, this isn't working at all.' P-J held Iris screaming in his arms and I did my best to get Willow to sit in the kitchen while I shut the door.

I turned round and took Iris in my arms and hugged her tight. 'I know, I'm so sorry. Iris is fine with Indy and she is so bouncy. I just don't understand why this is going so wrong.'

'Maybe it's because it's all the time. Iris doesn't get a break.'

It was true: Willow would get so excited and didn't know when to leave Iris alone. And she loved water so she would roll in the wet grass and make herself smelly, which Iris hated.

'And the licking! It never stops. She just licks Iris as soon as she sees her and doesn't take any notice when she gets pushed away. And you said you would do the walking. That was the deal.'

'Oh, come on! Iris hasn't been sleeping at all since Willow came and it's been so hard during the day. You said you would rather go out. It's been me dealing with all the meltdowns.'

I settled Iris with her favourite alphabet book and went through into the kitchen to talk more to P-J alone. I didn't want Iris to feel this was her fault. I stroked Willow, who rested her chin on my knee looking angelic. I wanted so much for it to work, but I had to admit P-J was right. Our lives had become much more complicated and difficult with her around. Iris seemed upset all the time; she wasn't sleeping and now avoided any room that Willow was in. Willow would seek her out wherever she could. It was a completely one-sided relationship and Iris was sick of the relentless attention and being covered with licks. So we rang the gamekeeper and took her back that afternoon. As I shut the boot of the car and looked at Willow through the window, her eager happy face and those gorgeous eyes, I felt terrible. I was sad to see her leave. It felt like I had failed at yet another part of life and I felt guilty for what I had put Iris through. How had I got this so wrong? The only upside was that I think Willow thought she had been on a holiday and bounced happily over to the other dogs at the farm while P-J apologized to the gamekeeper and explained why it hadn't worked out.

I hated it when my plans didn't work, but I was getting used to the feeling. I would create elaborate activities and feel so disheartened when they were completely ignored. Then we would have a success and it felt glorious, spurring me on to try again. The ups and downs were draining at times, to the point that I just wanted to give up, but when P-J told me that he thought that we should leave the animals idea for now, the stubborn streak in me couldn't let this idea go. 'It will happen when it's meant to happen. Remember how Meoska came into our lives, and the horses in Venezuela?' That expression irritated me. I didn't believe that any more. I believed you had to work at creating opportunities.

Over the summer before Iris's third birthday, I had read many stories about children on the spectrum, some more powerful than others, and *The Horse Boy* moved me to tears. A boy called Rowan, who sounded very much like Iris, had been transformed by his affinity with horses and then by an epic journey on horseback in Mongolia. His parents, Rupert and Kristin, took him to see shamans and they saw a reversal in their boy's autistic tendencies. His connection with horses, and his father's open mind, his ability to be able to see life through his son's eyes and adapt, made me wonder if horses would once more play an important role in our lives. I found an equine therapy yard not far from where we lived where people who had trained with Rupert worked and I felt certain this would help Iris. They didn't have any availability for a few weeks so we put some dates in the calendar and I couldn't wait to take her.

Looking through my photograph albums of our adventures on horseback in Venezuela I remembered how incredibly loyal our horses were. These creatures were highly sensitive, and I felt sure that they would work well with Iris, and that like me she would feel a deep connection to them. Horses might well be the key for getting Iris more used to social situations, maybe even a key to her communicating more verbally. I looked up to the wooden beams in the garden room where our Venezuelan saddles now lived. The brightly coloured pads and leather saddlebags transported me right back there. It was a fascinating country, and the malevolent murmurs from the unrest in the cities had been silenced for us by a land filled with majestic wonder. I trusted and admired Cantenero, a little horse that had totally changed the way I interacted with animals, shifting my approach towards gentler methods. It was he who had taught me never to underestimate what horses are capable of.

We had bought our horses from a hotel owner who had won the pair of stallions in a card game. He had no equine knowledge, and they were very badly neglected: thin, riddled with worms and both of them so broken in spirit that I made him an

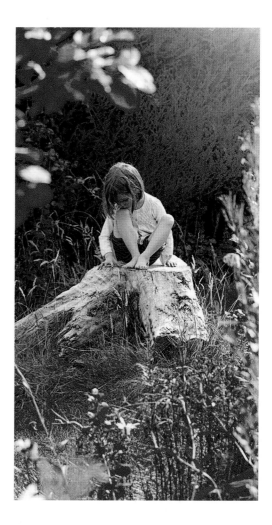

offer. I knew when we bought the horses that it was going to be a challenge but I couldn't just let them die. I didn't know how I was going to look after them in this beautiful but strange land but I knew about horses and they understood me; the rest I could learn along the way. A month later and they were already looking so much better. I had managed to find a vet that supplied us with wormers, and had travelled for miles to towns further south to find a store that sold shoes and learnt how to shoe them ourselves. We explored the tropical valleys and mountains, going for long treks each day, finding new routes and tracks. Cantenero was loyal, my best friend. He was fierce, a black beauty, but so badly treated in the past it took a while to gain his trust. Most days while P-J was trying to get some work done I would take Cantenero out and we would go on adventures together, my camera in the saddlebag on one side and map and snacks on the other. We climbed steep mountain sides and waded through rivers when the tracks were blocked by fallen trees. Like a mountain goat he always nimbly found a way. To my surprise on many occasions he would enter our home, just walking in as if to say, 'How's it going? Tea ready yet?' It wasn't a party trick: he genuinely thought he belonged with humans.

But then Cantenero started fighting with our other horse, Bonito, and since we hadn't been able to find a suitable field for them yet the young man who had been helping us learn how to shoe them said that he would take him for a while until we got everything sorted. I trusted him and he assured me that everything would be fine.

After about a week we went over on a surprise visit since we had heard nothing about how it was going. As I clambered out of the Toyota Land Cruiser I saw P-J glance over and he couldn't help but laugh – the sight of me trying to get out of this ginormous vehicle always made him smile. Although it was a monster I had become very attached to its overpowering presence, with its pumped-up suspension, huge metal bumper guard, tinted windows, snorkel exhaust and pull-up tent on the roof rack. It was as if we were surrounded by a fortress, a welcome feeling in this South American country on the edge of civil war.

I heard Cantenero whinny, and saw him tied up tightly to a fence. He pawed his hoof and tried to make his way over to us. There was no shade, food or water that I could see and I started to feel upset.

It turned out he had been fighting with their stallions too, so they had separated him, but had cruelly not looked after him properly. My heart was racing. This animal was my responsibility and I loved him as if we had been friends for years.

'Don't get angry with the guy,' P-J whispered to me. 'It's not worth it. Let's just get Cantenero and go.' He knew how quick-tempered the men here were. The atmosphere had changed since we had first arrived in the Andes. Life was becoming increasingly difficult with fuel strikes and shops closing, and food was becoming hard to come by as the supermarket shelves emptied. The laid-back, jovial manner of the locals was gradually turning, while the students protested, burning tyres and blocking streets, and the miles between the city and our safe haven seemed to be shrinking. Looking at my horse tied up, dusty, hungry and standing in the sun, my mind was made up: I would ride him back to our house that afternoon and P-J would drive back, meeting us along the route to make sure that we were safe. Luckily I had his saddle and bridle in the Toyota from when we had dropped him off, so we told them we would take him back with us. It would be a long ride back and we would have to go quickly to make it back before dark. We could keep Cantenero in our garden until I found another field.

'Take it steady and be careful. Don't talk to anyone and keep going. I will meet you at the top road just here.' P-J pointed at a wiggly line on the map.

I had never known Cantenero move so fast. His short rather uncomfortable stride was extended, and we were flying through the tropical valleys and there was a joyful bounce in his every step.

As we climbed in altitude the air got cooler and we took a break in the forest by a stream among the banana plants. Cantenero drank the fresh water, and black butterflies with turquoise patterns took flight in the commotion caused by his long slurps.

Row your Boat, acrylic, April 2013

Just beside me, perfectly camouflaged, I saw an insect in the shape of a leaf and I could hear the familiar buzz of hummingbirds swooping by in search of their favourite flowers, fuelling up and then on to the next. The noises in the forest were changing and everything was becoming louder as the light faded. Strange sounds that I hadn't heard before echoed around me. We cantered up the valley towards the road where I met P-J.

'You will be back in no time. Don't worry, there's plenty of light left.' His unfailing optimism could be rather unrealistic at times, so I took a shortcut through a more cultivated area filled with small farms. With very little light left and knowing how dark it got there with no light pollution I raised my reins in a little short upward motion so that Cantenero knew we had to pick up the pace again. The familiar smell of the grapefruit orchard near our house told me we were getting closer.

Suddenly I was aware I was not alone on the track. I could hear voices approaching and the smell of tobacco. Figures appeared round the corner with little burning lights from their cigarettes. Cantenero felt my legs tighten round him, and he raised his head high, arched his neck, trotting in a menacing fashion, snorting, plunging his hooves hard on the ground. We were on this adventure together and he was now taking his place as the protector. He had learnt to be careful of men: some you could trust and others were cruel. His hooves pounded the ground, the noise reverberating across the valley, and the men that we passed were intimidated by the stallion's presence and gave me a wide berth. I didn't hear a word from them: none of the usual jeering I had become accustomed to.

I was so relieved as the distance between us and them increased. Tensions were running high all over the country and there was no telling what you could expect from the locals. I knew that they were confused by the outsiders who loved horses and above all I was a young blonde English girl, just twenty years old in a foreign land. I was a potential target so always tried to be as careful as possible but the realization of my actions hit home: riding alone at dusk seemed ridiculous. I felt like I could breathe again once I saw my favourite tree covered in Spanish moss that was gently blowing in the breeze. For some the silhouettes of these trees would be a haunting sight, but for me they meant I was safely back home. P-J was there to meet me and as I slid the enormous metal gates shut I realized how dark it now was. Cantenero was tired but very happy to be with us and settled in immediately, grazing in the garden.

On a trek down the valley some time later I was approached by a student who was studying in the nearby city of Merida and had been visiting his parents in the country for the holidays. He was so excited that at first it was hard for me to understand his Spanish and broken English, but I understood enough of his story to learn how our faithful Cantenero had come to be. He had been raised by this young man's family in the hills, and from being a foal he lived in their humble home with earth floors and a tin roof. He was surrounded by the family and dogs so began to act just like them, protecting his owners. They trained him with gentle techniques and in turn Cantenero was kind. Sadly they had to sell him years before as one year their crops had failed but they all hoped he would still be safe and well.

Thinking about all our adventures with horses and how they helped me it felt like a natural progression to introduce Iris to horses and I felt confident this would bring much happiness into her life. At first our sessions at the Equine Assisted Therapy stables that were set within woodland were successful. Iris liked riding in front of me on the western saddle. She would look up at the canopy above and felt relaxed in my arms as we were led through the trees. We were only out for short rides and my back

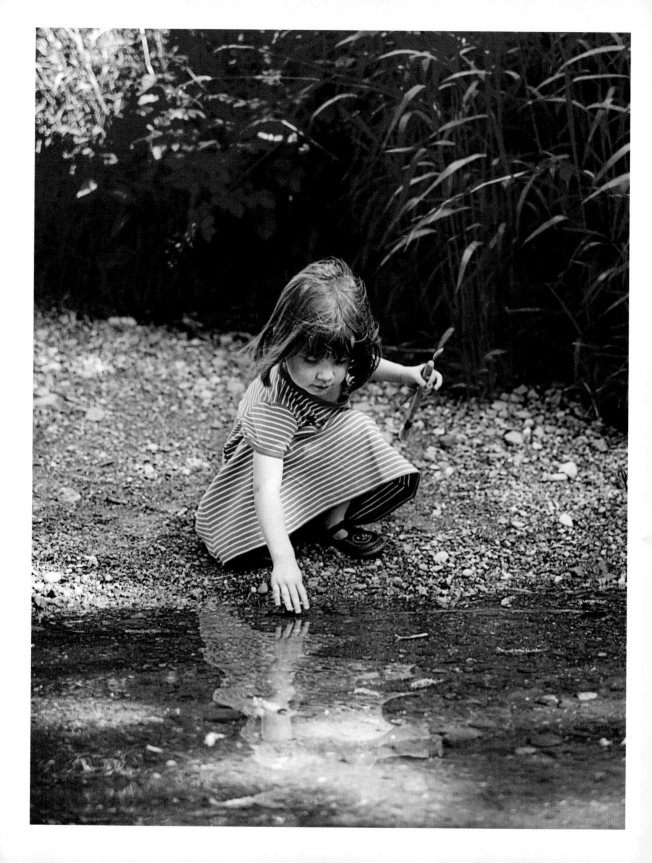

seemed to be OK – a little painful but worth it to see Iris happy. There was a large trampoline at the stables that she also liked.

But as the weeks went on it became clear that she had no interest in the horses themselves; they were just a mode of transport to take her through the woods so she could be in nature. Some weeks, if the horse wasn't ready for her to go straightaway, she would become distressed and impossible to calm and we would have to make our exit. She didn't want to stroke the horses; in fact, she wasn't interested in any contact. And it was hard for me to watch as once again I realized that I had been pushing my own agenda. It was my love of horses that had driven this latest therapy. I so badly wanted more developments – to hear her talk, to see her play with others – that I had pushed an idea which hadn't come from Iris but from my heart.

It sounds like the simplest of ideas to follow your child, to use their interests to build on their strengths to make connections, but the reality is very different. It's a continual learning process: constantly observing, taking yourself out of the picture and focusing on what is motivating your child, thinking fast and outside the box. I had believed so strongly that Willow and horses were going to help Iris, but it was too early at this stage in her development. I needed to give her time.

It was time for me to think again, to go back to what I knew Iris was interested in, to stop trying so hard, to stop rushing her into more therapies, to stop desperately trying all these different techniques. Instead I needed to concentrate on what was working, and most of all have some patience. So I took Iris to places where she could be immersed in nature. We visited gardens, forests, streams, lakes and rivers, always encouraging speech through play. The outings provided some relief from the isolation for all of us. Water play became part of every day and incredibly useful with her speech therapy.

By the end of the summer I felt happy about the idea of Iris starting preschool, although I didn't think it would be easy. I felt certain we would have some sleepless nights, but was hopeful that Iris would settle in well. She would have a support worker with her every day, whom we had already met, and she had been kind and accepting, making me feel that we were in safe hands. She seemed so interested in Iris and her condition; she was going to attend a short course on autism and she wanted a great many details from me, such as how I communicated with her and how Iris communicated with us. I believed that she had the best of intentions and as she answered my questions and assured me I would be allowed to stay with Iris for as long as she needed, I felt calm and confident that this was all going to work. I was concerned about the noise levels when the children first arrived in the morning or while they were leaving so she said that we could arrive later and leave earlier. She also wanted Iris to start her term a little later than the others so that most of the children would be settled by the time Iris was introduced. It was all looking very positive and my worries were eased by the school's flexibility and willingness to understand and help us.

As we approached her third birthday Iris gradually came out of her shell more and more. For her birthday we had a small intimate party. This time, I didn't wrap her presents in paper; instead I packed them all up in an owl rucksack that was to be her school bag and she excitedly pulled each item out one by one. They were all small toys with her interests at the core. She enjoyed herself immensely and I felt I was getting into my stride.

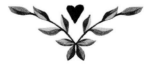

Darling Iris,

We are very proud of you. Over the last year you have achieved more than I could have imagined. My precious little girl, you have taught me so much. We are learning together and now that journey continues. Today is your first day at preschool. I don't want you to worry. I will be with you every step of the way. I know at first it might seem frightening, but remember we are all here for you. I understand that change is hard but sometimes change can be good, exciting even. You love to explore new places in nature and I hope in time you will enjoy being around other children and exploring with them too. Good luck, Beanie Deux, on this special day xx

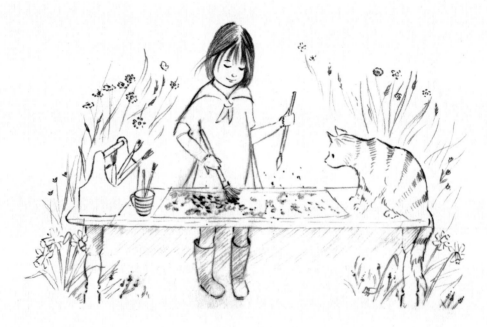

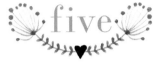

five

For the first time at preschool I saw her smile. Her pale face was transformed: happy rounded cheeks and beautiful bright eyes with long eyelashes. At three years old she looked unusually tall alongside her peers. She picked up a jug with one hand and filled it with water. The other hand held a green wooden disc, a part from a puzzle that had become a treasured piece. She poured water slowly over one of the half-submerged toys. Bending down close to watch how the water moved, she observed every ripple and drop with fascination. I heard her short intakes of air as the last drops fell. Then her hand was resting lightly on the cool surface of the water, happily feeling the sensation and the pressure against her palm. I took the chance to step back for a while and watched her in this rare moment where everything had gone quiet. The other children had moved away to the other side of the room to have their mid-morning snack, but Iris had chosen to stay at the water table. The guilt I had been feeling so heavily for the past weeks lightened as I watched her – maybe everything would be OK. We would get there and Iris would be able to manage preschool.

A little boy, having finished his snack, was on to his next mission, and with the carriages attached they were off, knees shuffling speedily from one side of the room to the other and the plastic wheels of the train running noisily across the hard floor.

Iris reached out to me immediately and wanted me to join her, but before I got there she started to cry, unable to bear it any longer. The noise from the train obliterated the progress we had made that morning and I could feel her pain; she was shaking, gripping my arm so tightly that it hurt me too. Her heart was beating fast and she had gone strangely pale, in contrast to my hot flushed cheeks. Failing to prise off Iris's limpet-like body, which had no intention of ever leaving her rock, I explained to the teachers that we needed the train to be put away so Iris could settle. They didn't understand. Why would they? Iris had a complex condition and in any given moment she moved along that spectrum with varying sensitivities and autistic traits. Sometimes these were predictable but at other times you had to open your mind wide, thinking like her to understand. She perceived the world differently and had very weak communication and social skills, withdrawing into herself when around others. With no experience of autism or how certain sounds can be a living hell for children on the spectrum, my request was not taken well – in their opinion the removal of any toy wasn't fair on the others. I wanted to stand up to them and fight our corner, to fight for my child who couldn't yet speak for herself, but I had run out of energy and could see there was no point. The noise, the chaos of free play and the mess was closing in on us. Those rare moments of happiness were fleeting. Even the lighting was a constant irritant: the strips of flicking light that sent peace on its way, and that train with carriage after carriage being dragged, pushed and bashed along the floor. I took Iris out into the playground and breathed in the cool air, trying to find some strength to carry on with the morning. How could I make this work? How could they understand when there were no clear answers and no format to follow with this complex condition?

I began to sense my presence was no longer welcome in the preschool class. I had already stayed for three weeks now to try to help Iris adjust and manage life in a class filled with other children. It was not going well. Whenever she moved away from the others to try to find a quiet space they followed; it turned out she was rather like a magnet. Just as Willow had loved following Iris about, so did the other children. They were curious about the intensity with which she played with toys, her interest in textures, how surfaces felt on her skin, how pouring water can become an art form, and they sidled up beside her trying to join in. Iris's gentle nature was pushed to the brink as her personal space shrunk by the second. If kept at an arm's length, she could tolerate them, but any closer and there was trouble. She would either burst into tears and be inconsolable for a long period of time or push the child out of her space. Repeated patterns drawn on to paper with a crayon by me or the support teacher helped. She would follow our zigzags or swirls with interest and jump on her tiptoes with excitement. We used the exercise to try to gain eye contact and encourage speech. First she would guide our hands, wanting more patterns to appear. Then as soon as she looked up at our faces we would make our move, drawing patterns on the paper. After that we would say 'more' and pause, waiting for her to attempt the word. When we heard an 'm' the page would be filled with more to reward her efforts. I was grateful to have found such little pockets of interest that allowed us to get closer. These activities provided a sanctuary, but not for long; before you knew it she had got so obsessed by the activity that it was nearly impossible for her to move on, and we would be stuck with the snail-shell swirls. She grabbed these predictable formations and held on until our time was up and we could make our way home before the other mothers arrived, avoiding the inevitable mayhem.

Our attempts at getting Iris to have fun in the playground were challenging too. While the others played, Iris followed the white perimeter line off to a tree far over on the other side, away

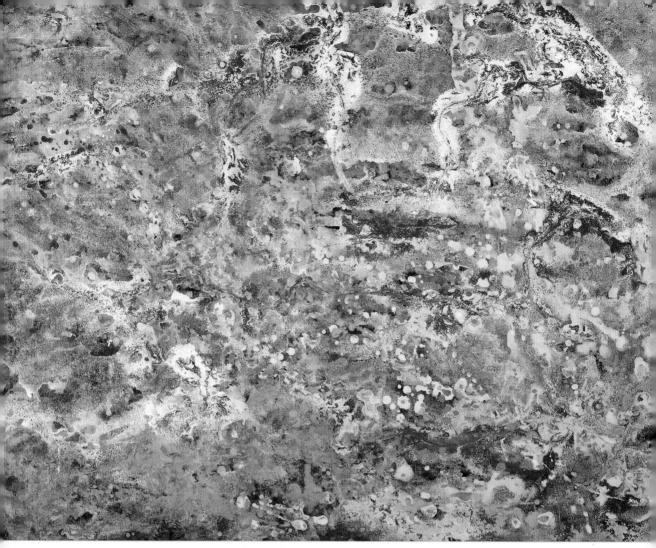

Separation, acrylic, April 2013

from everyone else, and sat alone to inspect a cracked area of the ground under her feet. She craved solitude and her eyes glazed with a faraway look. I knew she wanted to be back in our garden in the swing chair. I could see she was finding some peace by letting her mind wander but she was unresponsive to the outside world. She would not turn if we called her name or even look at us when we approached her. She avoided all face-to-face contact and wouldn't ever hold our hands. I felt like we were taking backward steps. Actually they felt like huge backward leaps. At home, even when she needed space, she was with me, in the present moment, experiencing life and enjoying it. She was more responsive than she had ever been, but at preschool it was like seeing her a year before. And the more she slipped away, the more I felt my heart break. All that work, for what? To see her crumble? For our lives to return to those earlier days?

Every time I took her in, I dreaded the walk through the corridor between the buildings to her classroom. Iris would spread her arms and legs out wide as I carried her, trying desperately to grab anything she could to prevent us going in. It was like being on holiday in Cornwall again when I was trying to take her into shops. She was making her feelings clear and I was ignoring them and that just felt so wrong. I had promised I would listen, take more care and consideration, and here I was breaking that promise. As soon as we were through the door she wanted to go home. I hated myself for putting her through it, but at the time it seemed like the only option. This was what we were advised to do to prepare her for what came next: the transition to school five days a week. Our options were very limited. All the other preschools were bigger, with larger class sizes. While the private schools conveniently had closed waiting lists once the 'autism' word was mentioned, and specialist schools and nurseries were too far away.

The goal for Iris to happily attend preschool and then school was fading, and I felt out of control, with no pattern to follow. But looking into Iris's face I suddenly decided I couldn't go through with it any longer. Her lips were cracked and bleeding from her latest anxiety-driven habit of picking them endlessly. She had lost weight from not eating properly and had dark circles that resembled sunken pits round her eyes. Her sleep patterns since starting preschool had gone from unpredictable but improving to ridiculous, and I was starting to suffer too. P-J tried to help but Iris just wanted me. It was difficult to watch him continually being rejected and our tempers were frayed. His relationship with Iris was falling apart and she rarely wanted to be with him any more; even music didn't help. Nothing I said or did made any difference. She had been pushing him away, which was a regression, and with me too she didn't want to play. She would still hug me but in a more desperate manner, clinging on, squeezing me tight. P-J and Iris had made such great progress with their relationship during the summer but Iris was now shutting down to everybody. Everything we had worked so hard for since her diagnosis was disappearing fast, being replaced by a monotony of fear and frustration.

Her autistic traits were at the forefront of everything, controlling everything: our relationships, our life, our work and our health. Her senses, emotions and feelings were never in harmony; they were always fighting, and for Iris this was devastating. Her obsessive and controlling nature was pushing all of us to our limits. P-J couldn't keep up with all the different ways she liked to have things. For example, she had to be fed from the same side and have her water cup given to her a certain way otherwise she wouldn't have any of it. She also liked to be put in the car a particular way and put into bed the same way each time. When she was at home she got stuck on certain parts of cartoons and wanted them playing constantly. She wanted one book open on a particular page and for us to read it to her over and over again. The one customary item that she liked in her left hand had turned into a collection. This caused enormous frustration: there were too many things for her to carry and her hand eventually resembled Edward Scissorhands, with items wedged between each finger and clasping a couple in her palm. Every aspect of our day became ruled by a set routine that fluctuated on Iris's terms. And as her communication skills broke down and she rarely looked at us any more, these tendencies were becoming very difficult to handle. The only way we knew we were getting it right was if she didn't cry. But if we got them wrong, she would get distressed really quickly. It was trial and error as we tried our best to understand what she wanted.

As I left the school that day with Iris looking shattered in the back seat, the car stalled with a big bunny-hop – completely my own fault through tiredness. I checked my mirror and noticed the other mothers all chatting at the gate. Their carefree happy manner held my gaze. Jealousy ran through me and I began to feel angry. Anger at what, I didn't know. I couldn't blame Iris – this wasn't her fault – and I certainly couldn't blame the other mothers for having an easier time of it than me. I imagined what their lives must be like, dropping their children off at school, having some time for themselves – even if it was just a few hours – how refreshing must that feel. I stopped myself: there was no point in comparing lives. This was mine and that was theirs. Even if they looked like the picture of perfection right now with their freshly ironed clothes and beautiful hair there was always something hidden behind those smiles and happy chatter. Everyone had hardships to deal with and wallowing in mine wouldn't help. Driving home felt like we were breaking free – down the hill and then on up the country road – there was such a sense of relief for both of us.

I wanted to hold on to that feeling for ever: the freedom, that glorious freedom. Before I knew it I was making a vow to Iris that we would not return, and I could see Iris's reaction in the mirror: she was happy, and that gave me the courage I needed to go through with it. The decision to take Iris to preschool had been down to us. It wasn't a legal requirement and I could take my time over the next year to prepare her for school myself. We had asked too much too soon and plunged Iris into the deep end with people who didn't fully comprehend her condition. As I parked up in our driveway and unbuckled Iris from her seat she hugged me. It was a beautiful hug, calm and sweet, her face tucked into my neck, and I could feel her breathing

Namazzi Blue, watercolour, January 2014

steadily against my skin. I don't know if she understood what I was saying to her about how we weren't going back there or if she just sensed my relief, but that hug made me not question the decision. It stopped all negative thoughts in their tracks and reversed them, shooting them into the positive. Surrounded by people that didn't understand in the preschool, I had felt so alone, but at home that day the loneliness disappeared.

I would teach Iris at home for the next year and hopefully regain all that we had lost. My head filled with ideas, fuelled by the hope that I had to cling to. I was going against advice and making our own way. I knew that P-J would be one hundred per cent behind me but I was worried about Iris's grandparents. Every time we spoke on the phone or in person they would all ask eagerly after Iris and preschool, their hopeful tones and faces wanting the answer to be that she was settling in just fine, that we were over all the difficulties and that things were OK. The disappointment that came with my replies and their hugs of support made me emotional. But to my relief when I told my mother we were stopping preschool she was totally supportive. She couldn't handle seeing Iris like this any more either and suggested that I find some private therapists to help me over the next year.

With winter approaching my aim was to research and find professionals to help me in four key areas. An occupational therapist to help me with Iris's sensory needs and some of her more challenging behaviour, like her problem with transitions between activities, play skills, responses to certain stimuli and her ability to self-regulate. A speech therapist and a music therapist to encourage communication, and a dietician to help me assess Iris's diet and see if there were any improvements we could make to help with her behaviour and sleeping problems.

There was one cartoon that Iris loved called Dipdap, in which a drawn line created endless adventures for the little character. He was an almost alien-like creature with two huge eyes, but no other features – all very plain. I could see the attraction; it reminded her of our game together when I drew stories, and the character had a simple face, with nothing confusing to figure out. So for the following weeks I followed suit and simplified our lives, creating spaces that Iris could relax in. With all the turmoil of preschool over the previous month, the house had got increasingly untidy as I had struggled to manage our lives. So the busy, cluttered alcove in her playroom was emptied, decorated and organized to give her a fun creative space. I drew a tree on the wall with a pair of owls and flowering branches with Iris's colouring pencils. Her books were neatly put away on the bookshelf and I bought pieces of furniture to display her toys. Her playroom was no longer a chaotic space but had some order to it.

I think the whole process was therapeutic for both of us. I needed to feel like I was getting some control back in my life, that we were working towards a positive future, and Iris found some peace in the order. She would line up her toys, and play fruit would be taken out of the bowl and neatly arranged along the edge of the sofa. The same was done with large gravel stones from the driveway; she brought some in one at a time and lined them up on the windowsill. The more organized I got the better I felt. I could tell Iris felt it too and her hand slowly emptied until we were left with just one last item: a pink spoon. My mother suggested that we came over for lunch during the week, a quieter time where Iris could learn to be at theirs and relax again. We decided to go on Fridays and to stick to that day as best we could to give Iris a sense of routine. Generally Iris would still only interact with me but the lunches provided opportunities and security for her. Some weeks she would settle well, exploring the garden after lunch and then going off upstairs. My mother and I would follow her and let her discover all sorts of treasures in the other rooms. There were certain ornaments and perfume bottles from my mother's dressing table that she adored, so they became part of a new routine. When we arrived Iris would fetch the bottles from the dressing table and come back downstairs to be with us. My mother would remember and put them closer to the edge so she could easily reach them. These details were anchors in Iris's world and it was a technique that worked well to encourage a smooth transition.

Planning was well underway for Iris's home education. We didn't want her to miss out on any of the opportunities that she would have had at preschool and we wanted to prepare her for the following school year. I found out about all the activities that were on the curriculum. I would need to teach her numbers up to twenty, her alphabet, learn about shapes, colours, some basic phonics and a whole lot more. And, of course, I also wanted to get her speech going. Financially the thought of hiring private therapists to work with Iris once a week was a worry, to the point of me not knowing if we could afford to go ahead. I will never forget the kindness from my aunt Celeste who lightened that load. Her generosity meant that we could pursue my search for the right therapists and I could photograph fewer weddings, giving me time with Iris to educate her at home. Celeste was there not just for Iris but for me too. She wrote to me, reminding me to look after myself and that she was there for me, and whatever I needed to ask for help. I needed to hear that; just knowing that she was thinking of me helped me not feel so alone.

By the end of October I had found a brilliant local occupational therapist. Becky was just what Iris and I needed – strong, knowledgeable, positive and a realist, but behind all of her strength she was as sensitive as they come and knew exactly how to be with Iris. How to hold her, what movement or pressure she needed to calm her. An expert in the senses, she taught me so much about how to help Iris regulate her system. Iris needed to effectively use all the information from her senses –

vision, touch, hearing, taste and smell, as well as signals from the inside of her body: movement and her internal body awareness. Sometimes these could be confused and, therefore, were disorientating for her. All this input has to be registered by sensory receptors and processed in the brain, which stimulates a response. But at times we could tell this wasn't happening and she became overwhelmed or frustrated. She would experience both under- and over-sensitivity. Our aim was to try to allow Iris's system to respond in an adaptive way that wouldn't cause her stress. With Becky's help we developed a series of exercises called a 'sensory diet' to help Iris with various issues at different times of the day. Sometimes she

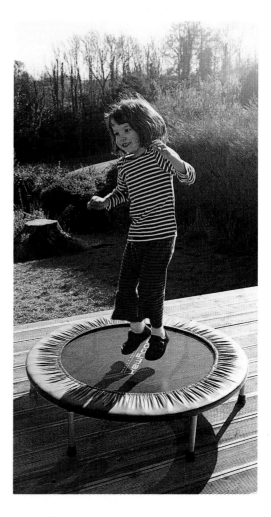

would need to bounce on the trampoline or on the therapy ball, to have deep pressure sensations through bear hugs, massage, joint compressions, brushing and rolling; while at other times she would need to be held, wrapped up or lie under a beanbag. All of this had a remarkable calming effect upon her. I learnt how to use these exercises and when Iris needed them. Becky showed me all sorts of ways that I could use different sensory play with rice, pasta, water and bubbles to help with Iris's sensitivities.

She also brought games to play that would gently desensitize her from louder more unexpected noises and other games that encouraged joint attention. We worked on transitions between activities, rewarding Iris for her good behaviour and ignoring the bad.

Becky worked with me on a gradual plan to develop Iris's abilities to follow my requests, to be more flexible towards tasks and transitions. Iris had become rigid in her behaviour, and things were sliding out of control, so every week Becky would work with her, moving from activity to activity – all the time encouraging her speech with basic speech-therapy techniques and motivating her to ask for 'more' or to count as they played together. She also wanted Iris to practise blowing bubbles through straws, to help with breath control. Iris had no problem with fine motor skills so some of the games would be more about other issues like noise. Becky would bring toys that made noise but give Iris something in return, all working towards getting her to become more flexible with everyday life. Through these various exercises her senses gradually calmed and she started to self-regulate her system. At first, sometimes in a whole session Becky would only get snippets of time, little bursts until Iris pushed her away and needed some space. In the gaps between, she would talk me through techniques and hear more about what had been happening, how Iris was doing. She was so in touch with Iris and her current situation; it was incredibly refreshing for me. I felt like we were in this together, working harmoniously on the same goal. And when Iris was ready Becky would continue. I was no longer alone and it was a fantastic feeling. For many months I hadn't properly understood why Iris was so sensitive or how to help her, so to get the help she needed felt wonderful.

Becky did also have a tougher side, a more realistic outlook on life that I needed to hear. She made me realize that Iris needed to manage in the world, that I needed to prepare her and that meant going out more and helping her achieve more independence. I needed that reminder. When you are living it you are in so deep, so totally consumed by it that you lose perspective. The isolation would creep in once again if I let it. I hadn't been going out with Iris very much as it had become difficult again. Our weeks were based predominately at home or at my parents', and I was starting to feel the effects of cabin fever. Iris had become so controlling that for most of the day we let her decide what was on the agenda, what was on the television, what toys she played with, what activities she did. I needed to turn things round to be more balanced. It was one thing following Iris's interests and building on her strengths, but we had fallen into a pattern that was unhealthy – not good for Iris or us. The series of short-term fixes – letting her watch the same cartoons, listening to the same music over and over, and her insisting on keeping certain objects exactly where she put them – had become habitual. These would lead to much bigger problems if we didn't work with her on this and help her become more flexible. We needed to move forward, to keep moving forward no matter how hard life got, to keep control of Iris's behaviour and not to let it rule our lives.

Iris's reaction to music in her therapy sessions changed over the weeks. At first she was transfixed as our talented therapist Elizabeth played, mimicking Iris's mood, copying sounds she made and improvising a tune to encourage Iris to respond. It was as though Iris was transported into the music, her fingers feeling the music like she did with the wind. Over time she became more responsive and interacted with the instruments, copying a tune or joining in with Elizabeth, who would create a game from the interactions and encourage Iris to play with the selection of percussion instruments she had in a bag beside her on the sofa. Some weeks Iris would need to cry and Elizabeth used the music as an emotional outlet; she would respond to Iris with her violin or the piano to let Iris know she understood her

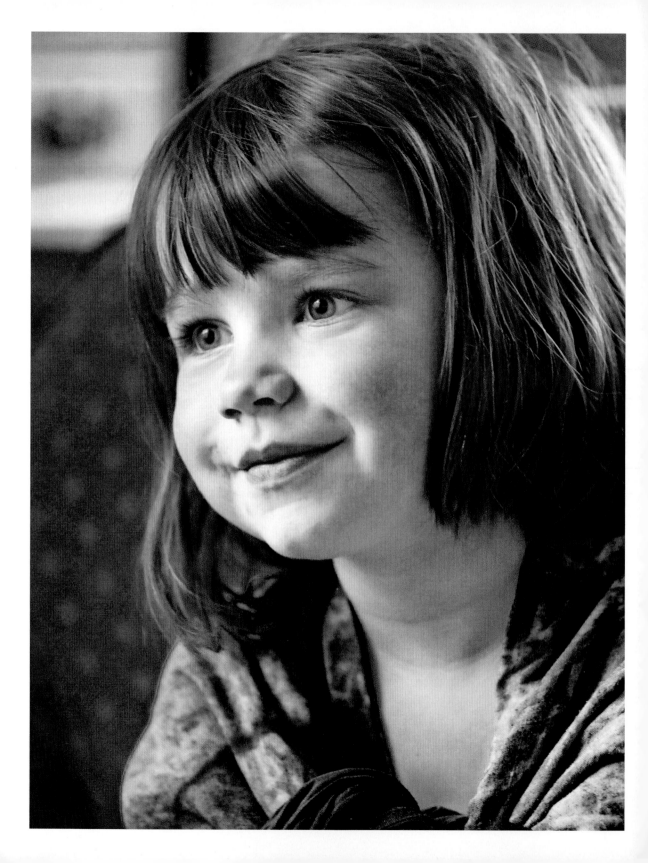

feelings and that it was OK to let them out, but then she would make her tune more comical and lively and Iris's mood would follow. It was incredibly interesting to see how powerful the music was and how quickly Iris responded. Iris would hum in response, and after a while she even said some sounds and words, which would then be included in the song. So if Iris said 'bee, bumblebee', Elizabeth would repeat it, then tell a story about a bee with her music and sing a song.

Iris didn't want me to leave her at first so I sat quietly at one end of the sofa with Iris at the end closest to the piano. It was hard not being involved when she started to say a few words; I wanted to give her a giant hug and a kiss, but Elizabeth needed me to stay quiet so I wouldn't distract Iris. My heart would fill with pride to bursting point as I heard these words. They were few and far between at first but as the weeks went on we heard more, which was so exciting. It always seemed to happen when Iris was relaxed and swept away with the music. It was like a conversation but with instruments, singing and words and without the pressure of a normal face-to-face interaction. There was no right or wrong way and Elizabeth quickly learnt when Iris just needed to have some time to listen and when it was OK for her to move closer and encourage speech, movement and music. She could pull Iris out of the darkest of places at the end of a long week and some weeks Iris would dance in delight as she played her fiddle, but there was always the same effect afterwards. Her mood would be improved and she would be easier to work with, and I started to love the music too.

In December I found a dietician, and I learnt so much from her about what foods to give to Iris and how to balance her blood glucose levels. I had been giving Iris too much wheat and fruit in the later part of the day, even a banana in the evenings, which wasn't helping my case at bedtime at all because Iris was so full of energy. She was on a healthy diet already but I needed to increase the amount of vegetables, keep up the home-cooked meals and be more careful about the positioning of her food throughout the day to encourage the behaviour that we desired. We began to give her more fish as there was a concern about a possible fatty-acid deficiency that was linked to her dry scalp, hyperactivity and poor communication. We also bought organic produce wherever possible. I lowered her wheat intake and cut out as many sugars as I could. Iris only drank milk or water so that wasn't a problem, but I was giving her too many biscuits, so I swapped to healthier options for her snacks. She became less erratic and her sleeping improved a bit, which I'm sure had a knock-on effect for every other therapy we were trying. She was more responsive and easier to work with if she had slept and was eating well.

We continued to take Iris out in nature whenever we could and gradually our happy little girl came back to us. She was still fragile; it didn't take much for us to see her bolting off to the sofa and picking her lips and she still found it hard to be affectionate with P-J and the rest of the family. A great many times she seemed to push everyone away, still needing her own space. She continued to hug me but generally only when she was frightened or very tired. It was going to take time for her to trust again and for us to regain her confidence.

But there was one new issue that had arrived so suddenly that I felt sure it was just a phase and would pass. Iris didn't want to wear tops any more. She preferred to be naked from the waist up. She would wear them when she was outside, which was a relief, but as soon as we were in everything was stripped off. It didn't matter how many times we put them back on, off they came again. I worked with the occupational therapist to help with Iris's sensory issues regarding her clothes, including using a technique called 'brushing' – the Wilbarger Protocol. It involved giving Iris deep-pressure brushing with a soft bristled brush followed by joint compressions, and the procedure was repeated every couple of hours. It really helped in regard to getting her top on but unfortunately it didn't last; Iris would just take it off again after about a minute. But with everything else settling I didn't feel too worried about it.

At Christmas I managed to keep my promise from the previous year. We made it all more manageable: wrapping paper was history and her presents were bundled in material with soft ribbon bows. I decorated the house over a few weeks, leaving some rooms as they were before to provide spaces where Iris could go if it got too much and focused on some key elements like a beautiful Christmas tree that we decorated together. I bought lots of Christmas books so she was prepared and understood what was happening. On Christmas morning she played with her presents under the giant Christmas tree, looking out into our garden. She could see her old friend the tree stump, and with music playing we took a much gentler approach in our pyjamas. The fire was lit and we snuggled up on the sofa with duvets while Iris showed us what Father Christmas had brought her. I didn't have the pressure of entertaining or cooking, and there wasn't a distressing catalogue of disasters that I had to fight against like the previous year, so we could enjoy ourselves and I was rewarded with the most precious gift of all: the three of us together, laughing and giggling, snuggled up under those oak beams. We went over to my parents for lunch, but didn't stay too long and we made sure that we considered how Iris was feeling; if she needed space and quiet, we gave it to her. By taking the time to prepare and to understand we were able to make it a magical holiday.

The damp cold days before spring the following year were brightened by the obstacle courses that still reigned supreme in the corridors and the garden room. Every surface low enough was covered with paper, pencils and crayons that were always out and ready to be used. If Iris couldn't express herself yet through

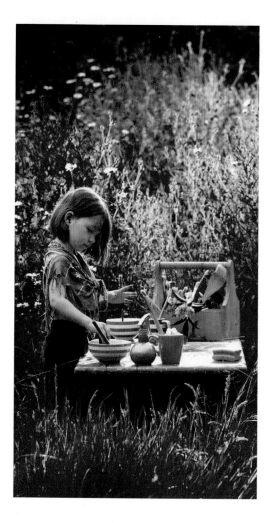

language, then art would be the answer. Each day we saw Iris becoming more playful, more engaged, but even with my very best efforts her speech was not improving as much as we had hoped. Time was marching on and Iris's lack of verbal skills at three years old was increasingly worrying. She had made some improvements in her music therapy when she said the odd word, which we celebrated, but the impatient side in all of us was starting to show. Her speech was unreliable; sometimes she would say some sounds and respond with a word, but mostly she was silent apart from her humming noises. She still communicated with us through her body language and by pointing at what she wanted. She was able to use those skills with people she knew well, but she didn't react well to people she didn't know. If we really encouraged her, we might get a 'more' for more bubbles when she was working with Becky or counting up to three as I pulled her down the mattress slide but it was slow progress compared with her peers. Most children at three years old know up to one thousand words and are able to tell simple stories and recite nursery rhymes . . . Iris could say around twenty words and even they weren't on command. We all had to work so hard to hear them, including Iris. It was frustrating as I could tell they were all there: locked inside, just waiting to come out. But there was somehow a blockage, a crossed wire, something . . . We didn't know what and nobody did. We saw a few more speech therapists and they always suggested the techniques that we were already using so we carried on, focusing on her play and activities linked to the curriculum.

• •

We had just had a very successful day with sand, when I drew letters and Iris started to say the letter out loud. Next was painting, so I prepared the easel that had been given to her by her grandparents that Christmas. I had high hopes for this activity; she had been having so much fun with her crayons and all the stories I told through my drawings that I felt certain she would enjoy herself and that it would provide many opportunities for me to fit in some speech therapy.

As I mixed the colours in the children's plastic painting pots Iris was getting very excited. She was bouncing up and down on the trampoline in the garden room and darting back and forth to the easel. She had been fascinated by the roll of paper that came with the easel as it was different from the one I had been taping on to the table, and of course we had an Andrex-puppy moment – Iris pulling at the paper so it tumbled across the room and I had to roll it back up and start again. I showed her by dipping a brush into the paint and making long strokes across the paper before us. She stood patiently beside me and then had a go. The moment the paint started to run down the paper she got furious, and the thin children's paper started to crumple and its shape distorted from the watery paint. She started to cry and threw herself to the ground with the paintbrush still in her hand. The blue paint splattered over the floor and on to Iris's arm. This made everything that much worse – she wanted the paint off immediately as she couldn't stand it on her skin – so I ran into the kitchen to get a tea towel and when I came back she was over by the window trying to open the door, crying. She wanted to escape from it all and I felt awful. This was meant to be a fun learning experience, not a tortuous affair that led to upset. I did my best to clean her up and then opened the door and she ran out into the cold air. I noticed she had also knocked over the red paint pot. Stupid pots, they were too light and flimsy. I put away the easel and paints, feeling disheartened. As I was clearing up some paint that had dropped on to the wooden floor I thought back to what had worked before – the large sheets of wallpaper liner taped on to the coffee table in the playroom for drawing with crayons. She had loved that: happy hours were spent at that table and I felt sure that paper wouldn't distort quite so dramatically under the weight of watery paint. And if it was lying flat Iris would have more control over the paint and it wouldn't dribble down the paper. I decided to change just one part of the activity – the medium – from crayons to paints, and keep everything else the same: from the position in the playroom to the wallpaper liner taped down so it was secure. Like the easel those plastic pots would have to go; I would use mugs instead: much more stable and familiar to Iris.

The next time, with the playroom suitably covered in old sheets to protect the furniture, I laid out some mugs filled with paint for Iris and I let her decide when to come to the table. I didn't need to wait long before the paper was filled with colour. She seemed so precise about the way she was painting: a quirky mixture between free and considered. She used lots of different techniques – swirls of colour, zigzags, splodges and dots – to make marks and I was surprised at how little ended up on the floor, and absolutely none on her. The colours were also clearly separated and not all smudged together. While the painting was drying in my office it occurred to me how attractive it was for a first attempt, so I photographed it to commemorate the joy we had found in this new activity.

The next few days followed a similar pattern. Her interest in painting intensified and the amount of time she would spend on each extended. This new fascination was opening up all sorts of opportunities for me to interact with her and she was so happy. The insecurities and defensiveness that usually surrounded social situations faded while the brush was in her hands. She bounced with excitement, listening to me as I talked to her about the colours and the formations of the watery paint. She didn't crave her cartoons or books any more. It seemed I had found another key into our little girl's world. We had been making wonderful advances but this was in a league all of its own. Feeling more motivated than I had in a long while, I made the decision to let her paint as often as she wanted to, letting her explore this new avenue of expression. I rearranged the furniture in the kitchen and made a space for the table.

By the end of the week, Iris was hopping about in the kitchen with anticipation as I rolled out a new section of wallpaper liner. As I taped it on to the table she disappeared into the garden room; she couldn't stand the sound of the tape as I pulled it off the roll. She waited until it had all gone quiet before she tiptoed back in and then she was by my side. With her small hand in mine she led me to the sink in the kitchen. Her finger was rigid and outstretched towards the blue pot, so I made some up, very watery this time as my hand was guided again and again towards the tap.

When the painting had dried I leant over as far as I dared, standing on a chair to photograph her work. What lay before me made my heart beat hard: layers of blue and green with repeated shapes and a wash of yellow. She was creating paintings in a way I hadn't expected from a three-year-old child.

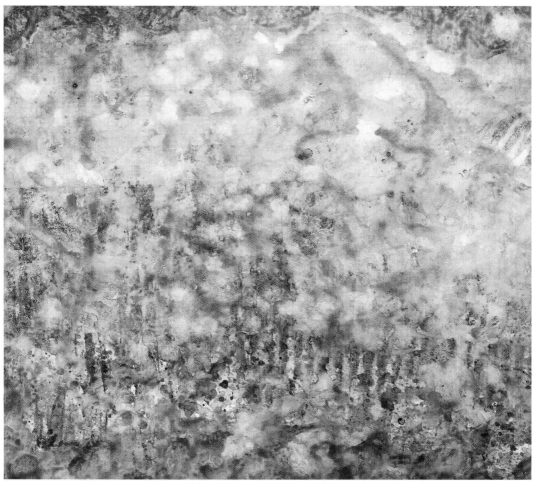

Sunny Day, acrylic, March 2013

'Have you seen the latest one?' said P-J, gesturing over to the painting. 'It's brilliant, seriously, come and have a look.'

'I know, that's what I thought. I've photographed it. Shall we get it framed?'

'Yes, definitely.'

'She seems so . . .'

162

'Grown-up.'

'Yes, different from before. I'm going to keep going with this. I know I have my list of activities but this is going so well.'

'Forget your lists! Go with what's working. At the moment that's her painting. You know she even hugged me this morning? Just came up to me and hugged me with a big smile.'

P-J looked incredibly happy. I knew how much that hug meant to him and how long he had waited for her to be comfortable enough to show her affection like that. It was spontaneous and genuine. Beautiful beyond words. There was an excitement in the air. The positive energy that surrounded the humble pine coffee table was having a massive impact upon our family.

As I watched her painting in her own unique style I realized that I needed to invest in some better paper as water poured off the table on to the floor. Luckily this was on the other side from where she was standing, but it needed to be remedied. So I bought the best-quality watercolour paper I could find in the exact size to fit the coffee table where she painted. Iris wasn't a fan of change and I was concerned that this paper with its rougher textured surface would not be appreciated. I did not need to worry, though. She studied it as if it was an experiment: first gently patting it with her palm on the paper, then looking at it so closely that her nose almost touched it. She appeared to kiss the paper but I could see that she was actually feeling the texture with the top part of her lip, just on her cupid's bow. With her head now turned to the side she rested her cheek and looked straight at me and smiled. This rare eye contact was a striking change in her behaviour. I handed over her favourite paintbrush. With quick flicks high into the air the paper was soon filled with explosions of colour and the cotton rag watercolour paper was happily soaking up all Iris's watery paint. After the colours were dry she added another layer of white – she didn't want any water added. By using a longer brush she drew the paintbrush over the paper in a wave-like motion, creating patterns, and then, moving round to the other side of the table and tapping the brush, she created dots of white. I slid her painting table under the kitchen table to let it dry and mopped up the floor. This had been a particularly vigorous session and little splats of colour were dotted all over the place. Then I heard the gate: P-J was home from his trip to London and as he came into the kitchen Iris was there to meet him, beaming at him, grabbing his hand and pulling him over to her table.

'Iris, what have you been up to?'

'Here let me get it out.' I moved the table back into its position and Iris shared all her favourite parts with her father. This process took a while as she pointed out all the white dots and wiggles.

As I made some food we chatted. Iris had gone through to her playroom and I could hear books being pulled off their shelf.

P-J was looking so proud. 'They really are amazing, don't you think?'

'Yes, but everyone thinks that about their child's artwork, don't they? I agree there is something very special, but do you think that it's just us seeing it? I mean, perhaps they seem special to us because of how she is while she paints, how it opens her up?'

The evening went on with more talk about her painting, why she loved it so much, how easy she was to interact with when she was painting, how it changed her. The more wine we drank, the more excited we got. It was fun to be focusing on something positive rather than talking about the latest problem. What I loved was that it was beyond our control. Iris painted when she

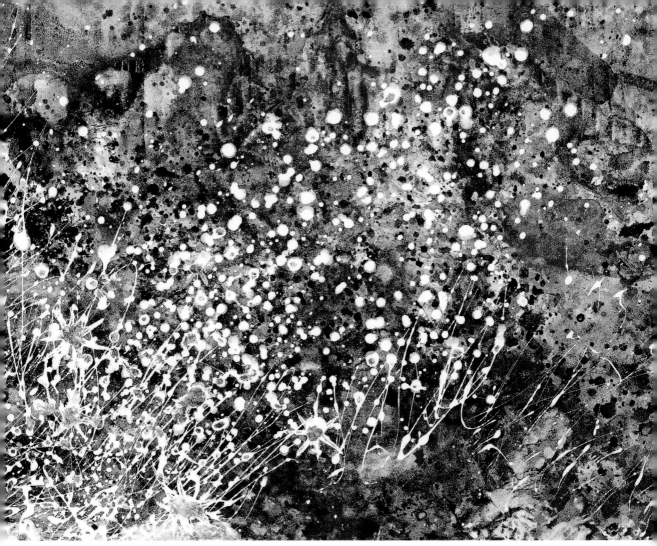

Explosions of Colour, acrylic, March 2013

felt like it; it was up to her and it came from her. I just needed
to stand back and wait for the opportunities to interact and be
useful as the artist's assistant. It was as though a pressure had
been lifted and I could breathe.

Unlike most activities where I eventually got pushed away, Iris
wanted me close by in the kitchen. I had become an integral part
of the process, helping make up the colours she was requesting.
I took the chance to use more words and she was responding so

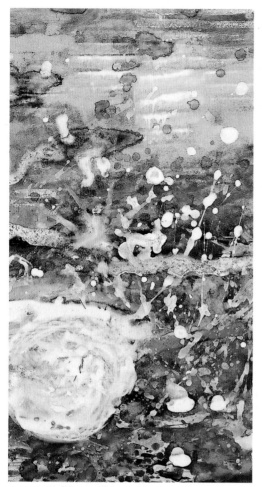
Rolling Balls, acrylic, March 2013

well that my mind was busily thinking about how I could harness this latest interest. I decided that I must make a sacrifice and forget about having a tidy kitchen. It had been my one space, a grown-up area that hadn't yet been a setting for our daily preschool activities. It was where we sat quietly in the mornings, prepared food, had our more grown-up conversations, and on rare occasions even entertained friends, but this was too important. This coffee table would be left out permanently, becoming her painting table for her to use whenever she needed to, even if it was early in the mornings or late into the night. This would be her space to use how she liked. The kitchen table was now squished right up next to the Rayburn looking rather put out and there were a few grumblings from P-J as he repeatedly hit his shin with the new furniture arrangement. I bought many more tools, sponges, brushes and paint, collecting as much as I could for her to experiment with. The excitement of having a new plan with a positive direction was so invigorating that I suddenly wasn't tired any more. I felt like I could do anything and Iris would do anything. P-J watched from the door as Iris darted this way and that, selecting colours, pausing, taking a step back, evaluating and then back to work on the latest piece. He couldn't believe how much purpose and thought went into these paintings.

The next morning my mother came with more supplies and a vase of flowers for the kitchen table. P-J had heard the gate and had come in too for his mid-morning tea break. We all looked at each other, smiling. Iris was busy at her table, where there was a wash of blue and another of red all merging, some areas pink and others purple. We heard her say 'ball' as she dipped her brush in the white and placed it on to the paper. With a stirring motion she created a circular ball on the far right-hand corner and another closer to the middle. She dragged the brush right across the paper, creating a slipstream of white. The painting stretched as far as it could, covering every part of the table – a massive one metre and twenty centimetres long. While we drank tea my mother interacted with Iris at her painting table. None of us were pushed away; she was content and proud of her work as we all talked about it. P-J and I watched, hardly believing it was Iris. She was so confident and assertive, so sure of herself, both of what she wanted and how to show us.

Iris and I quickly settled into this new routine. I could tell when she wanted another fresh piece of paper on the table: she would pull at the edge of the paper for it to be removed and run off to the office to get out another massive sheet. I would help get the mugs out and prepare the paints. Once that was sorted I busied myself with other duties in the kitchen, but always stayed on hand in case I was needed or saw opportunities for speech therapy. Iris looked at the four primary colours that I had put out on the table, considering each one individually, peering over into the Cornishware blue-and-white striped mugs, to see the colours within. She gently took the brush that was beside her and dipped it into the blue, stirring, inspecting, testing. She thrust the mug to me and took my other hand to guide me to the sink, gesturing upwards to the taps, so

I dripped some more water in and handed back the mug, which she put on the other side of the table away from the others, the large expanse of watercolour paper dividing them. Then she stirred the blue – still not quite right – and moved along the length of the table with brush in hand and dipped it into the green and then returned to the blue without making a mark on the paper. Once again she stirred, enjoying the swirling green dissolving into the blue and creating a different shade. She nodded once, lifted the brush up and with short sharp upward flicks again and again the paint flew in the air and droplets descended on to the paper. Her action quickening but perfectly in control, a mottled sea was emerging. Pausing, she examined the watery paint making its journey across to spotless paper beyond. Choosing another brush she made her way over to the yellow, wistfully stroking the paper along the sea. Her style of painting was constantly evolving as she experimented with all kinds of tools, household objects and materials. She mixed her own colours by swapping brushes from mug to mug, feeling her way and continually exploring. Sometimes we wouldn't know which way round the paintings were meant to be as she had painted from all four sides of the table, so we would get her to sit in a chair and I would hold up the painting. P-J would say, 'Is it this way round?' Then I would turn the piece. 'Or this way round?' She would respond with a frown or a little jig: a basic but effective method that we used many times. Once huddled away with her books deep in the sofa, Iris was now dancing in the heart of the home, with colours everywhere.

'I saw a secret seahorse deep down in the sea . . .'
And so the story begins to one of Iris's favourite
books. At first she would turn the pages with her
feet before her hands were nimble enough. She
would look at it over and over, again and again.
It was filled with colour, texture and fun. There
were mysterious coral-reef scenes, sequins stitched
for fish scales, beads and buttons for eyes and felt
for seaweed. So the appearance of a pink seahorse
character in the painting that was still drying on
the table in the kitchen didn't surprise me. It swam
in the sea of mottled green and blue among bubbles
with the sun shining above the sparkling surface.
It was a touching reminder of our happy hours
together reading the book, so that painting became
known as The Story of the Secret Seahorse.

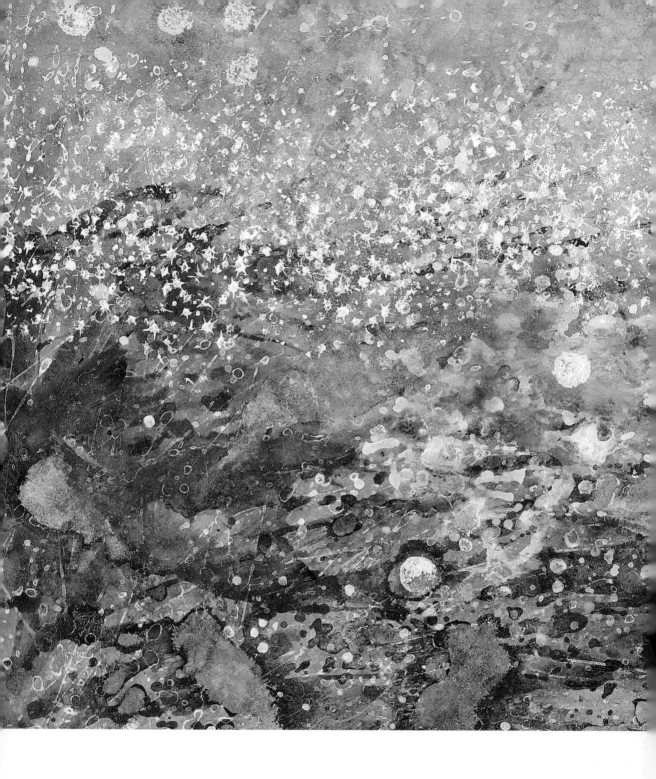

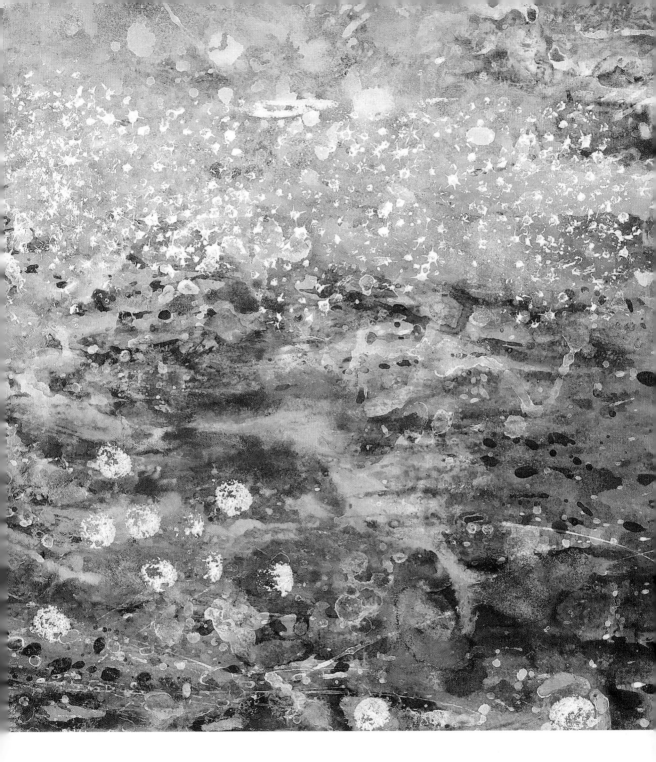

The Story of the Secret Seahorse, acrylic, April 2013

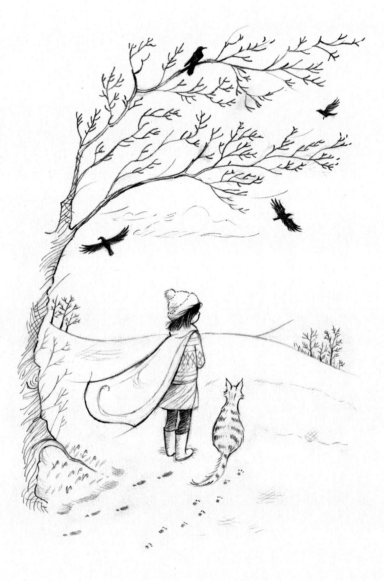

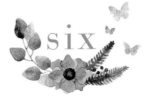

six

'Glass of wine?' I wasn't sure why he even asked any more; our Friday evenings always followed the same routine: some wine and a chat in the kitchen while I cooked and Iris was content with her books next door.

'Yes, please.'

P-J poured the wine and then stopped as the glass was half full. 'There is something I wanted to talk to you about, an idea I've been thinking of.'

I felt a sense of dread. I knew something was coming – an idea or an adventure – and I wasn't sure if I could take on something new. Life was for the first time in a while looking much more positive and Iris's confidence was growing daily. We had recovered from the preschool disaster. It was as if I wanted to keep still, not wanting to disturb the magic that happened every day in the kitchen.

'What?' I said with a rather tired tone.

'You know how much everyone loves Iris's paintings and how our friends thought they were amazing when you shared them on Facebook?'

'Yes, but that's our friends and family. Of course they're lovely about them.'

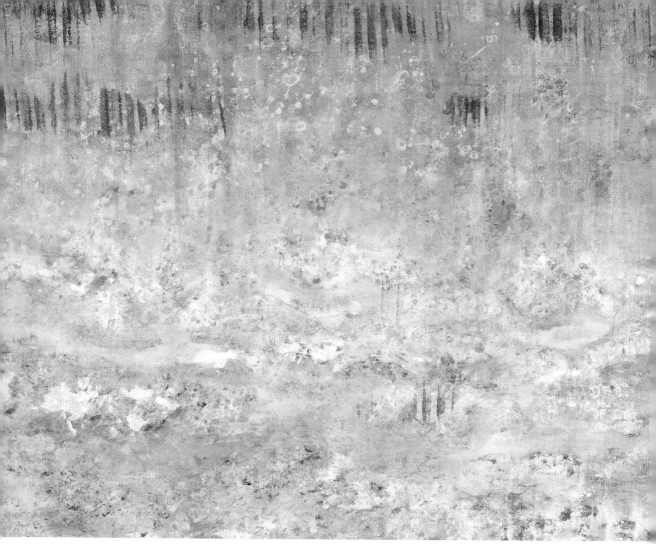

Patience, acrylic, April 2013

'I think it's more than that. I mean, the paintings are very good and that last one – Well, look at it.'

I looked, although I didn't really need to; I could see that painting in my mind's eye, with its soft pastels in many layers. It was a mix between a stormy sea and a bluebell woodland, magical and yet so powerful. It was subtle, with some areas of intricate detail and others that were more free. It was one of the most complicated pieces Iris had done up until that point, with many different colours and layers. She had learnt that you could let the paint dry and come back to it later, that a painting could take many layers and be completed over as much time as you wanted, adding more and more details and different colours. She did some and came back to it again and again over two days: at least six hours of painting altogether. She used different-sized brushes, rollers with texture and tiny star printers, splatting, dotting and dabbing. When she had finished she smiled and put down the brush even though there was paint left in the mug and did what I can only describe as jazz hands, grinning at me, and then she ran off, not returning to the table again. I had named that painting *Patience* as a reminder of how she had learnt so much within its layers of paint. Each painting came to have its own name that connected it to when it was painted: what we thought it looked like or how it had made Iris feel. I hoped that one day she would start to name them herself, but until then I would take on that job and I loved coming up with them.

I was starting to feel curious about this idea of P-J's. 'What were you thinking?'

'Set up a website and a Facebook page, almost like a Beanie gallery, but online, to raise awareness for autism. We could even get some of them made into prints to raise money for Iris's therapy. You can do the website; you did a great job on your wedding blog. What do you think?'

My mind was racing at the thought of all this. He was right. It would be such a beautiful site to encourage other parents, to inspire them to think of autism in a positive light. I thought back to when we realized Iris might be on the spectrum, how worried I had felt and how dark everything I read seemed to be. And then I remembered the diagnosis and the doctor's depressing manner: how I had wanted to read positive stories and to see other children with parents who had managed to find a way to connect with them. It would be brilliant to make others aware of how powerful using a child's interests could be, how there are gentler methods that work on a child's strengths instead of their weaknesses.

There was one niggling problem that stood out above all the others. The one that bugged me most was the thought that I hadn't actually told that many people about Iris's autism. Our social lives had diminished and the only time I seemed to see friends was at weddings or parties where it hardly seemed appropriate to launch into that conversation. I had compartmentalized my life, becoming rather removed from others because that was easiest. I didn't want to talk about autism; I was still only just getting to grips with it myself and my life was filled to the brim with it. And I didn't like talking about it with Iris around. It seemed wrong somehow. She would need to know about it when she was older, but she was still too young to understand, and it would be easy for her to take what I said the wrong way. She couldn't even ask me questions about it yet. Instinctively, almost before I'd mentioned it, P-J understood my worries. As we talked it through we realized that this could actually be a good way of letting everyone know: we could include a page about autism so they could read about it without asking us questions we found difficult to answer.

'It would be fantastic if our friends and family knew a little about it instead of us having to explain everything all the time,' P-J said as he poured me another glass.

I smiled. 'OK let's do it.' I got up and walked to my office and sat at my computer.

'Now?'

'Why not? It won't take me long; I have all the photos. I just need to write up some text. Don't worry, I won't publish anything tonight. I just want to get it started.'

P-J didn't say anything. He went to the cupboard, got out some snacks and came through with supplies and we worked on it together. I loved that about him, the fact that we fitted in that way. He wasn't made anxious by my tendency to leap into our adventures; he encouraged and supported it. Most people want to slow me down, make me consider things in more detail but he knows that then I worry, so it's best to let me run with it. He knew all he had to do was to sow a seed and I would be off soon enough.

The next day I had the site ready to go.

'Press publish then!' P-J was standing behind me grinning.

Bluebells, acrylic, March 2013

'Really? I'm not sure now. I know it's silly. I mean, probably no one will be interested anyway – I can't imagine we'll get that many visitors – but it will be out there for everyone to see.'

I could see how it might help other families and how inspired I would have been if I had seen a site like the one I had created that shined a light on autism, but I still couldn't press that button. Something inside me tightened, holding me back. Had I got carried away last night? What would everyone think? Why did that bother me so much? Who cares what people think . . .? Except I did. I didn't want to, but I did. That part of me that was still wanting our lives to fit, for us to be like everyone else in the life I had imagined before Iris had been born. Then I looked through the gallery, clicking from one painting to the next. The images were captivating, the colours alluring, and yet there was a prevailing sense of calm. My body and mind relaxed.

'Just press it. I know you really want to.'

I pressed it, the site went live and our story went out into the world. It was a surprisingly good feeling, exciting and liberating. The next stage of our plan was to find a printer who could take professional scans of the paintings and make Giclée prints. I wanted to print on demand, so we didn't have to hold any stock. I had no idea if we would be able to sell any at all. There happened to be an excellent printer only five minutes down the road from our house and they worked with me to come up with a range of different print sizes. At first they were amused by my request, but as the weeks went on and more and more paintings were brought in they saw Iris's style develop and they said it was only a matter of time – people would definitely be interested.

One day I had an email from a friend who was involved in a yoga charity in London. They offered special yoga for children on the spectrum and she wanted to know if we would be interested in donating a framed print for a charity auction that was coming up. I thought it was a fantastic idea and jumped at the chance to be involved. We decided on a print of *Patience*.

I stayed at home with Iris on the big night of the auction while P-J and my brother attended. There was a drinks reception and P-J overheard comments from the crowd as they saw and read about Iris's painting. They were blown away; there was so much interest and it achieved way beyond what any of us could have imagined.

Iris raised eight hundred and thirty pounds for a wonderful charity that evening. We were so proud of her and the excitement made me feel more confident to spread her story further.

Over the next few weeks we sold a few of her original paintings, some to friends and a few to some people who had found her on the internet. I was unsure at first about selling them but I knew how badly Iris needed her therapies, and this would be a way for us to get the help she needed. Some we would never sell; they were too special and Iris's favourites. But she seemed very happy about the idea of some going to other people's houses. I explained to her that they would be treasured and loved and looked at every day, and she smiled and giggled. The prints were also starting to sell as her story spread and the interest in her art gained momentum. It all seemed quite surreal. To me her paintings were a way for me to connect with Iris and for her they were a way of expressing herself, an incredible gift in itself. I had grown so used to them; there always seemed to be one on the go in the kitchen, but others were seeing a different side: a gifted child who created paintings that soothed their souls. People would describe how they made them feel, the extraordinary effects that her paintings were having on them. Emails started to come in from other parents saying how much it meant to them reading about Iris and seeing her paintings, how it had changed their views on autism, how they now felt positive for the future. Iris's story was giving hope and inspiration just like P-J had said it would. It was a remarkable feeling.

In June I agreed to have a telephone interview with our local paper, the *Leicester Mercury*, to encourage autism awareness. It was going to be a small article, probably hidden away near the back. But when P-J arrived back from collecting the paper he looked shocked.

'What's happened? Isn't it in there?'

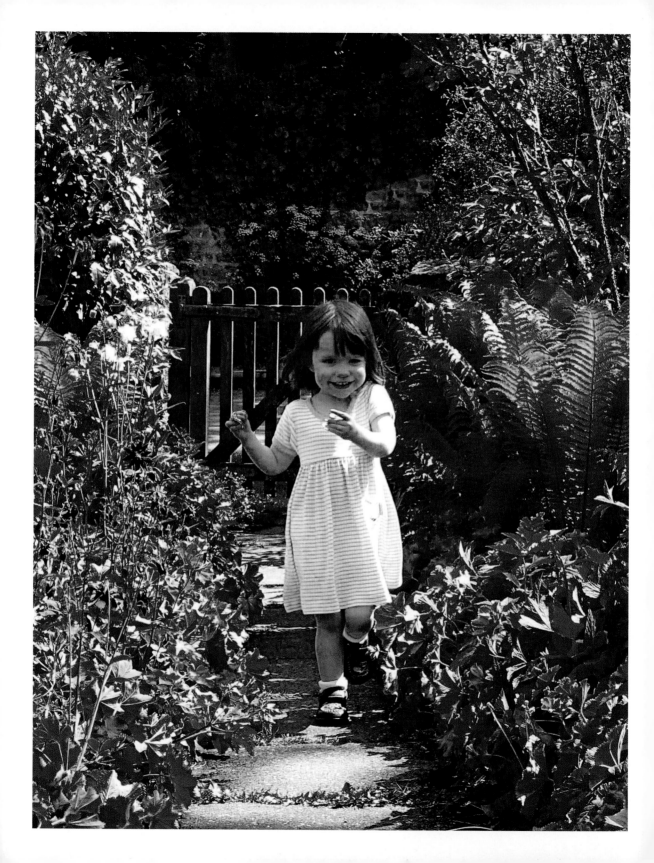

'It's there all right.'

'Is it awful?' I had been so worried about doing it. I imagined that loads of it had come across all wrong.

'I wouldn't say that, no. It's brilliant.'

P-J turned the paper round and put it firmly on the kitchen table. My heart leapt, there was our little Beanie running down her grandparents' garden path with her cheeky smile on the front page. 'Top artist aged 3' said the headline and then the full article was on page three. Within minutes of me reading the article the telephone rang and it didn't stop.

I had just wanted to raise some awareness locally, but I seemed to have underestimated things. Within a day Iris's story would be in all the major national newspapers. Above all I made sure to keep some normality for Iris at home. We tried to keep things as simple as possible: we didn't want any film crews coming to our home or doing any live interviews. We didn't want to go on television, but stick to emailed interviews and me sending out photos. I had no idea what to expect or how long it would go on for.

I tiptoed into Iris's room, kissed her on her forehead and whispered, 'I love you.' She looked so peaceful and blissfully unaware of the impact she was having. I went downstairs and settled in a comfy armchair in front of the glass gable end. It had been warm that day and the garden room was still hot so I opened the door and looked out at the calm beautiful dark sky, just a few stars out.

The next morning, the telephone rang first thing. I jumped out of bed and ran down the stairs. Iris wasn't up and I wanted to keep it that way for as long as possible.

'I'm bringing copies, be with you in five minutes.'

It was my father. I could hardly keep up with his voice; he sounded so excited. I held the phone slightly away from my ear to avoid my eardrum bursting. He always seemed to think he had to speak louder if he was in the car using hands free. It was as if he thought I was in a different country. In fact, he was less than a mile away. He was coming back from an early-morning swim and had stopped in at the newsagents to get the morning paper.

As I opened the front door he gave me a huge hug and a kiss. 'Have you seen them? Ahh, our little Iris. It's amazing, just amazing!'

I went into the kitchen to boil the kettle and he came in with the bundles of newspapers, putting them down on the table and one by one turning pages to the various articles, shaking with excitement and reading parts out to me.

P-J came down and we all peered over the papers. In one day Iris's story had gone from an article in the local paper to raise awareness for autism to national news. I turned on my computer. Emails were coming in by the hundred. Not just media requests but letters from parents, art collectors, teenagers, grannies, artists . . . It seemed everyone was touched by Iris and her paintings. Every few seconds there would be a 'ding': the sound of another email coming in. 'Ding, ding, ding.' I madly tried to find the setting to turn that off: the sound was driving me mad, but I couldn't figure it out without my morning cup of tea. Iris's story was everywhere, on a global scale. We were trending online and the telephones began to ring again at 7.45 a.m. and didn't stop.

P-J took my mobile, his mobile and the house phone and worked from his office to handle all the calls, while I was on email duty. Invitations to be on television and travel the world came flooding in. Everyone was enthralled by Iris, the three-year-old girl who didn't speak but who painted like an Impressionist. But the complete lack of understanding of what living with autism was like had never been more clear to us. This was what had inspired

me to open up more about
our lives in the first place, to
show what Iris's life was really
like through her Facebook
page. We had a chance to
make a real difference. My
theory was that if people
could understand Iris and
why she behaved the way she
did, and over time fall in love
with all her eccentricities,
then they would start to
care about her and celebrate
her achievements. Then,
when their paths crossed
with somebody else on the
spectrum, they would be kind
and understanding about
behaviour that was maybe
unexpected or different. It
would be fantastic for people
to look past the disability and
see potential. I wanted them
to look beyond a diagnosis, to
see that difference is brilliant.

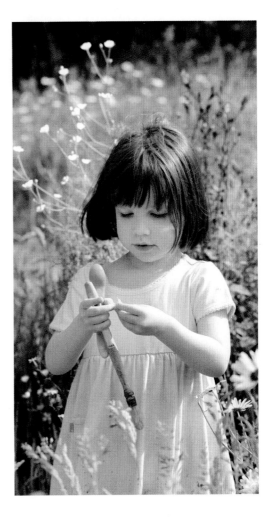

But I was also determined that under no circumstances would
Iris's life change, so whatever I did it needed to be from home and
to fit into our normal routine. It felt like I was finally on the right
road with her and I didn't want any more setbacks. For instance,
I would only read emails and letters from parents from around
the world when Iris was busy playing in the garden. They were
often incredibly moving and I no longer felt isolated or alone:
thousands felt the way I did and expressed their gratitude for us

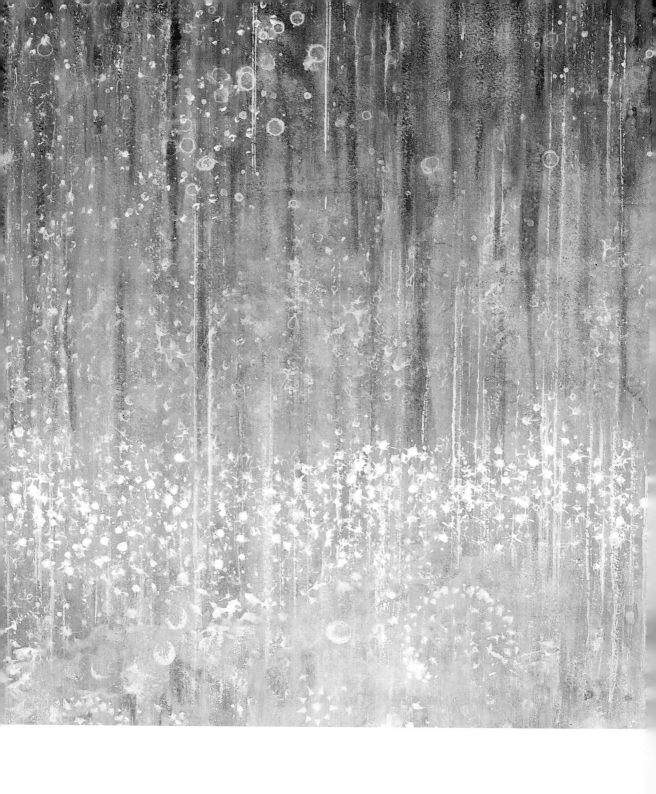

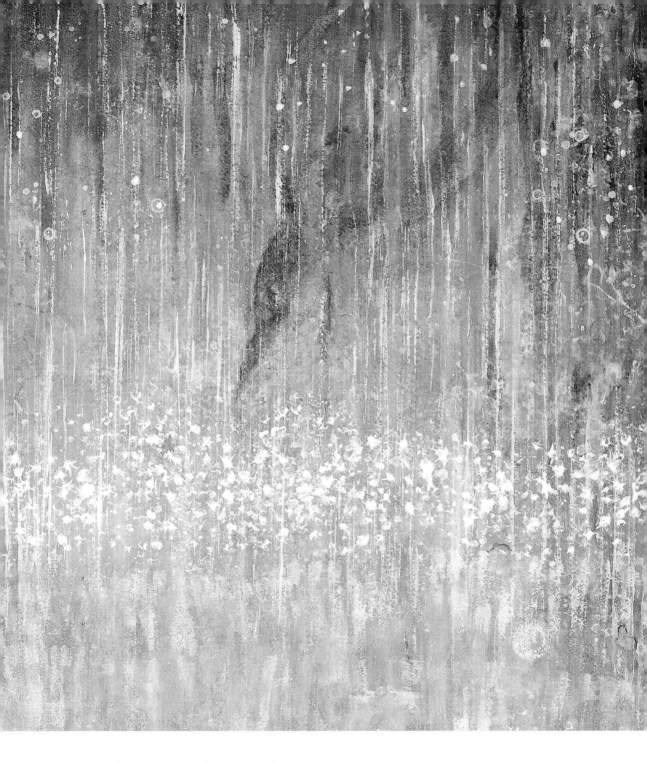

Water Dance, acrylic, June 2013

sharing our story. For parents who had just received a diagnosis for their child, reading about Iris seemed to give them hope. It was a powerful gift and I was so proud of our little Beanie.

As the weeks went on it was clear that Iris's story would continue to spread — it seemed to have a life of its own, a community that was growing through her Facebook page. We made the decision to manage it ourselves as best we could. We didn't want an external art agent, although there were many offers. We wanted to keep control of it all to protect Iris. At times I did struggle. I worked late into the nights to keep up with the flow but reading those emails made all those long hours worthwhile. The effects that Iris's paintings were having moved me to tears. One lady told me how she would visit her mother who was bedbound from her condition and that she had suffered badly from depression. After seeing Iris's paintings she felt joy and comfort. They had changed her life for the better, brightening up each day as she read about Iris's adventures. Her paintings weren't only inspiring those who were affected by autism; they were touching the souls of millions for many different reasons. Her story reached people in over two hundred and thirty different countries. Some said she reminded them of their happy childhood, others that she painted like Monet and many simply enjoyed looking within the paintings and telling me what they saw.

• •

As the paintings themselves began to pile up on my desk I realized that we needed to find a better way to store them. 'How about using my plan chest? You know, the one I used to store drawings in. It's just in the stable now with all the flower-arranging equipment piled on it,' my mother suggested. I thought it was a fabulous idea and we made arrangements for it to be brought over.

This meant that there was movement in the house. Iris shifted under her duvet on the sofa and started to cry at the sound of furniture being pushed across the floor. Change in the house still unsettled her. She had got used to all the obstacle courses, but the furniture generally stayed put and that, in her opinion, was how it should be. I went to comfort her but her look told me that I should back away, so I got the rest of my office ready for the new arrival.

We got the chest into position under my desk without too much trouble and I went about cleaning and preparing the drawers. This was the new home and protector for Iris's paintings: a plan chest that had been passed through my side of the family, the guardian of architect's drawings, photographs and now paintings by our dear little Iris Grace. I carefully positioned each painting inside and covered them one by one with layers of tissue paper, then shut the drawer to fill another. The whole chest was then draped with a red velvet throw that covered the peeling paintwork and out of the corner of my eye I saw Iris tiptoeing quietly in through the door. I gently opened the drawer again, exposing the painting on top: *Cinnabar*, a bright red painting with splashes of green. The painting enticed Iris towards the chest. As she looked, her agitation disappeared and was replaced with curiosity and delight. She placed her hand on it, gently patting it, and then gestured for me to push the drawer closed. She moved along the front, feeling the handles and kneeling down so she could feel the texture of the wood and metal on her face, then she climbed on top and laid across it like a cat, sprawled out and perfectly relaxed. She understood the intruder's purpose and it had been accepted into her world.

Iris was content at her table, busily painting, when my mother arrived one day with some lunch for us. As she put the casserole dish on the table she turned to me. 'Where's the pink spoon?' she whispered. 'Has she lost it?'

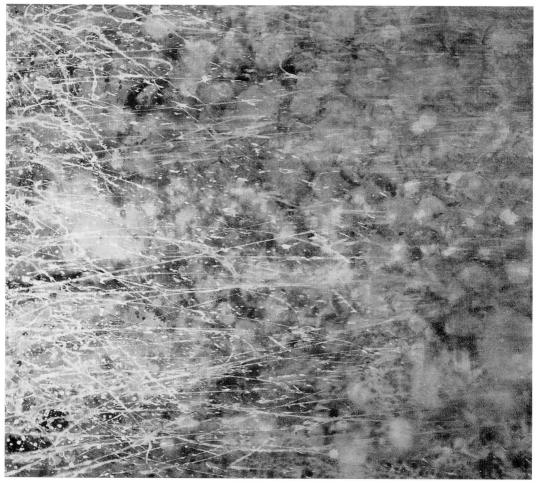

Cinnabar, acrylic, September 2013

'No, just doesn't need it any more. Brilliant, isn't it?'

The little pink spoon had been a friend to Iris like no other. It had been a year-long relationship that had endured bath times, activities and even the tiresome process of slipping through sleeves — tricky but possible. Nothing apart from deep sleep had broken this bond. The spoon hadn't been the first item that Iris had got attached to; there had been a long line of objects that had been carried constantly in her left hand. But the spoon had

had the longest reign. Then, all of a sudden, I had been handed her beloved like a golden chalice: she wanted me to take it and look after it for her. I had found a drawer in the kitchen where I placed it and she had been checking in now and again. To us, it was a symbol of her new-found confidence and greater sense of security, a sign of progression and independence like no other. I was sure her pink companion wouldn't be forgotten and it would be there for her when she needed it, but nothing else had replaced the spoon. For the first time since she had been able to hold on to objects, her hands were free – she was free.

Throughout the summer we balanced our lives so that as much time as possible was spent outside in the garden for Iris's education and her therapies. The sessions were going very well with Iris blissfully unaware of any stir she was causing in the outside world. On days when the weather was good her therapy would be taken outside and as I watched my heart sang. The joyful interaction between Iris and her music therapist made me smile as I moved quietly away. Iris was at ease playing the piano when she felt like it, but she was always more interested after her music therapy sessions. Her paintings hung all around and family photographs rested on top. From the stool she could see our garden through the floor-to-ceiling glass gable. The huge expanse of sky, the bank of trees in the valley and the rolling green hills beyond were an ever-changing landscape. There was pink apple blossom in the spring, green leaves dancing in the wind through the summer and an explosion of colour in the evening light throughout the autumn. Iris watched as birds swooped through the valley, following their flight, then spreading her arms wide with a long white feather in her left hand she would gracefully imitate their journey dancing around the room.

'I've been thinking,' I said to P-J as he came in.

'Yes . . .'

'Don't worry, it's nothing massive. I know we're busy right now, but I wanted to come up with something that we could do together as a family, something outside. But I can't decide what to do. You know how relaxed Iris is in the garden . . . Well, why don't we try to widen that to somewhere else? I worry that she's too isolated here. Any ideas?'

'How about going out on bike rides?'

'I thought of that but she's no interest in learning how to ride a bike. She hated that tricycle. Makes me a bit sad really. I loved riding around the countryside with my father.'

'No, I meant me taking her on my bike. I could get one of those seats that goes behind mine. That way she will be able to see the countryside and not have to worry about riding. It will be relaxing for her. Well, hopefully . . .'

With that decided we went in the next day with Iris to several bike shops, for a bike for me and a seat for her. It was stressful as Iris just went running off exploring, inspecting the most dangerous items in the shop. Our first bike ride was a little tentative, not knowing how Iris would react to such a new activity, so we paired it up with some music playing from P-J's iPhone that we knew she loved and hoped for the best. With Peggy Lee at full volume she immediately relaxed just as she had when she had first heard her voice. It had been a few months earlier that my father had been to an antiques market one Sunday morning before one of our lunches and brought home some CDs, one of which was Peggy Lee. He played it for her and she danced around the room on her tiptoes while she listened to the happy tune. The cheerful lyrics followed us down an old railway track and across the countryside, along canals and through the villages. Peggy soon became as much a part of our lives as Iris's books, being there for Iris when she needed a helping hand. Iris loved the bike rides from that day on and they became part of our routine.

Riding behind P-J I could see Iris ahead, her body leaning forward in the slipstream of her father. She looked at the countryside, the waves on the reservoir, trees and birds. She studied everything wide-eyed, with squeals of excitement and her hair flying in the wind. Every so often she turned to me with a smile that was so infectious that I immediately smiled right back at her. We talked to her on our journey together: 'Moooo, goes the cow' if we saw some cows in a field, for example. We hoped with all hope that our words were sinking in, but we knew that it might not be possible due to there being too much visual stimulation and sensory input. In traditional speech therapy you aim to have the child's undivided attention

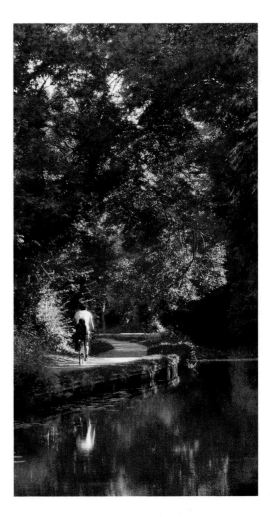

and to be in a plain room with just a few toys/activities that you are both focusing on. There is lots of repetition, encouraging them to say words like 'more' to get the toy. Out in the open countryside with fields and woodland to her right and water on her left, we couldn't have been further from that situation, but somehow it was working. On our journey home in the car Iris spotted some cows in a field and said 'Moooo, Moooo' repeatedly without prompting. She had listened and understood and now used the words in the right context all by herself. It seemed we had found an interesting combination therapy: painting for peace and relaxation, music for the soul and freewheeling speech therapy on the bikes. I wondered what would be next.

Connecting and interacting with a child with autism can sometimes be like tuning into a radio, but once you get through the whirring fuzz you are there, clear as can be. It might only last a few seconds but you have it and my god as a parent it feels great, emotions flying high. Two little words from Iris after a bike ride – 'bye-bye' to the bikes as we put them away – helped me forget my tired legs, and filled my heart with joyous pride. Words up till then had only seemed to come sparingly when she was happy and relaxed and doing some sort of activity, playing in the garden, drawing, painting, listening to music, but now we had found another 'spark' – the bike. Iris riding on the back of PJ's bike, hands stretched out, feeling the wind, free from worry, didn't fret about her dress and cardigan or worry about things having to be in order and under her control. This sensation seemed to unlock something, so that a word could find its way out.

But there was something creeping up on us that I couldn't ignore any more and that was the decision about which school Iris was going to attend. She was due to start in September and we needed to find a suitable place. She would be young for her year but after speaking to some of the head teachers and describing where we were at with her, they felt it was the right time. I was fearful of what was to come as we had once again made so much progress and for that to be destroyed would be heart-breaking. Iris was proving to me how much she was learning in this gentle natural environment and I was nervous about what a school would do to this.

Finding a suitable school was one of the hardest challenges I had to face. I mostly went alone to visit them while P-J looked after Iris, but I couldn't see us sending Iris to any of them. In the eyes of the schools and teachers, having looked at Iris's diagnosis reports and listened to where she was in her development, she couldn't be placed in a mainstream school as it would be too much for her. I agreed with that. So that left the special schools that were dotted around the counties surrounding us.

I visited them all and never felt that she would fit into any of them. Iris's problem with wearing certain clothes concerned me greatly. The advice from schools was that she must wear the set uniform no matter what, because they wouldn't allow her attendance without it. They described how she would be in what they called 'sustained distress for many weeks if necessary, while they dealt with the problem'. Knowing that Iris must have reasons for her anathema to clothes, and horrified by their suggestion, I did the opposite. I wanted her to want to wear her clothes, not for me to force them on her. I believe that every time you treat another in such a way, animal or person, you take a piece of them away. There is always another way, a different road to travel; it usually takes longer and it may create doubt and uncertainty at times, but the end result is pure.

Most schools just replied to any question I had with, 'Don't worry, we will take care of everything.' Those words made me worry more than ever before. I left every car park, one after the other over many weeks, crying at the steering wheel. How could this be right for our girl? It certainly didn't feel right and in my heart I knew it. It didn't seem to matter how fantastic the facilities were, how many soft playrooms, sensory rooms, swimming pools . . . The sound of meltdowns from other children on a regular basis scared me. This was apparently 'normal', but for us it wasn't. Yes, Iris went through meltdowns but they now happened rarely and only when things had spiralled out of control. Usually we could see the signs before it got to that point and managed to calm her; we would lower the lights, turn off televisions and sit quietly, focused on a book she loved, and in time the anxiety passed.

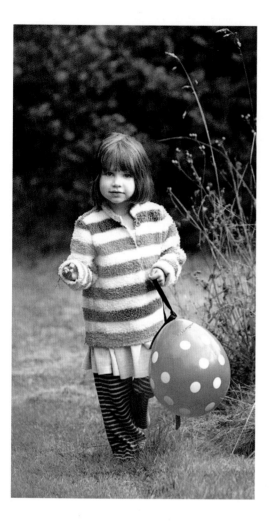

She was so vulnerable, only able to speak a few small words, and unable to tell me how her day had been or what had happened. I needed to trust, to feel safe in the place where I was to leave her every day. The reality was I felt terrified. It's something I feel teachers and therapists may over time take for granted, the leap of faith a parent of a non-verbal child must take to trust another with them.

We settled on one school that seemed to have a more flexible approach. The headmistress was kind and listened intently as I told her about Iris's paintings and how much she had learnt over the past months, how I had been engaging her in activities. She was a breath of fresh air to me, with assurances that they would do everything possible to accommodate our needs and support us, even if that meant flexi-schooling so Iris could work partly at home.

But then the teacher I had met moved on to another school and the new head wasn't impressed when I talked about our previously agreed plans. Iris was placed in a different class to the one I had been expecting, all non-verbal children with severe disabilities. As I watched her play with toys and wander around the room with the others in their wheelchairs I worried how she would develop. How was she going to interact when there were so many difficulties? Iris even started to copy some of the more challenging behaviours in the classroom and it just didn't feel right for her. I expressed my concerns, adding that I didn't want Iris to have the sugary snacks that were on offer at breaktimes as we had been working so hard on her diet. None of my requests were taken seriously and I felt uncomfortable. We did a trial week at the start of September, but by the end it was clear that it wasn't the school I had thought it was. I found their expectations and aspirations for Iris deeply depressing. They didn't seem to listen to me as I spoke about how she could paint and the way I had been using her passions to teach her and open up doorways to communication. They didn't see her potential, and I knew we hadn't found the right school so the search went on.

•••

There was a clicking noise from my bike tyre; something had lodged in its treads, so I stopped. As I pulled out a rather large twig, a loud hissing reached my ears and a long sharp thorn made an appearance. I rang my bell four times to alert P-J to stop and we quickly exchanged keys so they could go on home and rescue me with the car. Trying to keep calm so that Iris wouldn't get upset I smiled at her and off they went. I was by myself, walking the bike home along a narrow country lane with the warm wind swirling around me, and the thump, thump of the wheel. As I looked down I realized how much it resembled my feelings that afternoon, going flat and losing energy, out of luck and going round in circles. For the past week I had been speaking to more and more potential schools. Some were full and others had only a couple of places left for the following year, with many children still applying. Had I left all of this too late, with the excitement of Iris's paintings and the media storm? Maybe I had got too distracted from what I should have been doing, finding a school. Was this all my fault? I had visited some more, each one making me feel like I was being backed into a corner, making do and compromising. Words from one of the teachers rang in my head as I walked home: 'We train the children.' I had always believed that the best teachers show you where to look but don't tell you what to see.

I wanted to find teachers that wouldn't suppress Iris's creativity or break her spirit: she needed to be happy in order to learn. I walked on, enjoying the peace of my unexpected time alone, considering my options for Iris's education. With a rejuvenated, powerful sense of freedom the idea of homeschooling returned. She was still very young and so much might change in the years to come, but right now, I realized, this was the best option for Iris. I had only planned to educate her at home this year but things were going so well, why stop now?

In that moment the rescue team arrived over the hill and as the bike was fastened safely to the back of the car, I kissed Iris on the cheek. What followed can only be described as our own special handshake: a combination of hand movements and sounds as we both giggled in the back of the car.

That evening after the bike was back with its tyre mended, I made a list of some fun activities that Iris and I could do the next day. P-J and I discussed how we would make it work and we both felt confident about the decision. I couldn't help but feel grateful for that spiky thorn for giving me the time alone to think.

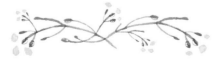

September brought mixed feelings, Iris turned four and she had a wonderful birthday but I was reminded everywhere of our different life. The new school year had started and photos of our friends' children all dressed in their smart uniforms had been proudly posted. It made me wonder if I had made the right choice. Sometimes it was hard to be so far removed from the norm, the feeling of not fitting, remote and alone. Our daily struggles and challenges felt like a cruel reality while we saw everyone seemingly cruise on by. In those moments I realized how hard I had to work for the simplest of interactions: to hear Iris's voice, to see her smile and for her to look at me. That realization hurt and then it was washed away with the thought of how we had started to connect with her and I was grateful for that. We had been blessed in ways no one could predict and our lives would not be ordinary; they would be extraordinary and that was something to be proud of and to celebrate.

•••

A few weeks later the atmosphere changed quite dramatically, I looked for Iris in the garden and saw a white mound by her favourite tree stump. She was under her duvet, which she had taken outside so she could sit comfortably in the cold air with some loyal friends. 'Fimbo' was a character from a cartoon that Iris had loved the year before. The plastic toy was clutched in Iris's left hand, his striped yellow-and-green arms resting above her forefinger, which was curled round his tummy. Her play had been evolving; she now interacted with her little friends instead of performing a daily inspection line and they went on adventures together, getting tucked up into bed after a long day. This development was like a keystone in a social world, making progress possible. But today even Fimbo wasn't comforting her. I called her to come up to the house, but she turned and then

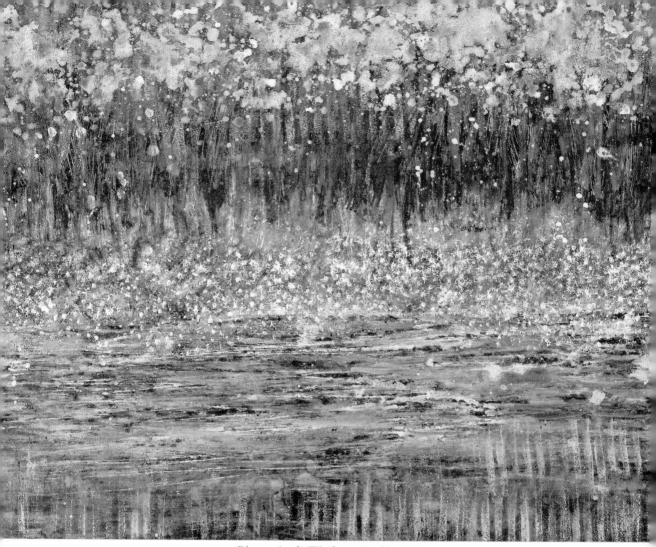

Blossom in the Wind, acrylic, May 2013

buried herself underneath again all cocooned in white. For the last few days a sadness had overcome her. Autumn had arrived so suddenly that it shocked her mind, body and soul. Change was never easy. One day she had been dancing in the warm sunlight in the garden, then the next a cold wind had made her shiver, damp grey air surrounding her. It was as though when she woke in the morning and looked out of the window her heart broke. She cried and stormed outside, determined that she might change this unwarranted shift in her world.

Painting, drawing and music lifted her spirits so I would start the day by using those to gently coax her into a better mood. So I cleared all the surfaces in the kitchen, laid out Iris's music books and instruments, and played music from a CD. I encouraged Iris to dance, to move and to use the instruments in between her painting sessions. Gradually we saw our happy Beanie come back to us.

• •

'Let's go for a bike ride.' P-J had finished his work for the day and was ready for some fun.

'Good idea. It's going to clear up this afternoon. The weather forecast said sunshine.'

'OK, I'll wrap her up for the ride and she'll be all warm and cosy. Even if it's sunny, the air will still be cold.'

The wind was blowing, but the sky was blue and the sun was out, so the three of us were happy as we rode along the towpath. The water of the canal shimmering in the light and the beauty of the autumn colours were having a delightful effect upon Iris. She was incredibly relaxed and happy, a relief after the unsettled week. As we passed under a bridge and out of the other side, leaves fell all around us. Iris lifted her arms up high, her fingers stretched out wide and she turned to me smiling with her hair wildly dancing.

In the evening I tried to settle her for bedtime but I could see there was no point, she was far too awake, still buzzing with happiness. We stayed up deep into the night. At midnight Iris was still full of energy. She led my weary body off the sofa and took me to her favourite nook in her playroom, where interlocking mats covered the floor, removable alphabet shapes within each one. The mats had been bought in the hope of them being educational but I also loved the safety aspect. She guided me to the letter 'A' in the far left corner. Carefully she took the letter out of the mat and said 'A', then put it back into position. She pushed on my leg to move me over to the next letter and picked it up, saying 'B' and so on until we got to 'H' when she wanted me to say it. I was shocked; this wasn't a game we had practised. I didn't feel tired any more: I was flying high on the back of this new discovery. Iris didn't only know her alphabet but she could also say the letters to me unprompted. As she finished she was calm and peaceful but her face was pale with dark circles round her eyes. I could see that this had been a massive effort for her and she was exhausted, so I carried her over to the sofa and a few moments later she was fast asleep.

I could hardly believe it. Iris had managed to learn her alphabet, I knew that it was expected for her age at four years old but being able to do so without being able to talk and easily converse with others was an amazing achievement. She had been memorizing the sounds and shapes, teaching herself through the iPad apps and books. Like the golden leaves, language was gently falling into place, forging pathways like a network of branches, each leaf falling and leaving behind a path that was now free.

Over the next few days sounds of alphabet letters filled the air. There was a melody following me from room to room. Iris was speaking and I could not stop smiling. Over that week following the midnight alphabet session she had immersed herself in language, finding it where ever she could: books, games, iPad apps, television, the piano, art and us. Her tenacity and strong-willed eagerness from the moment she woke till when she fell asleep took my breath away at times. For someone so young to be filled with a determination that could be compared with an Olympian was incredible. Of course there were ups and downs, quieter days and frustrating days, but she was gaining momentum and growing in confidence all the time.

Her vocabulary was expanding quickly, she was soon able to say hundreds of different words and then one day I found a more reliable way of hearing them. Iris leant against me with her arms draped round my shoulders as I knelt before her work table in my office. I picked up a stack of cards adorned with short words, which we spelt out carefully one by one and I heard her voice saying words like 'at', 'on', 'up' and 'see'. I wrote them on a piece of paper and she repeated the words. She was learning to read. I could not believe how quickly we had been transported out of her almost silent world. It felt like a dream. There was a mountain of catching up to do, and so much for her to overcome, but Iris loved it. Through getting Iris to read, I could now hear her voice and the delightful daydream of one day chatting to my little girl and hearing what she thought and felt was so close I could almost touch it. Her communication skills improved dramatically after that day, not to the extent of actually being able to chat to me, but she was verbalizing names for objects, textures, colours, animals and some small linking words. It was still frustrating at times; when she was upset all those skills seemed to disappear and she would just repeat a word that she had been using, but it would have no relevance to what she wanted. But when she was relaxed and happy we saw great improvements. She would comment upon things, the life around her, the wildlife down at the canal: 'Duck, moorhen, bird, tree, good to see . . .' she would say. If we were about to leave the house, I would say, 'Let's rock 'n' roll!' She would repeat this as 'rag 'n' roll' and add 'bike ride'. She said 'night-night' in the evenings and 'goodie' in the mornings and started to copy some lines from songs.

The sun was low and the bike shadows danced on the wet road as we rode along, and Iris watched the shadow shapes change as we turned to the left. She twisted round and frowned at me if my shadow touched P-J and Iris's ruining the perfect outline. Their separation seemed important to her so I stayed a little behind.

Her long legs were dangling down, occasionally being nudged by P-J rotating the pedals, but she didn't seem to mind; she was completely relaxed. A row of neatly clipped yew hedges lined the road like soldiers standing to attention and one of them caught Iris's gaze. A robin was jostling its feathers in a pool of light right at the top of the column. He cheerfully viewed the world in the warm sun on this wintery morning. After our bike ride and a hot cup of milk Iris led me into the kitchen to get the paints out. This was already a good day and as the paint flew all over the kitchen I knew most people would be disgruntled at the prospect of the clean-up but I didn't care: colour was everywhere and happiness filled the air. She was in a state of elated relaxation after such a vigorous painting session; I took advantage of that and we did some puzzles that she sped through, then some alphabet cards and numbers. She leapt from one number to the next along the sequence of large foam numbers that I had laid out on the floor, saying them as she jumped. On days like this one the decision to educate Iris at home seemed like the best in the world and I felt like that robin in the sunshine. Of course, it wasn't always that easy and the enormity of what I was taking on and sometimes all the work ahead felt overwhelming.

Late that evening I turned the lights down in the playroom and encouraged Iris to settle with me on the sofa. The hall light was on and she noticed her shadow against the wall in front of her. I realized in an instant that adjusting the lights had triggered a new game and bedtime was sailing off into the distance. With some simple manoeuvres of her body she tested the shadow: a wave, a jump, hand on head and hand on hip. Then to my surprise she imitated a bike in a sitting position, using her hands to rotate like a wheel or the pedals. Imaginative play and copying wasn't her strong suit, so it was a joy to watch, and we both giggled at the shapes being created on the playroom wall.

Our lives were filled with so much joy and happiness – in nature, out on the bikes and with Iris's art – but as if to balance all this new problems were arising. Iris started to find bathtime very difficult. Washing her hair became a distressing event and sometimes I couldn't even get her in the bath tub. In fact, as soon as I placed her in the bath she scrabbled at me madly, scratching and screaming, and then as I tried to wash her hair it was as though I was causing her pain. She became like a wild animal: frightened, desperately trying to get away, and many times it was a battle that I just couldn't cope with. Afterwards when Iris was dry and calm again with her books on the sofa I would cry alone upstairs. I struggled to manage those feelings. I longed for the days when she loved having a bath to come back, and I daydreamed about how it had once been – us having a warm bath together, her lying against me with her head resting on my chest – a peacefulness that now seemed so far from us.

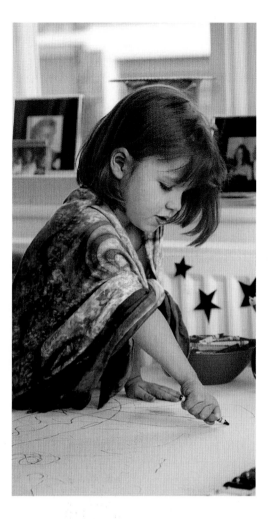

She also obsessed over keeping her socks and shoes on too, which added to my challenges as I tried to slip them off after she had fallen asleep. We tried our best with all sorts of techniques to help but most failed. It was as if we had stepped forward in one direction, then something else fell apart in another. But when things fell apart it would have effects upon the other advances we had made. She wouldn't sleep as well, for instance, so I was more tired and struggled to manage everything. That's why it was important to try to deal with the small issues as soon as they arose as they could so easily spiral out of control. But some things needed time and I needed to be more patient. There had been improvements with the clothes on her top. She tolerated wearing a blue cape, a beach sarong that my mother had given her in an attempt to keep her warm on one of our Friday lunches. We had been trying all sorts of materials to see if any were more acceptable to Iris than others, even resorting to my old dressing-up box with its velvet capes, silk scarves and many other tried-and-tested clothes.

'Try this. It's soft and she might like the colour. I just found it with my holiday clothes and I don't need it. There's so much blue in her paintings . . . It might just do the trick,' my mother had said, draping the cotton beach sarong over Iris's shoulders.

'Blue,' Iris said as she rubbed the tassels in between her fingers. She watched the frayed tassels twizzle backwards and forwards for a while and then pulled the fabric round her more so the two sides met in the middle.

'Well, that's working! Well done, Mummy!' I said, tying it into a loose knot, but as soon as the words came out the cape came off. I decided to take the blue cape back home with us anyway and to give it another try. After a few weeks it was more successful and eventually it turned out to be a real favourite.

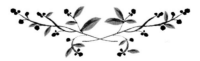

A row of seven plastic frogs look comically at me while I soak in the bath. They are the last in a succession of toys that I have used to try to coax Iris into the warm water. All have failed miserably and as I lie here my mind mulls over some other ways to try to rectify this sudden bath phobia: sensory play – done, massage with moisturizers – done, stories about water – done, water play with bubbles – done. What to do? Autism has a way of suddenly creeping up on you when you least expect it, like a thief in the night, swallowing up something precious and stealing it away. The unfairness of it all and the never-ending questions about why or how it happened are exhausting. Some children regress, some lose language or have sudden sensory issues that are difficult to control, and some retreat into their own worlds, almost out of reach. Even when you have rescued your dear little one, it's still there like an ever-present shadow and again, without warning, it is back in a different form, overwhelming their senses with uncontrollable feelings and obsessions. Relentless but rewarding, the love for our children drives us on.

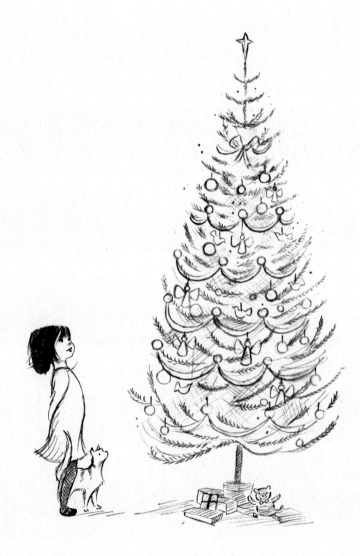

seven

It was December again and I was on another slightly panicked pre-Christmas phone call. Only this time, for a change, it wasn't me who needed help. My extremely capable mother was in the middle of preparing their Christmas Eve party but also seemed to have inadvertently filled the house with animal guests for the duration of the holidays. Not only had she promised to look after several dogs for a friend, but my brother was bringing his girlfriend's cat, Shiraz, to stay as Carolina was spending Christmas with her family over in Sweden. The cat, a beautiful Siberian with a kind temperament, was more than used to travelling, but the thought of the mayhem that might ensue was causing my normally calm mother to envisage all sorts of disasters.

It felt good to be the one offering a solution: 'Why don't we have the cat at ours over Christmas?' I was naturally concerned about how Iris would react, as I didn't want a repeat of the Willow incident, but in my mind a cat was different, more self-sufficient than a dog, and everything that I had heard about this cat sounded fantastic, a perfect match for Iris. Maybe Iris might actually like this animal. She had developed so much since we had last tried and we were keeping the holidays very low key. P-J and Iris would stay at home for the drinks party to avoid her becoming overloaded and I could take the cat home afterwards. It could be a lovely distraction, taking the pressure off Christmas Day.

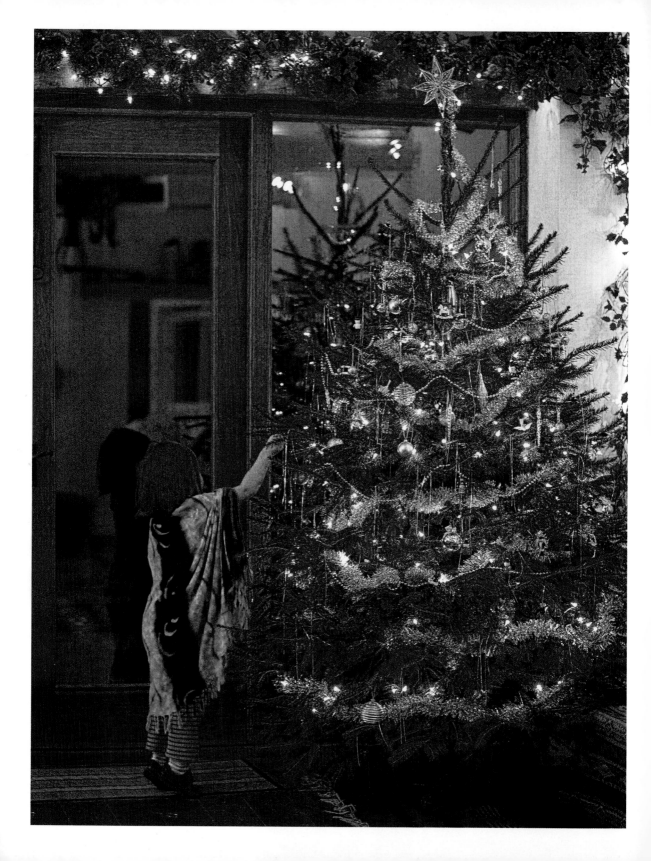

The party itself started as they normally did. When I arrived my mother was busy in the kitchen, the fires were lit and my first job was to light the candles. My father was having the usual debate about where the drinks should be and my brother was calm, managing to deal with our rather frantic father, who settled down enough to pour us all a glass of champagne. Peace was restored before the first guests arrived. We gathered in front of the fire with carols playing in the background and my father gave me a hug, squishing my head up against his colourful bow tie, a trademark that goes back as far as I can remember. As a child I used to love going through his bow tie drawer; there were so many fantastic different designs and colours. Why on earth someone needed so many was beyond all of us.

Every beam in my parents' house was decorated with garlands, and there was a beautiful flower arrangement on my father's desk in the corner and one on the mantelpiece with candles glowing. Their warm golden light transformed the old farmhouse. The house was the epitome of Christmas and the tree over by the French doors made everyone smile: it practically burst out of the space. All the old family decorations were hanging from its branches, including the fragile fairy that had once been my grandmother Iris's. It was somewhere where everyone felt at home, packed full of character. Every room seemed to be on a different level, such as the kitchen that was through a stable door and down a step. The door frame was painfully low for some but the warmth from the Aga and my mother's homely cooking would cheer up any bumps from the architecture. I had been looking forward to the party: for me it was a chance to see friends whom I had grown up with, and going out had become so rare that it was a real treat. My parents also invited many of their friends and it had become a tradition, a time for us all to get together and catch up. I did feel a little nervous. This would be the first time I would talk openly about Iris and autism. I wasn't sure what people would say, how much they knew about her story and if any of them had even been following what had happened over that past year.

'I know we always say this, but this evening is the start of Christmas for all of us. Your parents have done it again! Brilliant party! How's Iris doing? We've been following her, you know. I loved that latest painting. So much energy . . .'

As I chatted to the guests, surrounded by people from my past who all now knew about Iris, our challenges and triumphs, I felt relaxed. There was no need to awkwardly explain, to make excuses for her not being there or to anticipate a hasty retreat. Everything was out in the open and people were being so kind. Some were interested to know more about autism and how Iris saw the world, and I explained what I could and then moved on to welcome more guests and hand around canapés. Later, as the party wound down, my thoughts were with my new responsibility, our Siberian house guest.

My brother took me through to the laundry room to introduce me to her. 'James, she's beautiful!' I cried as I looked inside the pet carrier. 'Look at that coat and those fluffy paws. She's got snowshoes on.'

She was a tabby cat, her eyes bright green with a knowing, intelligent feel to them. She had small ears, a full black-and-white tail, and a thick coat that was longer around her shoulders and back legs. It was as though she was wearing breeches. To my surprise my brother was very protective over his girlfriend's cat. I listened carefully as he told me about her daily routine, her food and what she liked to do. He even gave me a jacket of his that she liked to sleep on. I drove home after the party with Shiraz in the back and I was looking forward to seeing what Iris would think of our beautiful guest.

As I turned towards the house after shutting the gates I could see Iris's face at the window, obviously still very much awake. I had talked to her about the arrival of the cat and made it clear that she was only staying with us for the holidays but that had been many hours ago and I wondered if she had remembered what I had said or if she had even listened to me. Sometimes it was difficult to know what was sinking in. But it turned out she had listened carefully to everything. She was extremely excited as I came through the front door carrying the box and couldn't wait for me to let the cat out and to meet her.

Iris was immediately drawn to Shiraz's luxurious fur, long white whiskers and stripy bushy tail. This was no ordinary cat, she was magnificent, and Iris followed her around the house on Christmas Eve with great interest. 'C' 'A' 'T', 'CAT', 'More cat' she said as she walked after her. Words never came easily but as soon as this pedigree feline entered the house Iris had no trouble saying what she wanted in regard to the animal, even to the extent of spelling out the word for good measure. Eventually Shiraz turned to her and settled on the carpet, waving her tail into Iris's lap as she knelt beside her. Iris lay down alongside her body and stroked her tummy, her hand weaving into the soft fur and smiling.

Over the Christmas holidays Iris tried to firm up her bond with the house guest by offering her water and then even wanting her to join her for a cup of tea with the egg cups that she had especially climbed up on top of the dresser to get – a curious and adorable show of affection and kindness.

If Iris wasn't feeling well, Shiraz curled up by her side and immediately Iris forgot about her frustrations, her illness and her lack of sleep. Iris hated being ill; she couldn't stand not being able to breathe properly and it was hard to explain to her that it wouldn't last for ever, that it would pass. Luckily she was very rarely unwell but I did dread it. Shiraz, however, seemed to be the best medicine. As I looked at them together, Iris stroking her fur, I couldn't believe how quickly they had bonded. Our Christmas guest had become like a nanny over just a few short days. She would soon have to go back to London, but she had opened up a door that I had no idea had been unlocked. Maybe my efforts in getting Iris involved with animals in the past had all been premature: she had needed time to develop. Iris hadn't paid much attention to animals before: it was as though she didn't see them. Now it was a different story. Shiraz had given her comfort in times of need, calmed her senses when she was overloaded and provided friendship. Timing is everything in life, something I am reminded of every time I pick up my camera: picking the right moment can make the difference between success and failure. Living with autism can be a game of timing too. My New Year's resolution was not to try to forget those experiences with Iris that hadn't gone well in the past – you never know how time can change everything.

Even before we had taken Shiraz back to London I had made up my mind. I would start searching for an animal once again, but this time we would be more focused about what we were looking for and open our minds to the fact that the traits we desired may come from the most unsuspected source: a cat. Could a cat provide all that I was looking for in an animal for Iris? Shiraz certainly seemed to know what to do. Had I overlooked cats all together due to their reputation of being more aloof and less loyal than dogs? Shiraz had changed my perceptions. Her company was missed after she left. Iris had been prepared for her departure and knew that she was only with us on a visit but she still wandered around the house asking for 'cat'. This made me more determined than ever to find Iris a cat of her own.

I had some experience with animals behaving in surprising ways. By giving them opportunities, patience and kindness they can fulfil roles that you wouldn't expect. This was what had

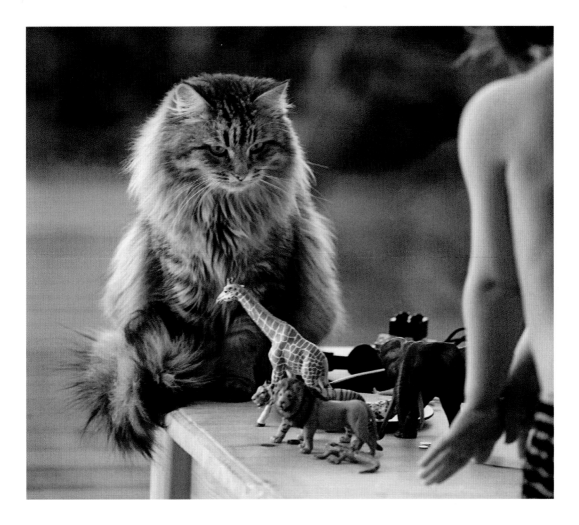

happened with Baggins, the faithful Percheron horse in France. During my recuperation after my accident I heard from a friend about some horses that needed a home: they had been caught up in the sale of a chateau. P-J thought I was a little crazy as at the time we were trying to sell the horses we had, but one of them interested me greatly. It was a breed that we had seen at the local stud called a Percheron. A heavy horse known for its strength and loyalty, now a carriage driving breed, they were once the original warhorse bred for their courage and intelligence as well as their immense power. Her gentle eyes pulled at P-J's heartstrings too and we ended up buying her along with her carriage. We nicknamed her Baggins and she helped me in so many ways. I had a long recovery ahead of me and at first neither of us were in a state for riding, so I would take her for walks as you would a dog. She followed me around and before I knew it we didn't really need to fence her in. We would shut the main gate to our farm and she would roam around. Every time the postman arrived there would be a thundering of hooves as she galloped up the hill towards the house to find out who was there; she really was a horse-dog. Many times when I was walking her and tired she would lower her head for me to use her long mane to hold on to. She was the gentlest giant you could ever imagine. So perhaps Iris's animal friend wasn't going to be the faithful loyal dog I had always wistfully imagined, following at her heels and riding in her bike basket as my West Highland terrier had done in my childhood. Maybe it would be a cat instead . . .

The thought of taking a cat on a bike made me chuckle. Wouldn't that be something? There were times out on bike rides when having an animal with us might be hugely beneficial, perhaps when Iris had to wait in the car while we sorted out the kit when she would sometimes get frustrated and start to cry. She found these transitions hard to deal with and while we waited at gates for the other to open them or at the bridges over canals she wouldn't like that we had stopped. These moments worried Iris; they were when her anxieties rose. To have a friend there, a faithful companion, would be so valuable. I started to think of our daily routines too, our difficulties in the car. Iris was fine when the car was moving but as soon as we hit traffic lights she became impatient and worried, she would start to fidget, then to cry and from that point it became harder to settle her. Would a cat happily travel in a car on a regular basis? Could it provide the security Iris needed to settle on longer journeys? Then there were her sleeping habits, which had improved quite dramatically, but when you compared them to others we weren't exactly in the same league. She would go to bed at practically midnight. When I was a child having my dog at the end of my bed in the evenings helped me sleep, and in the mornings I couldn't wait to get up and see her; could a cat do the same for Iris?

I could imagine a cat fulfilling all of these requirements but there was one massive difference between cats and dogs that I couldn't ignore and that was that therapy dogs are trained to do their duties for a child with special needs and that an adult gives them commands to behave in a certain way in different situations. For example, if the child needs to calm down, the dog is given a signal by its handler and it will put its head on the child's lap to give them some deep pressure on their body, providing a calming feeling. Many children on the spectrum are 'runners', a common issue where the child bolts off with no sense of danger or knowing where they are going. A dog in a harness can be attached to the child by a lead and, if the child tries to run off, the dog is taught to stand firm and stay on the spot, preventing the child from running into danger. If a child is self-harming or engaging in repetitive behaviour that isn't desirable, the handler can give the dog a signal to intervene to distract them. I knew that cats could be trained with a clicker for treats but that was just to do tricks on the odd occasion. I doubted it would be possible to train a cat to do all that I had imagined, to be there for Iris in the ways that I desired. That needed to come from instinct, a powerful interest and love for Iris, and that wouldn't be easy to find in a cat. So I focused clearly on what I was looking for, the character traits that would make a good fit: loyalty, an acute interest in humans and their activities, courage and intelligence. A love of water would be useful – but even I could tell I was getting carried away with that one. All that I

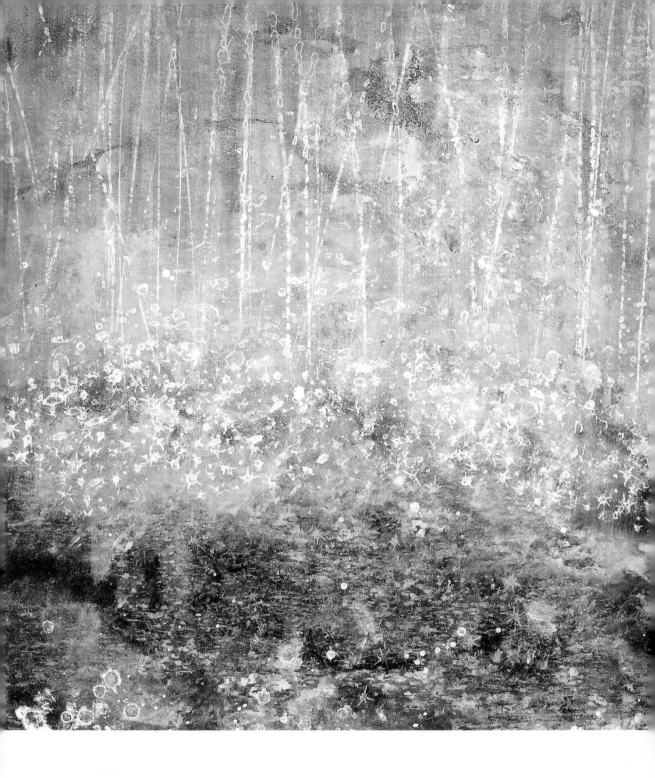

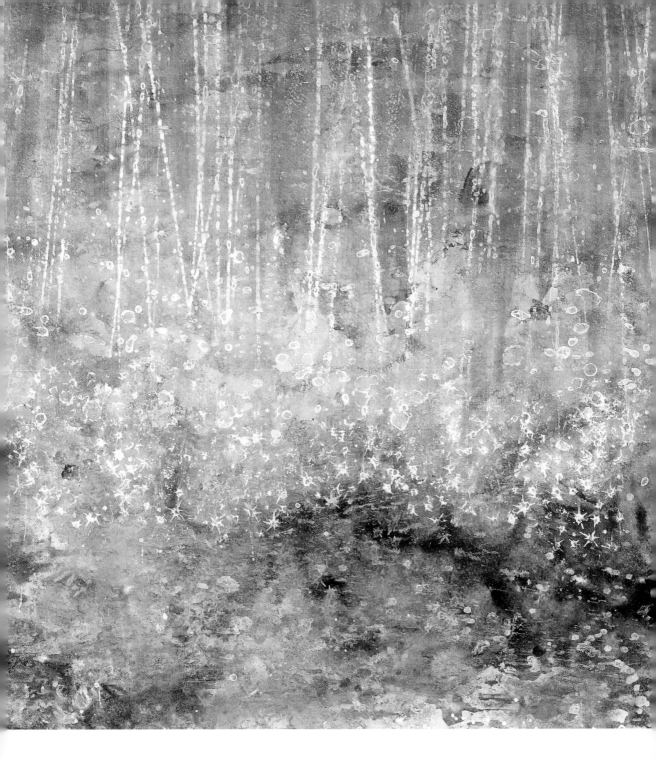

Raining Cats, acrylic, May 2014

was looking for was very unlikely but not impossible. I needed to cling to that – 'not impossible' – and believe in 'anything is possible'.

I had been in touch with various cat-rescue centres and one of them did have an older female cat who sounded like she was what we were looking for. They suggested we take her for a week to see if Iris got on with her but it didn't work at all. Once again it was as though Iris didn't even see the animal in front of her and the cat showed no interest in Iris either. In fact, she seemed to really dislike all of us and just wanted to go outside. She wasn't shy, rather boisterous actually, but she made it clear she wanted to be in any room we weren't in, and as soon as we went close to her she stalked off, flicking her tail, annoyed at our presence. I tried tempting her with treats and toys but after she hissed at me I could see it was a pointless exercise and that we hadn't found the right fit. This wasn't something that I should be forcing or even need to be encouraging; it needed to come from the animal and for it to be their choice.

'OK, maybe this isn't meant to be. After all, how many times can we do this to Iris?'

P-J was getting frustrated with my endless searching and felt like we were looking for a needle in a haystack. I did start to wonder if I had become so used to researching that it had become a habit. I was always looking for something that we didn't have, trying to find something that was just out of reach, that elusive component – maybe it was a coping mechanism, a need to keep my mind busy to block out my concerns about the future.

I decided to give this idea one last go and use everything at our disposal including asking Iris's Facebook followers for some help. I described what sort of cat I would like for Iris and asked if they had any suggestions for suitable breeds. A deluge of comments, emails and letters came flooding in. There was a breed that I hadn't heard of before, a large American cat called a Maine Coon, that was known for its loving, fun and loyal nature, which stood out from the rest. Some of the owners described them as 'dog-like' – they were incredibly interested in humans and they loved water. I couldn't believe what I was reading; it was as if I had unearthed the 'Baggins' of the cat world. This was the breed for us, surely the perfect companion for a child.

As luck would have it there was one breeder not too far away from us and as I spoke to the lady on the phone she described a kitten that sounded promising. She was a lot smaller than the rest but that was probably because she spent all her time with humans instead of her mother. As the breeder heard more about Iris she felt that this kitten would be the right fit as she was so incredibly interactive and loving for such a young kitten. The owner was very different to the other breeders whom I had spoken to. It was almost as if I was the one being vetted. She asked a great deal of questions about us, our home and what Iris was like. I loved how much she cared for her cats and that she took the time to get to know us first. I placed my faith in her judgement as she knew the cats far better than I ever could and we made arrangements to meet the kitten.

'She's just through here in the kitchen, mind your step. I don't keep them all in cages like some breeders do; they all live with us.' I tiptoed through a pride of ginormous cats in her home, which was a converted school. Magnificent felines sprawled across every ledge of the high windows. Some were sitting proudly on the sofas, others on the dresser. With a cat on every surface, the smell was quite overwhelming at first and I was pleased that Iris was waiting in the car with P-J. I had never felt like this around domestic cats before; I was in awe of their beauty. There was something wild about them: the lynx-like

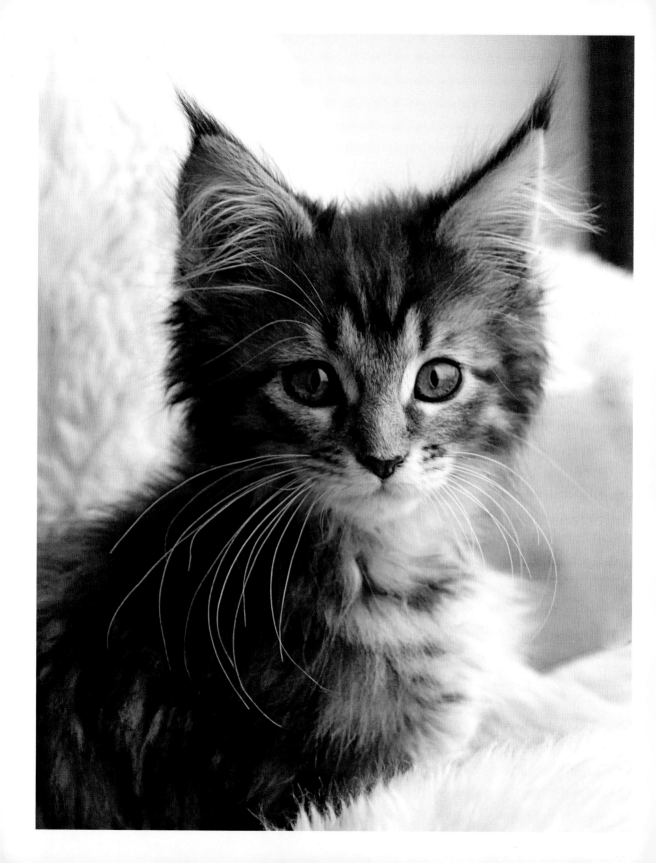

ears with long tufts at the tips, large round copper eyes and an almost human look on their faces. Stroking one of the males that stopped me in my tracks as I walked through the kitchen door was like looking into the eyes of Aslan. He had a shaggy mane and large tufted paws. He moved slowly past and then I saw the kitten playing with some newspapers on the kitchen table. When she looked at me I couldn't help but smile. Her enormous ears and long white whiskers were comical against her tiny tabby body. She was much smaller than the others but as I listened to more information about her and how she had been sleeping on the breeder's pillow and how she had become quite the sous chef in the kitchen, I fell in love with her and we decided to take her home that day.

Iris watched me carefully as I brought her over to the car in the pet carrier box. I placed her beside Iris for the journey and we stopped off at a pet store on the way home to get a few supplies. While P-J went into the shop I opened up one end of the box so our little kitten could meet Iris properly. They just looked at each other for a while. I encouraged Iris to stroke her and she giggled as her fingers touched the soft fuzzy fur. When we got home and they were both free to move it was as though they were already old friends as we watched them settle on the sofa. They sat side by side, the kitten's tiny body tucked in against Iris.

'Job done!' P-J said with a huge grin and patted me on the back as we walked to the kitchen. 'Well done, you did it.'

I couldn't believe it. Job done, he was right. It was immediate; they just clicked and there was no need to do anything else. I could stop searching.

The kitten was everything the breeder had described and more. We named her Thula, pronounced 'Toola', after one of Iris's favourite African lullabies, meaning peace in Zulu. Thula was at Iris's side from the moment she saw her and slept in her arms during her first night like a guardian angel. A true Maine Coon: affectionate, loving and intelligent. I watched them on the sofa, the kitten attentively looking at the iPad screen with Iris: gazing at everything and purring non-stop. When Iris was looking at her books she would delicately feel Thula's ears and her long whiskers. Iris would occasionally hold her tail right at the tip while she was thinking, casually twiddling with the fur as if it were her own. Thula never moved, liking the attention and she settled into life at home just as quickly as she bonded with Iris, although she was very different around us adults. She was a typical hyperactive kitten: naughty, incredibly inquisitive and a comedian. P-J took great delight in showing me how she would come to his whistle; but when I tried, not so much. Thula reminded me of Meoska in those times but she was different. Something intriguing about her, which always astounded me, was her level of interest in anything we did. Watching me cooking, cleaning and editing my photos, it was as if she was studying me. I had no idea what motivated that behaviour in such a young animal. Was she trying to learn, to fit in?

Our morning routine changed as a result of Thula's presence. Iris, once slow to stir and difficult to get going before 9 a.m., now seemed to have springs in her feet. She woke up with a wide smile with her new friend beside her and I heard her say 'More cat' as she followed her to the stairs. Thula's constant presence and gentle nature almost immediately had a remarkable effect upon Iris. I began hearing Iris giving instructions to Thula. 'Sit, cat,' she would say when Thula was trying to play on her iPad. She said it with such authority that the kitten obediently sat down with her striped legs neatly together. Unlike most children of

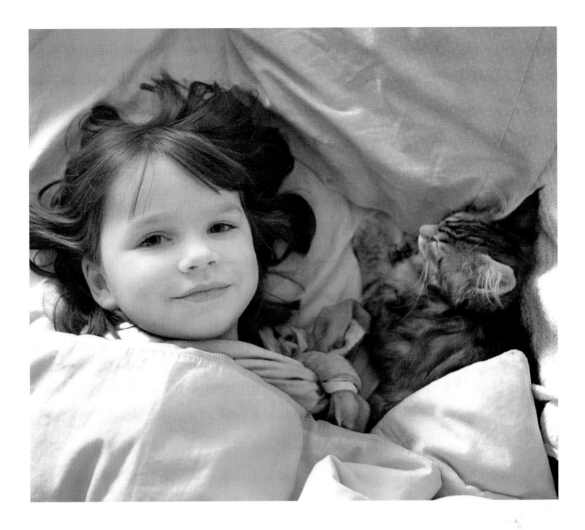

Iris's age, she didn't maul, stroke or pick up the kitten constantly. Their relationship was based upon companionship. Thula watched with great interest as Iris played, joining in whenever she could. Iris stood at her table playing with play-dough and Thula sat beside her, mimicking Iris's movements. I couldn't believe what I was seeing: this tiny kitten was implementing the basics of play therapy. The more I thought about it, the more I could see what a perfect companion a cat was for a child

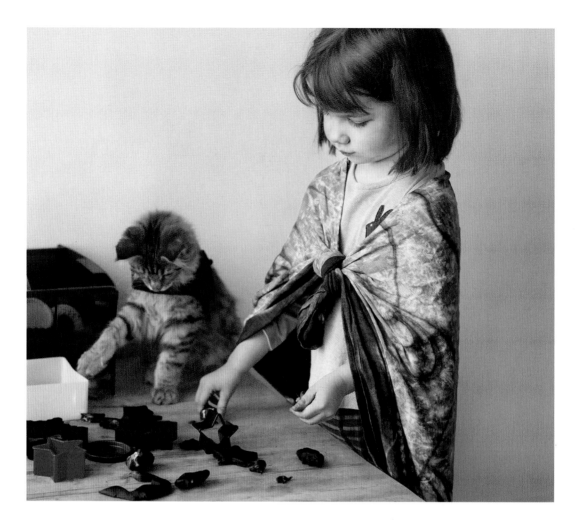

on the spectrum. They understood one another in a way that we would always struggle to. There was an undeniable bond forming between them, a powerful connection that we had been searching for all this time, and to finally see it was enchanting.

There was something about Thula's eyes that was bewitching and I wondered if that was why Iris didn't seem to mind holding eye contact with her or looking into her face. Sometimes her eyes looked greenish yellow, at other times blue, and they were circled with black in a beautiful eyeliner effect that swept out to the sides. Alongside her long whiskers she had extra long eyebrow whiskers to match. These whiskers, like her tail, seemed to have their own character and were so full of life; when she was interested in something they would move forward as if they were trying to grab the item.

If Iris woke during the night, Thula was there to settle her. It was as though she instinctively knew what to do. She would bring Iris a small toy in her mouth and drop it beside her. Iris would play for a while with the toy in her hands and the movement in her fingers seemed to release any tension. Thula would then snuggle up beside her and purr while Iris gently settled and fell back to sleep. I would watch them through the doorway; if I had gone in, Iris would have asked to go downstairs by raising her arms to be lifted and then guided me to the staircase with her own weight, rather like steering a motorbike by leaning into the corners. But with Thula there she was happy to stay in bed and be calmed down, not needing to move about the house. Then when Iris got distressed during the day Thula didn't seem frightened, but instead stayed by Iris and distracted her from her difficulties.

My past experience with animals had taught me not to assume anything and to give them opportunities as they may well surprise you. With this in mind I needed to put certain things in place in order to keep Thula safe if we were going to take her out more in the car and even try her in a basket on the bikes, so I bought a harness. It would be a way for us to attach a lead comfortably and it would also give Iris something to hold on to. From the moment I put it on Thula it was as though she knew its purpose. She sat in front of Iris letting her inspect the various attachments and Thula saw it as a sign that she was now working and she wore it with pride. The lead wasn't so simple. Every time I tried to attach it and get her to walk with me she just stopped, a perplexed look on her face. But with Iris on the other end it was a different story.

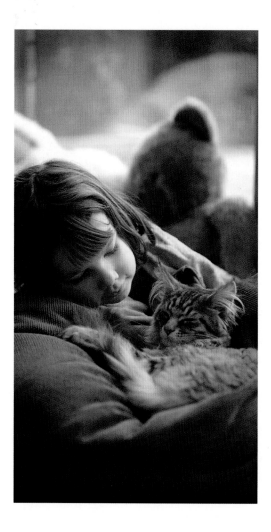

Thula walked happily around outside in the frozen garden. It was the first time Thula's paws had touched blades of grass and she walked along tentatively but never tried to stray away from her friend. I quickly understood that Thula's willingness to go above and beyond linked specifically to Iris.

With P-J and me she was as cheeky as they come. 'Thula, come back!' P-J shouted and a flash of Thula's tabby body flew past with what looked like a loaf of bread hanging from her mouth.

'Was that . . .?'

'Yes. Our breakfast. She's nicked the bread.'

Thula was busy booting pieces of bread all over the laundry floor, so there was no rescuing the situation from there. Thula had many such eccentricities. For example, she loved cheese. Just the smell of it would entice her from any situation. She also played fetch with objects, bringing them back to us for us to throw again and again, and she would hang out in a basket by the kitchen door so she could pat us as we went past with her giant paws. It wasn't long before she couldn't fit into the basket; she would try to squeeze in but eventually she gave up. It was no good: her body was growing at a phenomenal rate. She was already the size of a fully grown English farm cat and she was still a kitten.

The weather had been terrible, so when it wasn't possible to go for walks or be on the bikes we all went for a drive in the car with Thula curled up on Iris's knee and purring loudly. She became part of everything and moulded herself into every situation, helping whenever she could.

My vision of taking a cat out on the bikes started like any other adventure. Planning was, of course, essential. I found a comfortable basket box that was specially designed for small dogs and to be attached to the handle bars; I knew that Thula was

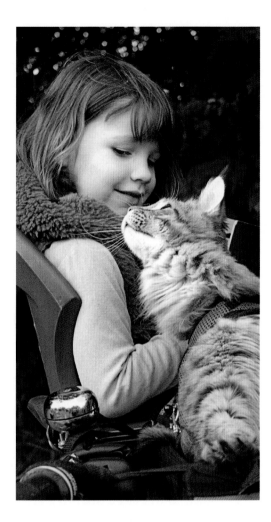

going to grow a lot more over the next couple of years, so the bigger the better. There was an internal lead and at first I got Thula used to just sitting in the box inside the house. Then I carried her around the garden in it, and the final stage was attaching it to the bike. But she adored riding on the bike. From the very first outing she was relaxed and enjoyed seeing all the wildlife along the canal and staying close to Iris. Right away I could see this was going to be a permanent arrangement.

She never tried to get out and was always keen to get in the car when she saw the bikes. From then on Thula was a biker cat, accompanying us on every bike ride and being a friend to Iris when she needed extra support.

When Iris looked like she needed help I would ride up alongside her and position Thula's basket right up against Iris's seat. Thula would stretch up as far as she could to reach Iris and kiss her cheek. The long whiskers tickled and got Iris's attention, pulling her away from her worries. Iris then placed her arm round Thula's body and we would just let them be for a while as she stroked Thula's head, delicately running her fingers along the symmetrical black markings in between her ears. Sometimes Iris would rub the long black tufts at the tips of her ears between her thumb and forefinger while Thula stayed still, watching the natural world around her with bright wide eyes.

As we rode along the canal towpath Thula's presence always left a trail of smiles, chatter and laughter as people saw a cat sitting so confidently with her paws over the edge of the basket, leaning forward into the wind with an eager look upon her face. Thula made them smile because she acted differently from what was expected of a cat, bringing something special to their day. I wished everyone could be as accepting and joyful in regard to differences that they encounter in their lives. Thula and Iris were sending out a strong message – that different is brilliant.

One day, cutting one of our bike rides short due to high winds, we returned to the house and I carefully peeled off Iris's snowsuit while she sat patiently on the stairs. Her cape was now a permanent fixture and I had it ready as usual. As I put the suit to one side I expected to see Iris desperately trying to get her top off, as that had been the case for the last year. But she was still sitting there looking at me, calm and happy. She looked at the cape and I gently placed it over her head with her other clothes still on. She then walked off to find Thula. P-J and I looked at each other and silently decided not to make a big deal out of it in case she thought better of it and wanted the whole lot off. But later that evening, with her clothes still on and Thula sleeping by her side, I thought about Iris's clothes issue. We had never discovered what had lain behind her sudden dislike of clothing. I felt that it had started as a sensory problem and then turned into her way of life. She felt free and happier minus her tops, more comfortable and confident. Was she now feeling that way due to Thula's presence and could therefore be more flexible? Whatever it was, it was a welcome relief that made life so much easier.

Storms had hit the south of England terribly that winter, with dreadful news of flooding and damage. We had been safe from the worst of it but the wind was blowing strongly and Iris had been uneasy all morning. The vocabulary explosion and all the highs that had come with it recently were inevitably counterbalanced with some lows. Iris had been working very hard on her speech, completely self-motivated using the iPad and her books. She was improving fast, but at times she looked phased-out and saddened by the pure effort of it all. It hurt me to see her feel this, and I thought again how unfair it was that she had to work so hard for something that came naturally to others. She paced around the house repeating words over and over: letters of the alphabet and a stream of animal names. It was amazing to hear so many words but there was a compulsive and rather uncontrolled manner in the way she was talking. I could tell she was anxious and wanted to go outside, so we ventured into the garden. The movement in the trees and grasses made her jump with excitement but it wasn't long before their rhythm generated a blanket of calm that swept through her as she watched the motion. Iris retraced her steps from previous happy days, revisiting her favourite trees and last of all her favourite tree stump, which rested in the centre. She stood perfectly still with her eyes shut, placing her hands together with her palms gently touching the soaked wood. I did not know if she was drawing strength and peace from her old friend or if she was comforting him, but there had been calm to be found in the storm and we walked back to the house together.

But despite this I was still concerned about Iris. The strain of concentrating so hard on her speech was beginning to show. Hearing her repeating animal names over and over had shown me the cost of making progress. She had obviously gained some relief and enjoyment from being able to say them, but then she couldn't control it and a new frustration would mount from that feeling of being out of control, as if she knew she needed to stop and rest but couldn't. Habits from the past, like picking her lips, started to creep back in, so I made sure we did as many of her occupational therapy exercises, the sensory play and the ones with the therapy ball, to relieve the tension.

I was thrilled Iris was making progress, but the effort of it all and the toll it took on her was noticed by everybody, and that included her faithful friend. One day Thula picked up a square piece of bubble wrap in her mouth and jumped up on to the sofa beside Iris and dropped it in her lap. Iris who was withdrawn and looking exhausted, smiled and said, 'Hi, cat.' She picked the bubble wrap up and started playing, then offered it back to Thula. Unusually Thula didn't want it to be thrown or dangled. She nudged it back to Iris and lay down purring loudly; she was prompting Iris to play with it and to feel the bumpy texture between her fingers. I watched from the doorway, amazed at what I was seeing. I had just been hunting for something to take Iris's mind off running through her words, a distraction from her current goal. How was Thula doing this? I understood she must be reading Iris's body language but to have the intelligence to find a sensory

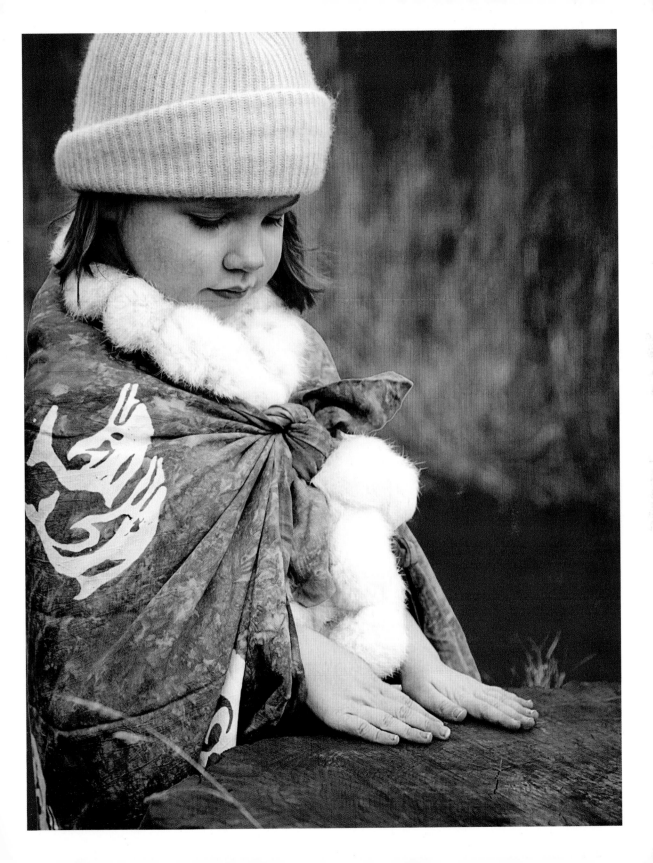

toy, not for herself but for Iris to play with to pull her out of this darker space was incredible.

I was seeing a change in Iris's behaviour towards the cat. Iris was more tactile and affectionate, massaging Thula's black paws and letting her fingers seep into her silky coat. And while she was on the iPad one hand was playing a game and the other was stroking her faithful cat who rested beside her. I felt certain that this has had an effect on calming her senses.

One evening P-J and I were preparing supper while our dynamic duo were playing with bubbles in the sink, using the painting table as a solid platform to stand on. Thula was by Iris's side, splatters of bubbles ran down the window, and there were squeals of excitement as yet more were blown off her hand against the pane of glass. It had been a while since I had seen Iris be this comfortable touching water with her hands. For months she had avoided it and used utensils to play with it. There had been times when even just one drop of water on her skin could cause turmoil; she would run at me crying, wiping her body all over my clothes to get it off her skin, and I could see it was painful for her. But gradually, as she interacted with Thula, stroked her fur and followed her lead with water and sand play, we started to see many changes. Turning to me with a huge smile and arms outstretched I received the most wonderful hug, a rare and beautiful show of affection. Then to our surprise she turned to P-J and did the same, and after that it was Thula's turn. I started to giggle and another hug came my way. Iris was pivoting on her painting table from one member of the family to the next and we couldn't believe our luck; her hugs were given so rarely and it was incredibly moving as I watched her open her arms and launch herself towards P-J.

We were seeing improvements in every aspect of our lives. The relationships between Iris and her grandparents had changed dramatically. It was as though her ability to show how she felt towards them had lain dormant. She used to dislike being hugged, kissed or even talked to at times, but that was changing. She laughed if my father caught her as she passed him, and he could tickle her and give her a hug and a kiss. When my brother picked her up and put her on his shoulders she didn't seem to mind at all and enjoyed riding around the garden. Before she would generally ignore these family members and it was difficult because I knew how much she loved them. Now, while my father relaxed in the garden, she was confident enough to go over to him, even grabbing his hand to lead him up to the top garden gate to go off on adventures into the neighbouring school field. She started to use her words around them: playing a game with her grandfather he started counting as he lifted up his feet and she would continue counting out loud beyond twenty. He was astonished and delighted in hearing her voice.

One Friday lunchtime my mother, Iris and I were all lying on the bed giggling. My mother and I held the blanket over us like a tent while Iris wriggled with excitement underneath and then leapt out. As she bounced around I realized how far we had travelled over the last year. Watching her tuck her body close to her granny and want a hug filled me with joy. After a lovely afternoon I got Iris into the car and my mother came over to the car door and kissed Iris goodbye. All of a sudden Iris waved and said 'bye' and then blew a kiss – perfection! I am not sure how it happened or when exactly, but something had stirred – like her speech the pathways were clearing and she was showing us how much emotion was locked away. The love for them had always been there; like the words in her head she just had great difficulty expressing it. Autism can be immensely cruel at times, hurting the people that care the most, but with patience and understanding you can be rewarded with the most incredible highs. The bonds that had retreated had come back

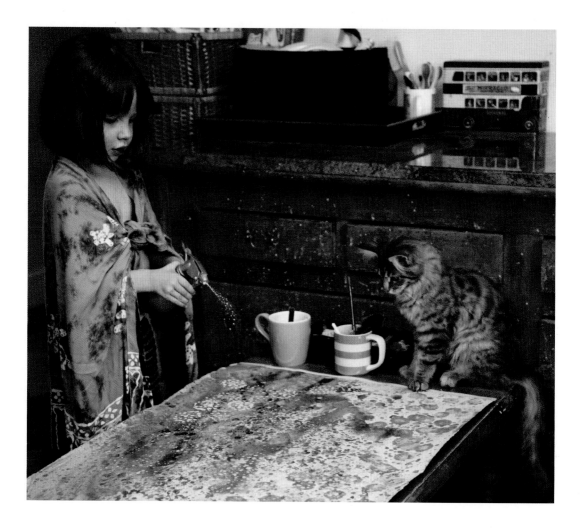

stronger than ever before. I was so pleased that my parents had never given up. Our weekly lunches and their regular visits to us at home had always continued, so Iris knew they were there for her when she was ready.

The new bonds Iris was forming with Thula were different to those with her first feline friend. Shiraz had been the mother figure, helping me like a faithful nanny over the Christmas holidays, whereas Thula was young and needed guidance, and this in itself altered Iris's behaviour. She trusted Iris completely and with that came responsibility on Iris's part to treat her with respect and love. One evening Iris was sorting through her paintbrushes. One by one a neat pile formed on the stool beside P-J, then she selected three of the smallest brushes and handed them to Thula. A little unsure how to deal with them at first, Thula began to play and Iris jumped for joy that her friend was sharing her passion. Every time Iris went to her painting table Thula would be there, sitting patiently in the left-hand corner of the table, watching and waiting, riveted, as the paintings developed. Occasionally the temptation to play would be too great and Iris would remind her to 'sit, cat' and she did. On days when the weather allowed it we moved the painting kit outside and there she was, waiting in position: Iris's faithful friend, confidante and artist's assistant. At first letting Thula out in the garden was a worry: would she wander off and go on her own adventures? But as soon as I put her red harness on she knew her responsibility lay firmly at home with Iris and she stayed by Iris's side.

Much of my planning at this time was done in one of the most unlikely of places, the bath. Iris's sudden issues about bath time meant it was somewhere she no longer wanted to go and so my bath times provided some rare time and space to think. One evening, just as I was mulling over what to do the next day, I realized I wasn't alone. I felt Thula's whiskers against my neck – she had silently jumped up on to the ledge at the end of the bath. I stroked her behind my head and resumed my plans for the following day. One paw, then two, then three and four were on my shoulders and then Thula walked down my body into the water and started to swim about, before settling on my leg. Her skinny neck was just above the water, turning towards me like E.T. I daren't move – her claws had stayed hidden away so far, but I was in a tricky position. I decided to stay still and see what happened next.

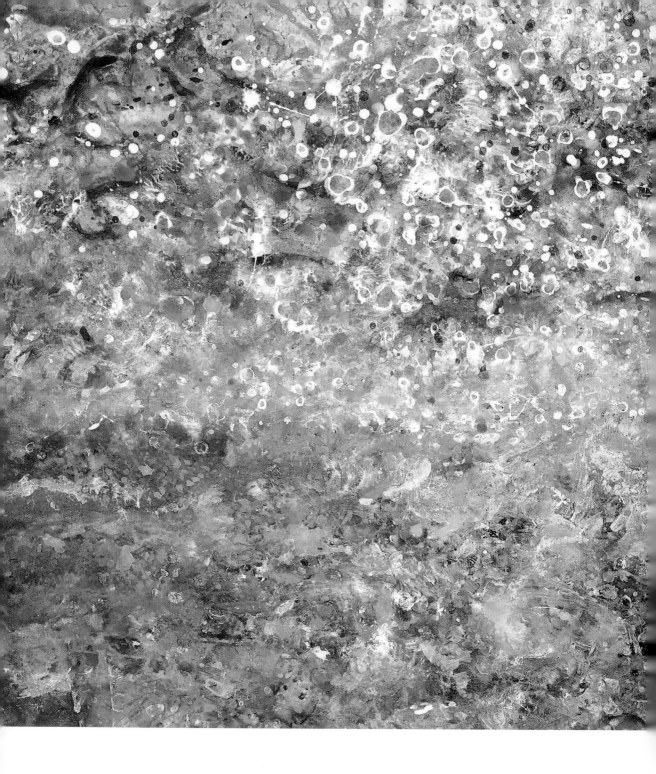

Blue Planet, acrylic, April 2013

Thula jumped from my leg neatly on to the side of the bath and then off on to the floor. She shook herself, and her long tail now looking stick thin and rather out of proportion, made me laugh. The cleaning, licking and drying then began and continued for quite a while until she looked more like the kitten I remembered.

My thoughts were no longer with schooling; my head was filled with this new discovery. Thula liked water; she really liked it. She had been amused with bubbles and water play at the sink, but this was taking things further than I had ever imagined. When we had first looked into the breed I had read folklore tales about their origins, how they were descended from Norwegian forest cats and had been taken over to America by the Vikings on ships. One tale tells the story of Captain Charles Coon, an English seafarer who sailed up and down the New England coast with a host of long-haired cats aboard his ship. Watching Thula so comfortable in and around water, unfazed, it was as if she belonged there and her ancestral past was clear to see.

My mind was thinking fast. Iris's bath-time difficulties had become increasingly hard to manage, to the point of it becoming very distressing for all of us. I hated seeing her so upset and we tried everything you could imagine to help her with this sensory problem but nothing had worked. Since Iris seemed fine with water play at the sink maybe this wasn't so much a sensory issue but a phobia that had been caused by a tiny detail I had overlooked. Could Thula be the perfect solution?

• •

'What's the plan then?' P-J asked as he listened to me, and to my surprise he didn't laugh at my new discovery. He was intrigued and could see where I was going with this one.

'I thought I'd just encourage Thula to be in the bathroom next time and see how things go. She might just get in like she did with me. It's worth a try. I don't think anything could make it worse and Thula wouldn't do anything that she wasn't comfortable with. And I know she won't want to hurt Iris.'

So the next time I had to bath Iris I tried it. At first my plan didn't seem to be working. I was struggling to keep Iris in the bath: as soon as her body touched the water she started to cry and Thula had come in and trotted out again. I tried to distract Iris with the supply of toys I kept beside the bath. Yet one by one they were discarded to the other side, lined up and given a very angry look in between

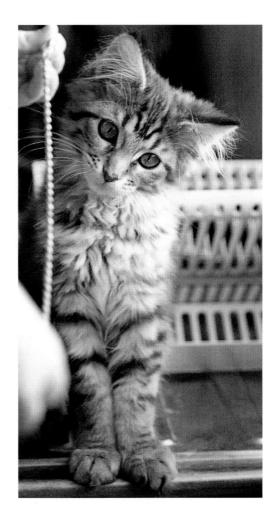

cries, and then she would turn to me again to see if my next offering was any better. But I had run out, and was all out of ideas too. As Iris's cries became unbearable I knew I would have to abort this idea for now. It just wasn't working and I was starting to worry about her safety as she once again nearly leapt out. Then Thula came back with a piece of jewellery that they had been playing with earlier. She jumped up on to the side of the bath and carried on playing with it. This distracted Iris for a moment and she stopped crying. Everything went quiet and I could think

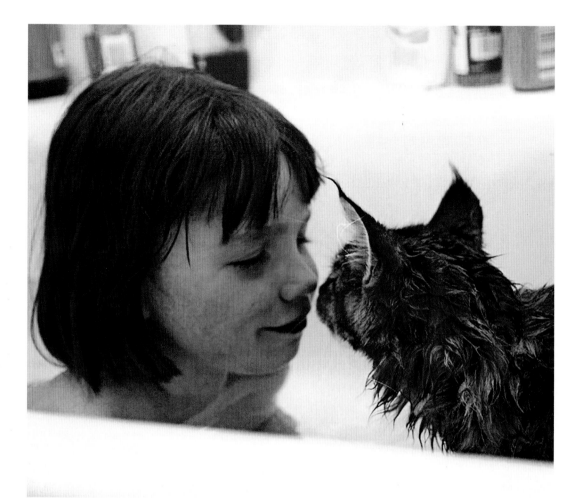

again. I sat back and took a deep breath, not wanting to break the silence, and then Thula got in the water.

I wasn't sure if I would ever get used to the sight of a cat so calm around water and then casually getting in. I loved Thula more than I ever had before; she amazed me time and again but this was truly brilliant to watch. It wasn't nearly as full as when I had been in the bath so she didn't need to swim, she was able to stand beside Iris, and immediately Iris greeted her with a 'Hi, cat' and I saw her smile. Seeing Iris smiling in the bath made me cry. I had wanted, waited and longed for her to enjoy our peaceful bath times together again; I missed them terribly. No matter how awful the day we were having was, there used to be a time where a warm bath with music would solve any problem and restore peace to our world. In that moment I was seeing that come back to us. She was so amused by her friend being in the bath she forgot about her anxieties and they played happily together.

P-J walked past the bathroom and I stepped out to see him: 'Come and see.'

He knew from my grin, which spread from ear to ear, that the plan was working. 'Oh, wow! This is amazing!' He went over to them both and stroked Thula, who was checking out some of Iris's sea creature toys. 'What's going to be next, swimming?'

'Funny you should say that. I was just thinking the same thing.' We hadn't tackled the swimming problem for a while and maybe it was time we tried again.

'I wouldn't rush things. Let's get her confident with this and then try.'

Thula must have become the cleanest cat for miles around, because she bathed with Iris as often as she could, even letting me show Iris how it was OK to have your hair shampooed. I used to dread washing Iris's hair. It was like I was causing her pain and I couldn't wait for it to be over, but then there was Thula. She sat still in the water as I washed her head and Iris laughed at the froth of bubbles all over her and then let me wash her own hair without a problem.

Cutting Iris's hair was also a continual problem for me. She was a champion squiggler, ducking, diving, running, jumping – doing anything possible not to have the dreaded haircut. It usually took days, sometimes weeks, of me cutting one part at a time.

When she was concentrating intently on something I had my best chance and even then I would have to have my hand skilfully positioned so that if she did move suddenly, her neck was protected. It was like painting bridges: once you finished it was time to start again. I had got rather lazy and neglected my duties that week and Iris's fringe was starting to move every time she blinked.

With Thula lying close and Iris playing a new alphabet game my chances were good. As I began, Thula put her paw up near the scissors and then placed it on my hand. She was so interested in what was happening that Iris followed her lead, looking up and to my surprise was now interested too. Instead of rushing off and crying or pushing me firmly away she stayed perfectly still and let me cut her hair without a problem. Thula moved close up against Iris's body and purred loudly, keeping Iris content. I stroked and thanked her for being my superhero and I really meant it; she was helping me through problems that I had lost hope of ever solving.

Swimming was another matter and a much bigger challenge we had visited in the past. We had never managed to get Iris through the door to the public swimming pool. Her old trick of turning into a starfish in my arms would return and Iris made it quite clear I was never going to get her through those doors and into the echoing chaos beyond. We had made a few enquiries into smaller, quieter pools, but never found one. And then a family friend in the village offered us their pool. It should have been perfect for Iris: quiet, light, a lovely swing chair in the corner, but after weeks of going regularly we realized that although she loved watching us swim we had no chance of getting her happy in the water due to her sensitivity to water and the fact that she hated taking off her shoes and her cape. However, many months later, after countless baths with Thula, Iris no longer had a problem at bath time. In fact, she loved it, and her shoes would come on and off easily. This was the moment we had been waiting for to try again.

'Wow, fish!' – a pair of very relevant and wonderful words from Iris that morning as she clung on to my body in the water of the swimming pool. All three of us were in. Thula, sadly, was at home; I felt it would be stretching the favour a little too far to bring her along as she would probably be up for going swimming too. After a while Iris was confident and happy to have her first swimming lesson with P-J and he encouraged her to start kicking. I was so proud seeing her little face beaming at me just above the water. We hadn't managed the armbands yet, because the sensation of squeezing her hand through worried her, but other than that she was doing very well and we couldn't believe the changes in her behaviour. Thanks to Thula swimming became part of Iris's life.

I began to lose count of the ways that Thula was helping Iris from day to day. When I told people about her I'm sure they thought I was exaggerating or that she must have been a cat that had gone through some special training. I could hardly believe it myself sometimes, especially when we were out on adventures in the countryside and Thula would stay by Iris's side, watching the water on the bridge at the stream or inspecting the bluebells in the woodland. The look in her eyes waimia when you talked to her. If we teased her, she would know it and stalk off. She had odd little habits – if she had been outside and her feet were muddy, she would go straight up to the bath and try to clean her paws in the leftover water by the plughole. Of course it was a very ineffective way of cleaning and there would be muddy paw prints everywhere, but her way of copying what humans did amused and fascinated us. Eventually she matured into a truly magnificent beauty with an almost regal look as she gazed down at us from the high wooden beams in the garden room. I didn't question it any more. I didn't need to know why she was doing the things she did or how she knew what to do; I just saw a friend, not only to Iris but to all of us – a member of the family.

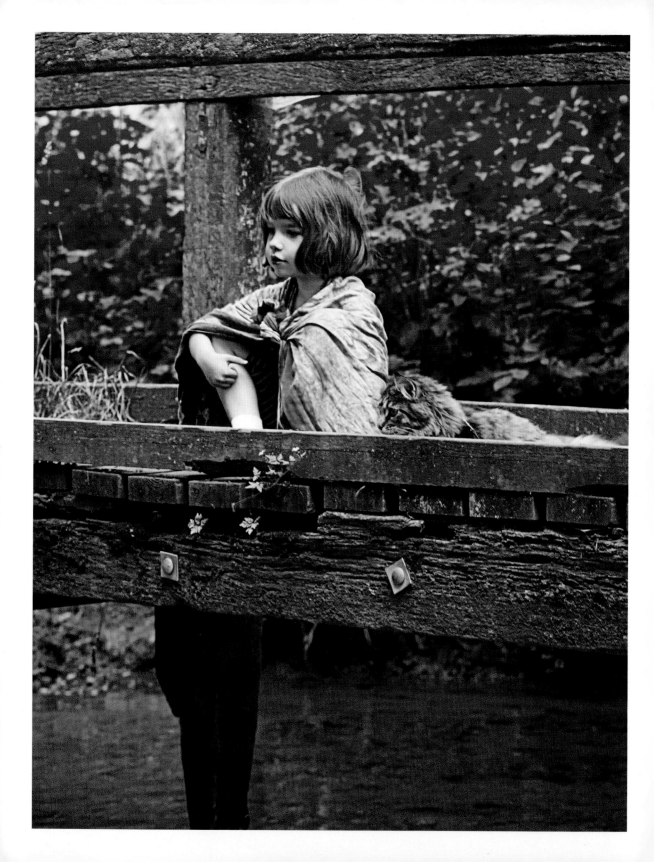

In the heart of the garden the three of them sit quietly together: Iris, Thula and Tree Stump. A place to think, to be still and to find peace in a busy and sometimes confusing world. With storm clouds fast approaching I call Iris indoors. Thula follows her best friend and gets into position on the painting table. She purrs as Iris starts to mix some colours on to the paper. The rain starts to fall heavily upon their kingdom out in the garden. They watch for a while from the window as the stump turns a darker shade, soaked from the raindrops. Back in the kitchen, the layers of paint deepen and delicate details emerge as Iris stamps, sponges and scrapes at the surface, uncovering bright colours beneath the dark blue. An image appears: a cat's face in the shadows. This connection is so strong that it transmits through Iris's art, a bond breaking through barriers, revealing the brilliance hidden within.

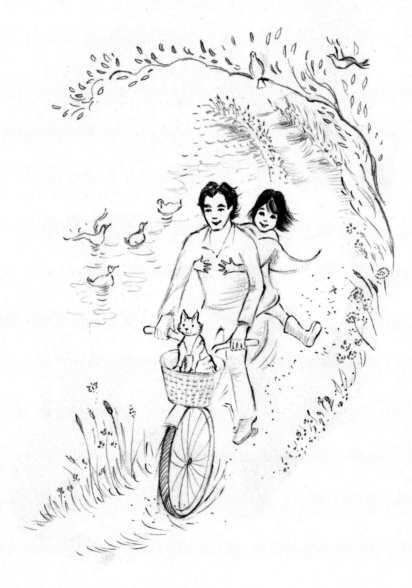

eight

For the third time since we had moved my office was been transformed. Formerly it had been my wedding editing room, then the painting storage area and now it was our home education room. I had everything so beautifully planned; there was a cosy area for reading in one corner, a desk for writing or more formal lessons and a play area. There was only one problem. I was alone. The pile of printed worksheets seemed to be mocking me, and my ridiculous attempts at teaching were failing miserably.

Thula came into the room and snuggled up next to me. I needed her more than ever before. 'Thula, how do you do it? Iris keeps on walking off.' I felt so hopeless and was starting to regret my decision. The past week had gone by without any successes and frustration was mounting on all sides. I was losing my way and needed help. Up until that point schooling Iris at home hadn't been easy but we were making steady progress. She now knew her alphabet and could say all the letters, knew her numbers past thirty and could read out some short words; she also recognized shapes and understood sizes and volumes. I had covered everything she needed to know under the preschool syllabus but now Iris would be turning five in a matter of months and we were venturing into reception-aged activities and I was struggling to hold Iris's attention.

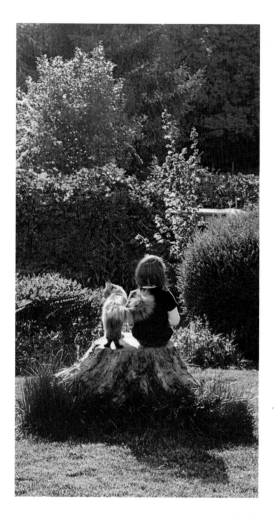

As I sat alone with Thula and thought some more I realized where I was going wrong. The room looked like a classroom and the activities and worksheets I was introducing meant nothing to Iris. She wasn't interested. That was the key to all of this. I needed to capture that incredible concentration span of hers in activities that would mean something to her. I had started to follow a generic formula set out by others that was outlined by the National Curriculum for reception but Iris wasn't like other children and I was quickly seeing that if I tried any more I would lose all that I had gained.

My heart began to beat hard. I felt hot and uncomfortable. Thula followed me out into the open air on the decking and we looked down to the tree stump where Iris was sitting. I began to feel better as I took deep slow breaths but I still felt uneasy. It was the guilt and I couldn't bear it any longer. For days I had been battling with it. It was like a sinking feeling within me. But I knew where it was coming from and it was all in my head: the knowledge and weight of responsibility that came with home-educating Iris alone, the realization that I might not be enough and that I didn't know what I was doing. I could see so much potential in Iris. It was there but just out of reach on so many days. In moments of failure I would question myself and debate the path I had chosen. I wasn't a trained teacher and before this had little interest in children's education. When we bought the house one of the perks in my mind had been that we were on the school bus route and how convenient that would be in years to come. I started to feel that loneliness creep back in, the isolation and the feeling of being so out on a limb and removed from the rest of society. Most of my decisions were made according to what I felt was right for Iris and by observing her behaviour, but I wasn't sure if that was enough any more.

We had a meeting with the authorities coming up and I would need to have a clear plan for her education and prove how I was going to put everything in place and teach her from our home. I knew if I had any chance of ridding myself of this guilt I needed to get things under control, but not in the way I had done before: no more print-outs from the internet. I had to design and create a curriculum for Iris myself that would centre on what inspired her. I would also bin the idea of educating her in one room and go for a free approach; I would teach her wherever she wanted to be, on the stump if necessary, out in the garden or on the bridge above the stream. If she needed to move, that would be fine; we would work around it, even use it somehow. But to do all this I would need some help. Designing my own education for Iris was a massive undertaking and without the knowledge of what Iris should be learning I wasn't going to get anywhere. So I asked my friend Charlie who worked in education for help and she very kindly offered to run through some options with me.

At first the curriculum plan in front of me felt a little overwhelming, but the more I read, the more I realized that I could create something like this for Iris but instead focusing on her interests. I was at Charlie's house and she was sharing her knowledge and experience from her years in education.

As I chatted to Charlie in her kitchen about what Iris could do, what she struggled with and what my plans were, it felt like this was the beginning of something truly wonderful and the heavy weight began to lift. I told her where we were at with Iris: her strong passions, her ability to read, all her achievements to date and what I had in mind for her for the next stage. Charlie's reaction was surprising. After a series of very specific questions she was incredibly supportive of my decision to educate Iris at home and felt like we did, that it was the best decision for Iris at this time. She showed me various options: different examples of curriculums used in both special and mainstream schools, and a topic-based learning format. I liked the theme-based method and in our mind it was the strongest option. We went through all the key areas I would need to cover. Schooling had certainly moved on since I was a child; there were many more skills within each subject that I needed to consider. To my delight what used to be information technology was now information and communications technology, meaning that it spanned all sorts of topics about collecting information with technology, and photography came under that bracket. It was so exciting to talk about it with someone who flew along with my ideas and guided me where I needed help. I left feeling excited about creating my own curriculum for Iris.

That afternoon I made a start. The first job was to decide what the theme should be. 'Cats' seemed the perfect choice and Thula soon sensed that something was happening and that her presence was needed. She jumped up on my lap and settled into a ball, purring.

'Just who I need, Thulie-Bulie. We are going to teach Iris using you, Thula. Isn't that wonderful?'

She lifted up her head and gave me a look as if to say 'Well, of course. What else, who else would you need?'

I wrote the word 'cat' in the middle of a piece of paper and put a circle round it, and then orbiting that I made more circles with the different subjects: English, music, art, ICT, science, maths, PE, geography and history. I started to brainstorm and plot out what we would do – the reading, the art-project ideas, the music – and the methods I could use with cat as the theme to teach certain skills, everything that I could think of including trips to zoos. I was running out of space on the paper and my writing was becoming illegible from all the Thula nudges. My neat plan wasn't looking so neat any more and that was before Iris came tiptoeing in and pulled the piece of paper off my desk and ran off. Not the best start.

A strong cup of tea later and I was back at my desk. I would need to become more cunning if I was going to win this one, so I opened up Photoshop and started working on the plan on the computer. It was brilliant; every time I ran out of space I just made my sheet bigger. This way I could adjust things easily and in no time at all Iris's cat-themed schooling topic was nearly finished. I had created far too many options and projects but I thought it was better to have some choice. I could never quite tell what was going to work with Iris and some days you don't only need your sleeves packed with tricks but bags full of them.

If Iris wasn't interested, she would just walk off and I would have to try again. Depending on her mood that could be disastrous. She could get so upset with me, confused and annoyed, pushing me away and saying 'back' or 'go away'. At those times she needed space and I would give it to her for a while. If I didn't, and pushed her further, she would get wildly upset, plunging her fist into her tummy and then shooting her arm and hand at me as if to say 'away with you' – all with the face of an angry bee.

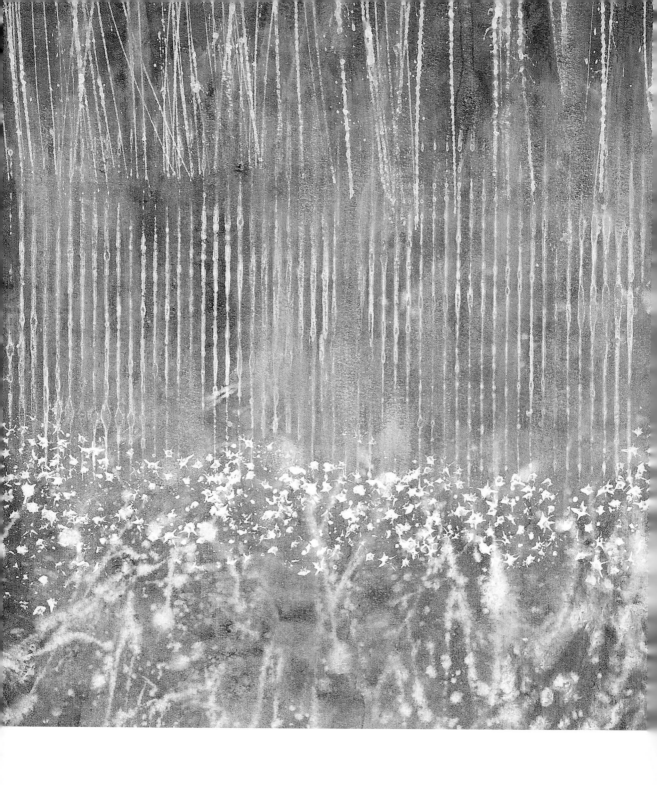

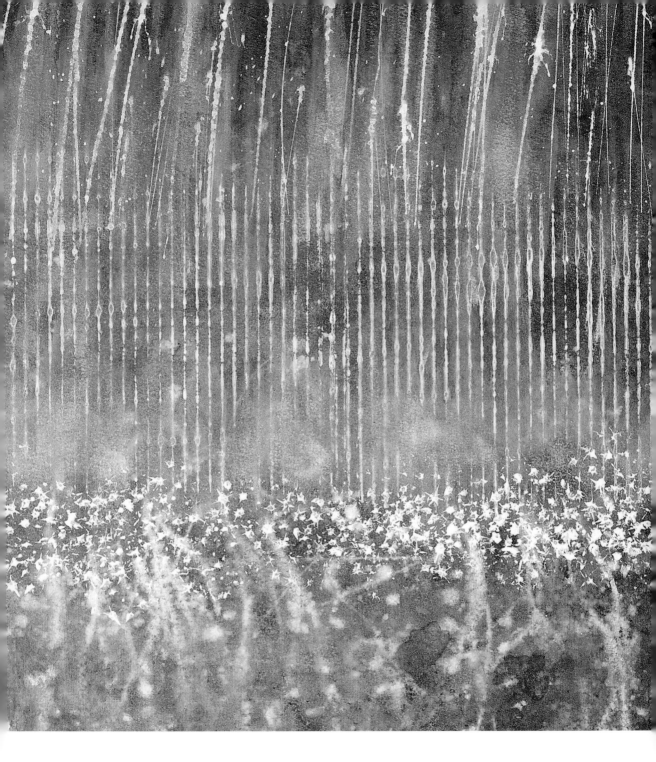

Kumbengo, acrylic, November 2013

It was then that I needed a breather too, and I would move into the kitchen to sit quietly, my mind busily thinking of how I could connect again and when I could try with something new. Then, later, something would work and it would be wonderful – a high like no other – and there would be pure joy through the simple act of working on something together and watching her learn. She learnt so fast; her understanding went way beyond what she showed on the surface and she would astound me by what she could do.

With each new thing I needed to start with something where I had seen a spark of interest before. There was a book out on the sofa, a heavy secondhand one that I had bought for Iris years before. I had read many poems and nursery rhymes from it that Iris had liked and I noticed she had the page open on 'The Owl and the Pussycat'. A plump brown owl sat with a tabby cat in a pea green boat in the blue sea with a pot of honey, some money and a guitar under a starlit sky. This is what I would recreate; we would make a boat from a cardboard box with props and, of course, Thula playing the part of the cat. We would then work on the vocab for the poem, practise writing some of the letters and saying the words. If that went well, we could move on to another one from the book, maybe 'Hey Diddle Diddle': a brilliant combination of cats, music and farm animals, which I had in my mind for the next theme.

I read through my plan once again, going clockwise. The English section was packed full of books, poems and rhymes. The arts section had all sorts of projects like making cat masks to encourage Iris to interact and to play. For ICT she would use my computer to practise typing simple words, her iPad with apps, and try out my camera to take photos of Thula. To add some science we would weigh Thula, compare sizes of cats, look at what whiskers were for and the other parts of the body. To practise maths skills we would count whiskers on the mask

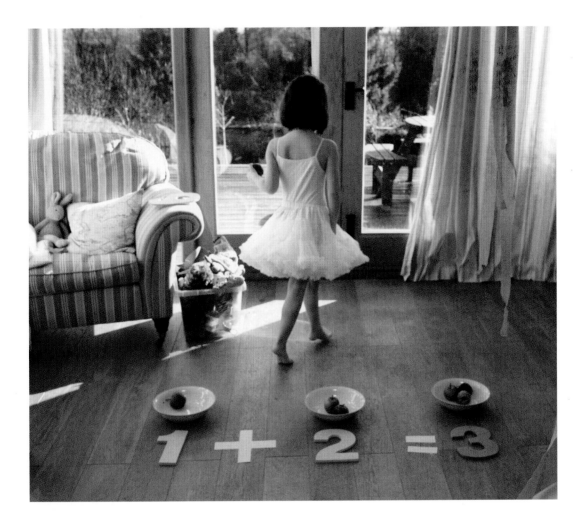

and maybe on Thula if she was sleeping, put the wild cat toys in size order, count them up and start to introduce addition. Geography was easy enough with the wild cats, and a zoo visit was essential for her to see them. And finally for some history I had a beautiful book, *The Cat: 3,500 Years of the Cat in Art*, which we could use, maybe looking into the Egyptians too. It was going to be an amazing feline journey. But to start we needed to make our boat.

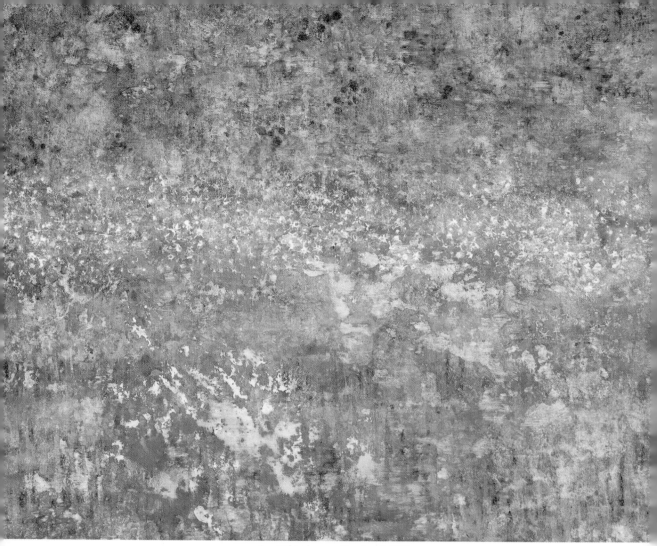

Sea Whistle, acrylic, April 2013

The paint had dried and as I took the cardboard boat out on to the decking Iris was dragging a bundle of blue fabrics that I had collected earlier. She knew that they must be an important part of this mission. I created a sea of cotton around the boat and added a few sensory toys: some sea creatures, a crab, some fish and a lobster. Then I hid a small bag of treasure inside, along with a jar of honey, Iris's pink ukulele and some binoculars to admire the view. I went to fetch some other items: an owl mask we had created earlier and a ring for the pig puppet. I put those in place and added a few silver stars to the hedge on one side – magic surprises that Iris could find and count. As I talked to her about the sea and the fantastic journey that we were about to go on, she looked at me as if to say 'Are you mad?' Then she ran off, returning with my iPhone and Thula trotting beside her. No adventure was complete without Thula and Peggy Lee. She navigated through the various settings to select her song and then we were off. Thula and I got in with her; it was a squish but Iris was grateful for our company as the vessel was still undergoing some inspection and not yet a safe place to be. As she explored she found the bag of treasure, and the golden coins and seashells glinted in the sun. She felt the texture round their edges, rotating them in her hands, then when she gave me a nudge I took my cue and climbed overboard. My plan was working; all those hours of finding the perfect box, painting it and finding the props had paid off. It felt very good indeed and I felt so pleased with myself.

But then Iris got out too and disappeared into the house. I had hoped all my efforts would have entertained her for a little longer. I felt disappointed. Had I gone too far? Was this all too much? Did I need to simplify things? After all, most of the advice I had received in the last year from experts and therapists who specialize in autism talked about teaching those on the spectrum with simple concepts and clear instructions broken down into stages. My methods were doing the opposite on many levels. But then through the glass I could see her coming back, this time with the iPad. Back on board Iris selected Google Earth, rotating the world, zooming in to South America, scooting over the Pacific Ocean and gently cruising her way around the planet, stopping every so often to take a look at the horizon through her binoculars.

This wasn't just playful antics. Iris was plotting her journey across the Pacific Ocean. It was way beyond what I expected. Her ability to understand and analyse a situation, her enquiring mind and intense focus, could still surprise me at times. Her autism meant that imaginative, pretend play was consumed by a curiosity about how things work and a fascination for nature and its beauty. It was a powerful gift and one I intended to use to help her understand new concepts. Iris was using her imagination but in a rather different way to what you would normally expect from a child of her age. To me it was brilliant. Thula played with the jewellery that she found in the treasure bag and Iris dangled a necklace in the sun as Thula batted it with her paw, making it swing from side to side. Iris happily hummed, watching the dancing splashes of light that the necklace created against the inside of the boat; it was like shimmering water reflections, adding to the magic. I read out the poem and Iris repeated parts and giggled at the part about dancing in the light of the moon. I used the puppet and the mask to encourage her to interact and that afternoon I wrote out the key words from the poem and Iris read them from the cards with ease.

Iris's education started to fill our lives. It didn't fit into set hours or days of the week; it took on a rather more spontaneous and organic feel. Every time we saw an opportunity P-J and I would take it. P-J took on the role of the storyteller; I made sure there were always plenty of books around on the current theme and he knew some of them so well that he could act them out, encouraging her to fill in the blanks. It didn't matter if it was late in the evening or early in the morning, in the bath or on the bikes; if she wanted to learn and explore or she was interested in a topic we went with it. It didn't even matter if I had already made a plan for another theme; I would put that to one side and go with what was most motivating Iris at that point. The freedom was powerful, although it did take some getting used to. P-J especially liked to go with what had worked last time, but we both needed to learn to see what was working on that day rather than to cling on to past successes. Once I

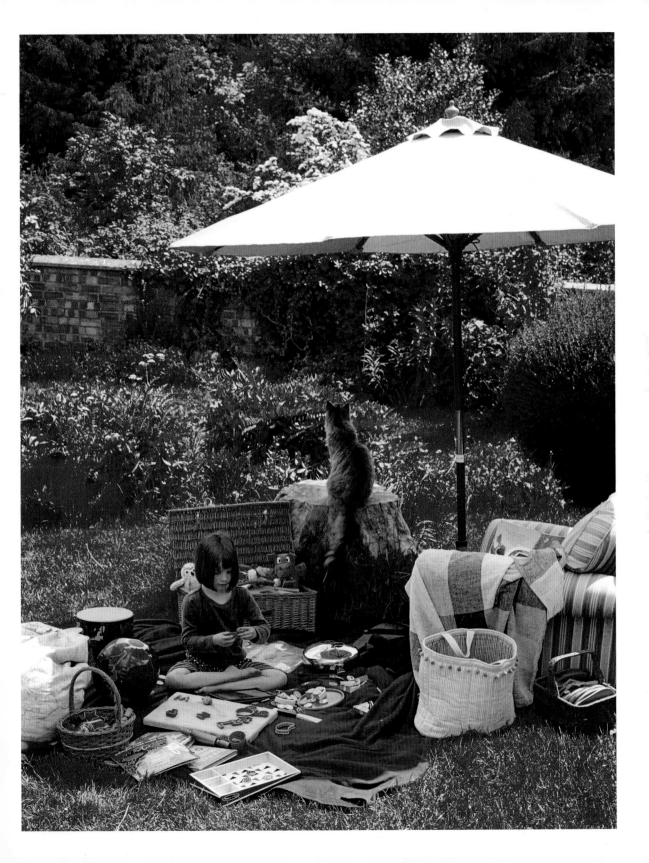

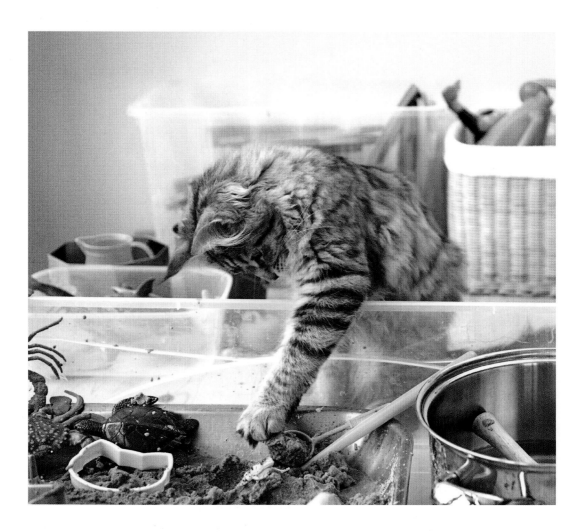

had prepared a topic and put all that effort in it was tempting to just plough on. Sometimes I tried regardless, but after some unsuccessful sessions I had to remind myself to stay true to my ethos of following Iris. Without a strong motivator she was very difficult to teach; in fact, at times it was almost impossible as she wanted me away from her. It was frustrating at times to be taken into another room, but if I didn't leave she would walk off, and if I forced her to stay she would be so distant I wouldn't achieve anything with her anyway. I would want to either burst into tears or scream with anger at why life had to be so difficult at every step and why she so often wanted to be alone. The thought that always pushed that negativity away was that it was harder for Iris. Her frustrations were so much greater. She needed us to stay strong and positive for her; she needed help and understanding. So I would take a deep breath, think hard about what I could use to reconnect with her, what lines I could say from a favourite book or song, or maybe which toy I could bring into the room that was on the theme that had inspired her.

Unlike most children Iris didn't have holidays or specific times when her education would stop. It was and is continuous, but we would constantly observe her, so if we felt that she needed a break, that she was tired or not in the right mood she would have some time alone with her books, listening to music or exploring in the garden. We learnt to gauge when we could work with her, when she just needed space and when we could use some of her relaxing activities as a teaching tool.

It was a magical time. Every day seemed packed full of delightful moments shared between us all and homeschooling became so much easier with my trusty teacher's assistant. Whenever I brought out a new activity Thula would be first at the table, leading the way and showing Iris that change is a good thing and how fun it could be exploring these new sensations and experiences. Iris then followed and I watched in delight as she grew in confidence.

••

Sometimes even our bike rides were transported into the current theme. After one week without our rides out in the countryside due to bad weather, we were all delighted to be speeding along the canal again, on our way to visit the black-and-white hairy pig, who played the part of the pig in 'The Owl and the Pussycat'.

So there in the wood where the Piggy-wig stood Thula tried as best she could. At first she shivered at the sight of the pig and Iris put her arm round her and did a little jig as we all giggled at the grunts and said 'hello' to the pig. Thula quickly gained confidence with her best friend beside her and looked down upon the beast from the basket on the bike with ears and whiskers forward.

There was just one last trip to finish our wonderful expedition into the cat world and to celebrate Iris's fifth birthday. The zoo.

Iris looked out of the window, she was interested in the cattle in the field, their huge horns and chocolatey-brown silky coat. As we passed by she nudged me to take a photograph. We were side by side in the back of the car for this drive-through safari, my lap covered in cameras, books and toy animals. It was a perfect introduction as Iris wasn't yet confident enough to manage the crowds at a zoo but with the protection of our familiar car she was handling the new experience beautifully. She laughed as I talked to her about what we might see next and picked up the toy tiger, rotating it in her hands, feeling the texture. We saw rhinos, monkeys, zebras, tigers . . .

As we entered the enclosure with the North American black bear Iris was happily eating her sandwich. We stopped to look at a very handsome and rather large bear right beside us. She looked out of the window and then hid her sandwich down beside me with a knowing glance. It made me laugh and then I got a nudge to take a photo. My purpose was clear; I was the image catcher, the photos reminding her of our journey once we were back home.

That evening while Iris was settling down in her playroom I gave her a hug. 'Happy birthday,' I said. 'This year will be wonderful, darling.'

'I'm five,' Iris replied.

One day a lady from South Africa emailed me. She had been following Iris's story on Facebook and wanted to tell me about a company that offered a rather different type of speech therapy, which she thought might help Iris. She had been trialling it out in her school and had been very impressed with the results. The program was called Gemiini. It was an online video library that had been filmed specifically for those who had issues with their speech. Each short video would focus on one word or even a short conversation and there was a choice to either see the mouth moving or the person saying the word with a picture of what they were saying beside them. It was really easy for us to use and I quickly started to introduce words on the current theme to Iris using the Gemiini platform. She would sit next to me at my computer and watch these videos avidly for twenty-minute sessions several times a day.

Iris and P-J were laughing hysterically at the kitchen table. I watched from the door as she asked him to do 'monkey'. She waited and giggled, looking straight at him. Again I heard the word 'monkey'. She paused, then she lifted up her arms and said 'ooh-ooh-a-a-a', trying to get him once again to do another round of monkey impressions, which he did. Iris got the hiccups from laughing so much and the game went on with other animals that she had learnt about from the videos. Her ways of interacting and playing with us were starting to change. She was now using her voice and enjoying it; it wasn't as tentative or as sporadic, or even repetitive, like it had been when she had got carried away before. When she had first started speaking she had got fixated with particular words, but after using Gemiini she was repeating words daily in the right context, constantly getting me to read words from books and studying my mouth while I said each word. I felt certain it was the positive impact of the speech-therapy videos because they focused so much on the mouth. A child with autism usually avoids eye contact as much as they can unless you are really encouraging it, so I think she was missing many of the skills she needed, just by not seeing enough of what our mouths were doing when we spoke. She would get my finger and guide it to the text that she wanted repeating, then watch my mouth intently as I spoke. It didn't seem to end at the words in the videos; they were a starting point, igniting her interest in different ones. It also seemed to help with her social skills and encouraged Iris to answer questions – just basic things to start with that she had seen on the videos. For P-J it was a real turning point because he had wanted for so long to have silliness, fun and games with Iris; his Peter Pan character had always been trying with Iris but she hadn't yet had the skills to be able to join in. Now that was changing.

Iris's new skills soon extended to the rest of the family as well, and when P-J's mother, Helen, came down from Lincolnshire to see us all I watched from the decking as Iris guided P-J's and her grandmother's hands together. Once they were holding hands she pushed upwards and positioned them in a bridge shape and then she ran underneath. Back and forth she went with her blue cape flying in the wind, through the tunnel and out the other side with squeals of excitement.

Since we were introducing so many other activities to Iris's day she was painting less than before, but the table, paper and paints were always out for her to use whenever she wanted to. There was a painting that sat in the architect's chest under a pile of unfinished pieces. It wasn't forgotten about and was often revisited but never finished until one rather stormy day. The wind blew so strongly that day that I worried we might lose some tiles off the roof. I stayed close to Iris in case she needed me, but Iris had her painting and with it placed on the table in the kitchen she worked fast, an array of colours splashing this way and that. While the paint was drying she used tools, toys and stamps to add texture. She jumped excitedly as she saw a

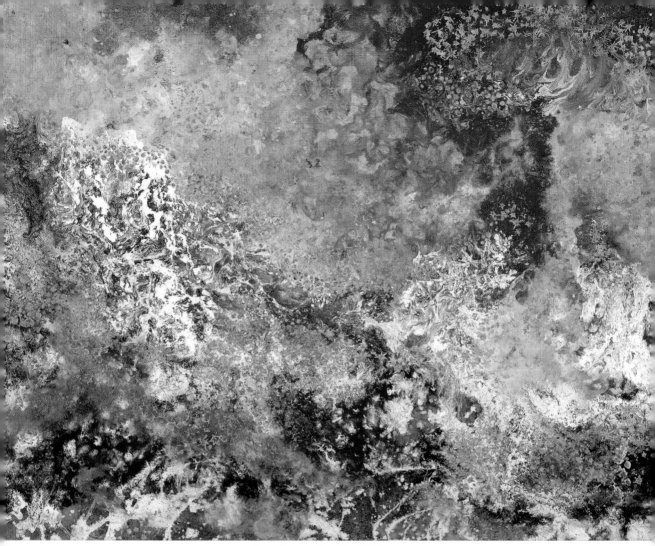

Octavia, acrylic, May 2014

pink layer below being exposed. I named it *Octavia* as a reminder
of its eight-month journey.

● ●

I had read about a study that proved the brain of a child with
autism creates forty-two per cent more information at rest
than the average child. Their brains are actually superpowered,

something that at first seems incredible and an overwhelming thought, but it makes you realize on a daily basis how much our children and adults on the spectrum are dealing with, and the importance of them being able to find peace.

An idea was forming, to start a global project through social media, asking anyone on the spectrum to answer our questions about how they experienced the world, to give us valuable insights that would help us and others understand our children. I called it 'Answers from the Spectrum' and every Monday for months I asked a different question and let others ask theirs too. The answers were enlightening and respondents always tried to explain themselves in ways that others would understand.

One Sunday evening a parent wrote to me asking if I could post a question about noise. One of the answers I received struck a chord with me and I could see how it applied to Iris too: 'Think of it like a photograph. For most people, only the object in the foreground is in focus. For me, it's like there's no difference between the subject and the background – it's all in focus. So instead of a well-composed artistic shot, it looks like a mess. I know I'm supposed to be looking at the person in the foreground, but my attention gets focused on the stuff in the background instead.' This helped me understand why Iris struggled so much in busy, noisy environments: why she needed help in those situations.

Another week we asked about stimming. Stimming or 'stims' is short for self-stimulatory behaviour. We all seem to do it, whether it be tapping our feet, a pen or maybe twiddling our hair. It appears to be a way of calming ourselves or aiding concentration. For those on the spectrum, stimming usually refers to specific behaviour, such as flapping, rocking, spinning or repetition of words and phrases. Sometimes they can be more unusual and surprising. Iris does this when she is excited or starting to get overloaded with sensory information. It can swing both ways; it can be a sign of pleasure or an indication that life is becoming a little too much for her. Now I can tell the difference and act to quieten things down for her if necessary. Many believe that stimming is an undesired behaviour and doesn't help the child or adult integrate into society; they will say 'quiet hands' to the child and make them sit on them if the child can't stop. To me this seems cruel; their bodies are doing this for a reason, to release energy in order to manage those feelings, and many on the spectrum have described it as a pleasurable experience and one that they need to do to regulate their own systems. I feel that by stopping this behaviour you may appear to be stopping a problem but are perhaps creating a much bigger one – all for the sake of appearing 'normal'.

The feedback I received on the topic from people on the spectrum was incredibly insightful. One person said: 'It is a release of energy for me, and I feel so much better when I rock my body back and forward, or swing my leg, which is crossed over the other leg . . . It makes me happy and it relaxes me.' Another said: 'I do this when I'm excited and overwhelmed (good and bad). It releases tension, rebalances my energy, and if I'm in a good mood and having fun, keeps that feeling going.' This information was so useful for me; it made all the theories and research real and I hope it helped many other families too.

It was exciting to see how this growing community was helping others understand autism and I was very grateful for their interesting insights. One comment stuck in my mind: 'Our imagination is stronger. We can see inner films and hear music, meaning that we may drift away if something fascinates us.' This explains many phenomenal autistic talents. Such intriguing revelations into the world of others on the spectrum were allowing me to understand Iris in ways that I couldn't have imagined.

• •

At this time I wanted to introduce some techniques that as Iris grew older she could use herself whenever she might need to self-regulate. So, in addition to Iris's other therapies, we were also having weekly yoga sessions. Though they were not always successful with regards to Iris joining in, she did always watch and I found that she was using the postures during the week by herself. On good days, though, she would participate and it was a remarkably effective way to improve her social skills. She would correct P-J's position, then climb all over him while I tried to concentrate on what I was doing and not laugh. P-J would try his best to stay balanced with Iris hanging off one leg. The yoga helped me in many ways too; it improved my ability to refocus when things were not going to plan, to breathe. I always had so much running through my mind and focusing during yoga helped me immensely. It was also helping with the back pain from my horse-riding accident and I found I no longer needed to see a chiropractor.

What surprised me was how quickly Iris made a connection with Kay, our yoga teacher, and the ways she interacted with her. Iris was so relaxed, smiling at Kay with wonderful eye contact and allowing her to come close and help her into the next pose, her body flexing into various positions. It was fantastic for her mind to concentrate on the present movement. What was planned as a short course of six weeks became part of our week.

Without trying to control everything there was a pattern forming. Our weeks filled and life seemed to be jam-packed with new and exciting activities. We loved the freedom of being able to use the good-weather days and take spontaneous bike rides when the sun shone or walk in the woodlands. I had never looked at home education in that way before: I had seen it as an alternative to the special schools that weren't suitable: the only option left. It had made me elated but worried at the same time – it was such a serious commitment and a heavy responsibility.

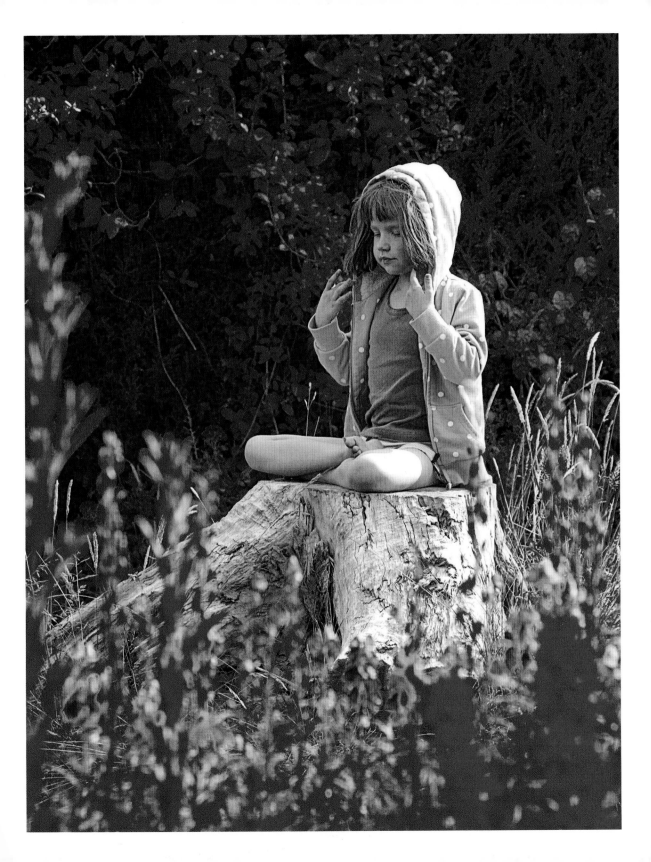

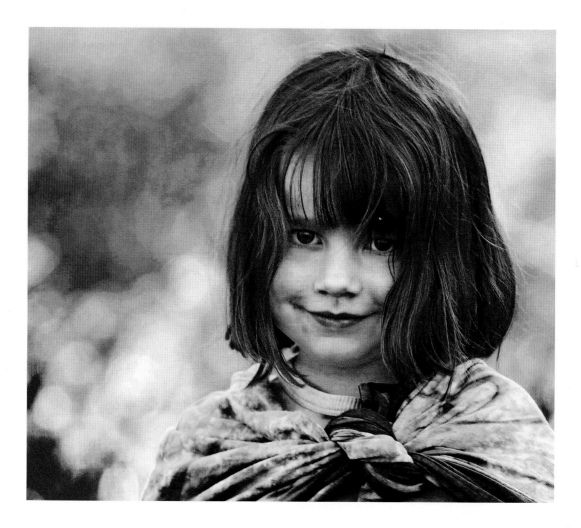

But now I was able to embrace the unexpected freedom and all the potential that our situation provided. It was an ironic twist in events when you think about it. Autism usually sits side by side with tight visual schedules and prompts, predictable routines and a firm structure, but Iris was starting to thrive on something different. She was beginning to relish unfamiliar environments and enjoyed exploring them as long as we were considerate of her sensitivities. These new experiences spurred on her language and other skills. We would see her light up just as she did when she painted.

Thula sits next to me on the side of the bath as I wash my hair. Suddenly I sit bolt upright looking down at the water: my bath is turning blue! Her bushy tail is half submerged and blue paint is leaking into my bathwater. I just knew there was going to be a time when that tail got it – the most tempting paintbrush ever to be seen. As I get out of the bath Iris is coming back up the stairs with a giant paintbrush in her hand, beaming. She runs straight past me and gets into bed. It's one of those moments when you can't quite decide how to feel: pleased that she is happy, relieved that she has an outlet for her emotions, frustrated that the artist's assistant work is never done and God only knows how much cleaning up there is to do downstairs and now more sheets to be washed. But seeing the painting makes up my mind. The energetic power from it gives me back my sense of humour and puts a spring in my step while I clean up the floor and sideboard. Nothing this beautiful could ever make you feel anything but pure joy.

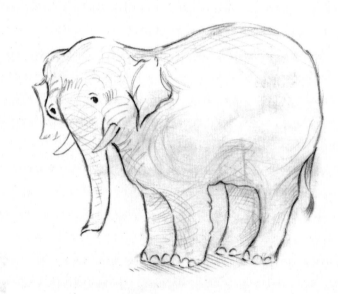
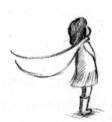

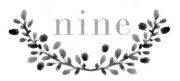

nine

Iknew we had to keep moving on. All our efforts meant that
we were teaching Iris the basic skills in social communication
that others pick up naturally, and having fun along the way.
But it wasn't enough. We wanted to open up her world to others,
encouraging her to interact with her peers, to see that it was OK
to be around other children and that it could be fun. Finding a
suitable children's club for Iris was another problem that didn't
seem to have an easy solution. Although Iris's relationships with
adults had improved and she was able to play and interact, she
was still nervous around other children. I feared this would never
change if we didn't step in. How could she learn and practise
those skills if we weren't providing opportunities for her to do
so? The tricky part was how to introduce her to other children.
We had tried play dates and they had never worked: Iris would
just hide away with her books upstairs or cry if I asked her to
stay. She was still very nervous in public spaces that were busy
with lots of children. All it took was a baby crying or a child
running chaotically past her and she would cry in my arms and
lean and pull me towards the door to leave. We needed to move
slowly and gently on this issue if we were going to get anywhere.

We were moved by a story from an inspirational mother in
America who had started her own children's club for children
on the spectrum. P-J was convinced it would work if we created
our own too. 'It will be easy,' he said in his usual jovial manner.

Whenever I heard that phrase from him I knew it would be far from easy.

The plan was simple in theory: an autistic-friendly club based at our home, where parents could stay and enjoy activities with their children in an understanding environment. Of course there were concerns about opening up our home to strangers, but I had made some connections with other parents through the autism courses that we had been to when Iris was first diagnosed so they were first on my list for new members.

We started off small, with only four children. Iris had been very interested in all the preparations I had made for our first session. We had named the club the Little Explorers Activity Club and I wanted each week to have a different theme. To start off with we went for a sea theme. At first it took some getting used to for all of us. Iris, in particular, wasn't sure what to do or how to be around the others and found it tiring. She was excited and intrigued by the decorations but that seemed to be the only reason she stayed in the room. She found noises from the others and their unpredictable nature difficult to handle and stayed as far away from them as she could while still still being able to explore the activities. After about half an hour she needed to have a break and she went upstairs. I couldn't help but feel disappointed when she needed to leave; the amount of effort I was putting in meant that when things didn't go to plan I didn't know what I was doing any of it for. Then I would remind myself that this wasn't ever going to be a quick fix – it would take time and I needed to be patient. It was the same for the other children too; they were allowed to explore the house and find their own quiet area if needed and that worked very well. I started to see that I would need to create more fantastical and inviting worlds if we were going to succeed in getting them all more engaged with the sessions and that the club would need to run regularly, every Saturday morning even through the holidays, to give stability and to build on relationships.

As each week went by Iris was able to be with the others for a little longer. Some weeks I felt like she was regressing: she would cry before the other children arrived and wouldn't come downstairs at all. Then the following week she would be fine again and enjoy herself. But at about six weeks in a change came over her. For the first time ever, Iris was waiting in anticipation for the other children to arrive. She was looking forward to it and rubbed her hands together as if to say 'I'm ready, bring it on!' It was a welcome change. Was the plan at last working?

Splashes of colour, shapes of stars, planets and a rocket were projected on to the walls from black card with cut-outs fixed on to the glass panels. Thula was convinced she could jump and catch the coloured delights on the walls and made joyful leaps from the dresser, which made Iris laugh as we waited for the others to arrive. I heard Iris say 'star' from the kitchen. 'Well done, Iris. Good talking,' I called out.

With African lullabies playing in the background, the morning was filled with making star biscuits, trying space food and jumping from the trampoline into a pool of balls, teddies and beanbags. And Thula wanted to be included in everything, especially when it came to cooking. The following weekend the kitchen was filled to the brim with miniature Italian chefs all busily squishing, pulling and kneading their balls of dough. The Italian-themed activity club was in full swing. The house was decorated with vines hanging from the wooden beams and a sea scene on the window with fish, seaweed and seahorses. Maps of Italy and flags provided an interesting game for James who wanted me to find particular countries in less than ten seconds. A seven-year-old boy with suspected Asperger's, he was verbal but had confidence issues and relied heavily on his mother. His behaviour at the club was normally fantastic but I listened to his mother as she described how when he experienced sensory overload the more challenging behaviour came to life. I had a soft spot for him; he latched on to me during the cookery sessions and I saw his passion grow. The more he could experiment in the kitchen, the more confident he got. His mind was inquisitive but he didn't know or understand the boundaries within social situations and often went beyond what is considered appropriate.

He would ask me what I was going to have for my lunch after the club.

'Sausages,' I replied.

'How many?'

'Uummm, two.'

'How many will Iris have?'

'Probably just one . . .'

Then he went on to ask about the potatoes, what sort of beans, what we would do after lunch and what we were going to have for the next few meals. I think he wanted to imagine what things would be like after he left.

There was another reason why this boy meant so much to me: his connection to Iris. He was so gentle and kind around her, always trying to include her whenever he could. Iris liked him too. He was older than the others, quieter and more predictable.

The pizza-making in the kitchen had lifted everyone's spirits to a great height and the bursts of laughter at our cookery attempts made me feel so happy. Our club was breaking through the isolation that autism had brought upon us all and as I looked at Iris I couldn't believe the changes.

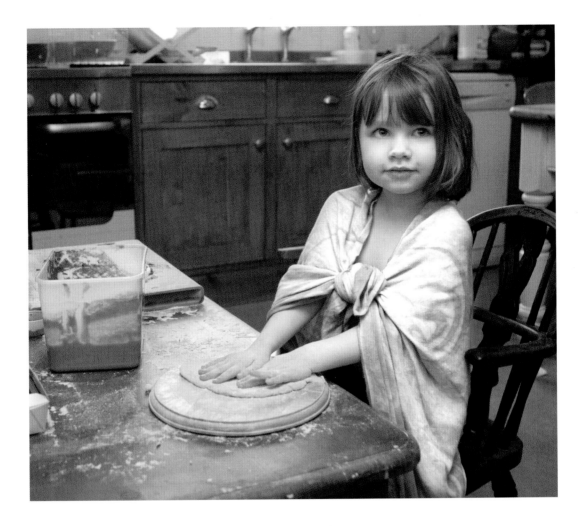

James carefully stretched his dough into an oblong shape. 'How do I get the right shape?' he asked in an agitated voice as he frowned at the ever lengthening piece of dough between his hands.

I showed him with mine how to shuffle it around to create a circle but he decided that, in fact, the oblong was by far the best way to go. His brother, Charlie, had already whizzed ahead on to the pepperoni while his mother valiantly tried to spin her base on the very tips of her fingers.

She grinned at me, then with the dough safely back in her hands she whispered, 'I can't believe it, look.'

As I looked around the kitchen my heart filled with joy. She was right, every member of the group was present, a rare achievement. 'They're all here,' I said.

'Brilliant, isn't it?' said Oliver's mother with a wide smile.

I didn't care about the mess or the fact that Iris had decided I was the new way to get her fingers clean, turning my clothes white with flour. We were achieving something great. For most families it would seem insignificant but for us it was spectacular.

'Oh, Thula!' cried Ed as she darted under the tables and chairs playing football with some fragments of dough, and then our cheeky cat created a new game of batting anyone who passed her way. She was kind to the others but not quite in the same way as she was with Iris. She was more boisterous on occasions and managed to deal with the boys playing with her and all the attention. She responded to each child in rather a different way; some she would play hide-and-seek with, while with others she stood still while they stroked her. I wondered if she knew how to be by instinct and wished so much we could open ourselves up to those feelings as well as animals still could, how much easier life would be if we just knew what to do and didn't question ourselves.

Oliver calmly sat on his mother's knee as they worked together on his delicious creation. To watch him so still and concentrated was a rare sight. After the first batch there were only two chefs left. James adorned his pizza beautifully and Iris stayed with the dough itself, enjoying the texture, patting, stroking and moulding it into different shapes. I heard her hums and little noises, a show of contentment. James talked every now and then to Iris but he didn't mind that there was no reply.

The plan was working – granted it was only for small fragments of time when all the children were engaged in the activities at once, but it was precious for every family. Later the group dispersed. Iris had retreated to her sofa with her new best friend, a rather aging piece of dough that now resembled the skin of an elephant, and in no time at all Thula was curled up sharing her blanket.

• •

But the following Monday I looked into Iris's watery eyes and I could see the familiar distant gaze I had hoped I wouldn't see again. The one where she wouldn't look at me, rather through me, and it was impossible to connect. She could stay like this for hours or days. With her face suddenly drained and pale I knew right away that life had got too much for her and she was retreating into her world where she had spent so long alone. It had been easy to forget Iris's autism lately with Thula's help and all the highs that came from her paintings. She had been doing so well, but with the excitement of the club and a social Sunday with family the day after, it had become too much.

She pointed at the lamp on my desk. I turned it off, then I saw her body curl up on the sofa with her legs tucked in and her head down. 'Iris, hold my hand,' I said quietly. She took my hand and I carried her up the stairs with her clinging on to me. With our arms linked we lay side by side under the heavy duvet for a long while in silence and she gradually relaxed. She turned towards me, looking into my eyes. She was coming back and her senses were calming. Thula joined us on the bed, snuggling up close to Iris, instinctively knowing that she needed her there. As she stretched her paw the long tufts of soft fur brushed over Iris's tummy and I heard her giggle. Once again Thula had found a way to lead Iris back into the light.

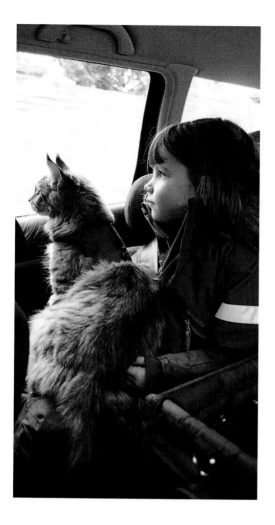

After that I began to adjust our lives to fit in more relaxing periods after the club or social events. I made sure that we wouldn't overwhelm her, but to gradually build on what we had achieved. It was going to take time but we had plenty of that; there was no need to rush. A new ritual began: after each activity club we would take Iris for a drive so she could settle down and have a snooze after all the excitement. It gave her a chance to relax with Thula curled up on her lap and by the time we got to the hillside with the bluebell wood they would both be fast asleep.

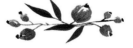

With some new funding in place for the club it was time to find some more activities. I wanted to give our Explorers every opportunity possible, to inspire as well as build on their existing fascinations, gently widening some of their more fixed interests. My passion for the club grew from week to week and although this project started out as a way for Iris to spend time with other children it became so much more. It became a safe haven for the parents attending and a magical world for the children. I adored creating themed kingdoms for them to explore, from rainforests with foliage from the garden to sea themes with painted cardboard boats and seas of blue sheets and towels. There was always an abundance of props, toys and books on the theme to enjoy. During the week, after Iris's therapy sessions, we would work on the next club theme. We would cut out shapes of creatures or letters to stick on the glass gable end. Iris would be 'helping', with Thula by her side, of course. My only disappointment was that I could rarely find another girl to join Iris, the majority of children diagnosed with autism seemed to be boys, whether this was because girls were more effective at adapting I wasn't sure. There didn't seem to be any concrete evidence as to why this was. Iris's behaviour was certainly different to the boys: she was so careful with her toys and her generosity about sharing her world and her things with them all surprised me at times. She was gentle and giving, not minding at all if other children played with her toys. As each week went by Iris was becoming more social; she could only manage small bursts with the others but they were lengthening and I saw more moments where she would play close to the others, not exactly with them, but by their side. She still wouldn't talk to them, though; she would stay quiet and watch them, humming with appreciation if something pleased or excited her.

• •

Animals started to become large characters in our groups, and we had regular 'meet the animals' sessions throughout the year. The children learnt about reptiles, falcons, owls, giant snails, hedgehogs and rodents from around the world. They were a wonderful talking point for the children, encouraging them to sit closely together to listen about the lives of these creatures, handling and spending some time with them.

Since all Iris's musical instruments were so popular at the club I also arranged for a series of music workshops with professional musicians. The children loved experimenting and learning about all different types of music. In these workshops we had electric guitars, pianos, drums, mikes and mixers. The light was bright and I had to work hard as a photographer to capture the scene before me. Happiness spread through them and to me. Iris danced by the window with the white ukulele, Ed with the mike and James on the drums, while Oliver bounced across the room on the big red therapy ball. The odd collision was inevitable as the musicians tried to dodge his moves. The music was loud but no one seemed to mind except Thula who had retired to the comfort of a duvet upstairs. Just as I took a photograph of James I felt Iris beside me, handing me the white ukulele that she had been playing earlier like a little rock star. Her hand guided mine into position. Bending down with her ear close to the instrument she waited there until I played. Satisfied, she moved on to P-J and got him to play the guitar, then she took one of the instructor's hands and led him to the sofa, presenting him the electric guitar. 'I'm not really a guitar man; I'm better on the piano,' he said, but the guitar was placed firmly in his hands and so he played it. Iris seemed satisfied and moved on to the next band member until everyone had an instrument to play and her band was complete. Keeping us all going was a whole new game and I watched her interact with each person in turn, including the children. The music was expanding her horizons. She was blissfully happy, confident and thoroughly enjoying herself directing, making everyone laugh. If only life could carry on like this but it wasn't to be. After this much intense interaction she needed a break, so she lay in our bed upstairs with some books and Thula while the others finished the session.

Our special Saturdays – from circus days to Viking warriors – became a source of so much, and my photographs that captured

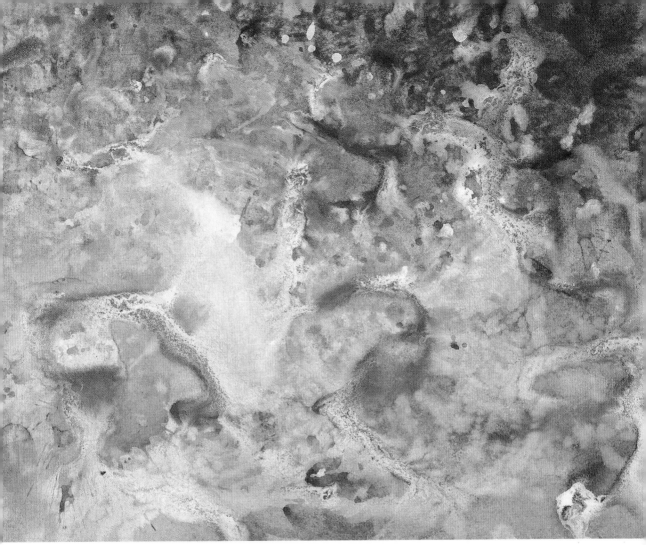

Koi, acrylic, May 2013

all the fun provided many opportunities for me to work with
Iris during the week. We would look over them, giving us a
chance to practise vocabulary and remind Iris what she had
achieved, building her confidence. We laughed and laughed
as Iris twirled around in her playroom, silk scarves held high,
doing little leaps imitating the morris dancing display that we
had watched at the weekend. The idea of a team of dancers with
bells on their knees and old English costumes might seem like a

challenging experience for children on the spectrum. In fact, I had had some doubts about how successful it would be and as more and more cars had pulled up outside our house and the garden filled with dancers I had begun to wonder if my idea was completely mad.

'Is this the activity club?'

'Yes,' I said.

'Good. Found it then.' The very tall man with a beard waved down another three cars filled with more dancers.

The gates opened and shut, and opened and shut, until my heart started beating hard. There couldn't be any more surely! I had completely forgotten to ask how many dancers would be coming over.

Iris, however, was intrigued by the layered colourful cotton on their clothes and her interest in them calmed my worries. With all the Explorers assembled, the music began and as I looked around at the happy smiling faces I realized that they were all looking at Iris. She was on the edge of the decking, copying the dancers' movements, her eyes fixed on them and the violin. She was immersed in a world filled with music and dancing, her troubles with social interactions melted away. Iris's enthusiasm was infectious. James sat down close to her and watched the different formations. Oliver and Iris both joined the team down in the garden and our new Explorer William was watching from the decking holding on to a dinosaur toy for comfort. I have had many moments while running the club when my heart filled with pride but I was almost in tears when I saw Iris surrounded by dancers having an amazing time.

In time William and his whole family became key to the club's success, motivating us and a driving force when I needed help.

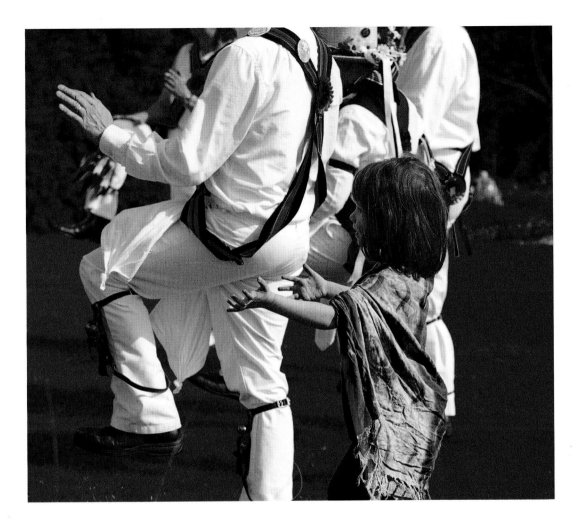

William's interests were firmly fixed on nature, animals and dinosaurs; he was a tiny encyclopaedia of natural history and entertained us all with his knowledge. I loved the idea of sharing the children's interests between the group and we decided to explore William's fascination with dinosaurs. I knew this would be more challenging for Iris and that I would need to prepare for this one, so William kindly offered to lend Iris a whole box full of dinosaur delights the week before the club.

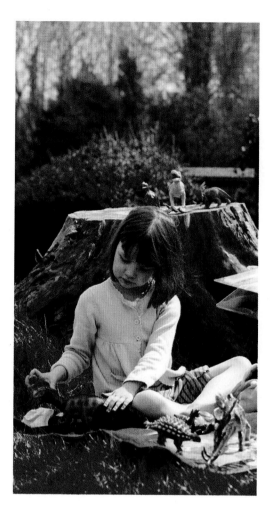

Iris studied the dinosaur toys and books with great interest on a blanket beside her tree stump. I had learnt when introducing new things it was best to pair them up with something she loved and somewhere where she felt comfortable, and the stump fitted on both counts. Watching Iris play with these rather terrifying creatures with so much grace made me see them in a different light. It was like a surreal Jurassic ballet as she tiptoed around the garden with the pteranodon carefully positioned with its feet between her finger tips and the wings resting gently above her rounded ballerina hand. She danced and cradled the triceratops, feeling the bumpy texture of its skin, the smooth long horns and the frill round the head. Iris has this ability to see the fragile beauty in everything, teaching me to notice details I might have overlooked: something unexpected, the exquisite texture or its interesting shape and form. I was delighted to see that the dinosaurs had captured her attention so beautifully and was excited about the arrival of the Travelling Natural History Museum, a company that provides exhibition workshops for children with fossils and all sorts of replicas.

The garden room went dark as the massive lorry parked up outside. It was early on Saturday morning and we were going to turn our home into a miniature museum complete with large model dinosaurs, bones, teeth and all sorts of other curiosities. Work was also going on in the kitchen to prepare for the plaster session where they would make their own fossils. The set-up was slow and as more boxes were brought in one at a time I began to have those familiar anxieties: what if we weren't ready on time? Even P-J was getting twitchy as he made the dinosaur expert some tea in the hope it would spur him on. Iris climbed on top of the triceratops and giggled, which did wonders

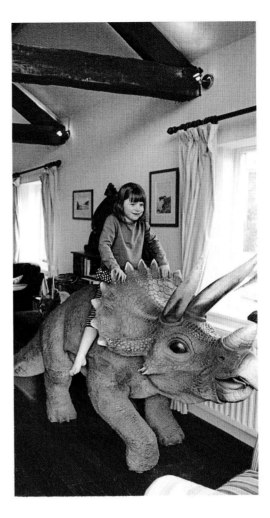

for my nerves. Everybody joined in, including Thula, for the meteor display outside on the decking. She took centre stage as the sabre-toothed tiger before the meteor plummeted into the bowl of flour, an explosion of white dust that made the children laugh hysterically.

After everybody had left Iris said goodbye to the dinosaurs in the lorry, still grasping her very own fossil. I carried her back inside, shutting the garden-room door behind us. She settled in the comfy armchair with her new dinosaur book and started to read out some of the words.

'Gigantosaurus!' she said in a loud voice. 'Stomp, stomp, stomp!'

●●●

It was an idyllic set-up for a while but things needed to change. We wanted to push the boundaries with the club too and start a new programme that would help the children even more, so we introduced a family of non-autistic children to the club who were friends with one of the families who had been before. My hope was that they would guide our children in times where they felt a little lost, encouraging them to socialize and be more involved with the activities. The new children were very sensitive around Iris and gave her space when she needed it but kept trying to include her and I was grateful for that. Later this developed into a buddy system of having non-autistic children enjoy the activities with the children on the spectrum. It was a move that made some of the parents uncomfortable. They felt it took away the support-group feel of the club but we believed it was the right decision. I started to realize how difficult it is to do your best for all involved, keeping everyone's best interests at heart given how challenging autism can be in the hard times. But this was the starting point of many adventures for our children and I am so proud of what we achieved.

As Iris's confidence grew we saw changes in her abilities to be able to go out. So during the week we started to take her to quiet places like garden centres where she could get used to being around more people in unfamiliar surroundings. At first our trips were short – only half an hour – but as each week went by we lengthened them to the point where we were going

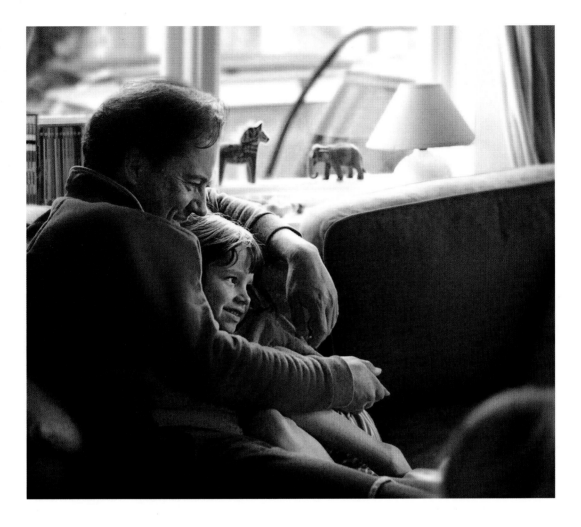

out for half a day. To make it possible we didn't push things too far: we prepared her for what we were going to see, she always had a good meal before leaving and ate as soon as we returned home. I didn't ask her to sit in cafés or expect her to eat while we were out as I knew she found that difficult – she still needed peace to be able to eat. There would always be something that she loved to keep her interested and many of our trips featured animals, water and nature. She gradually got

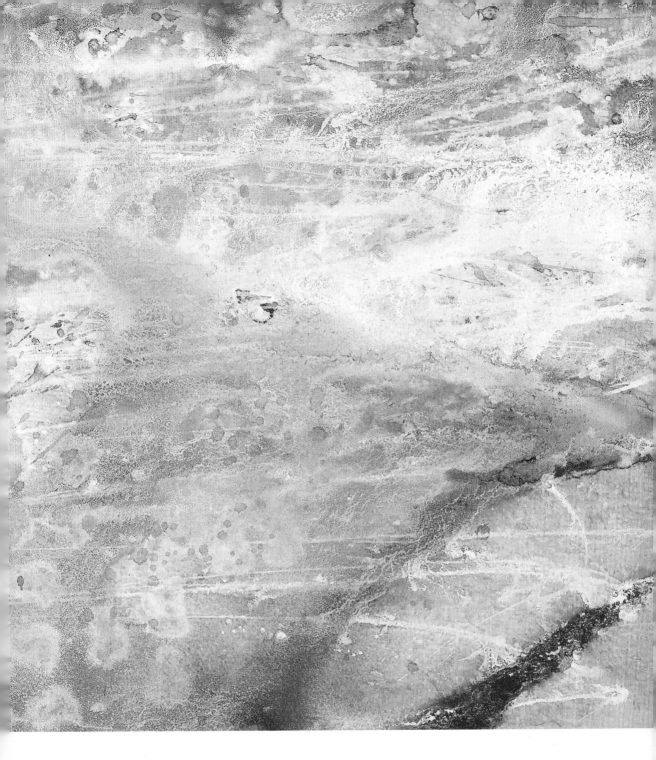

Aquilo, acrylic, September 2013

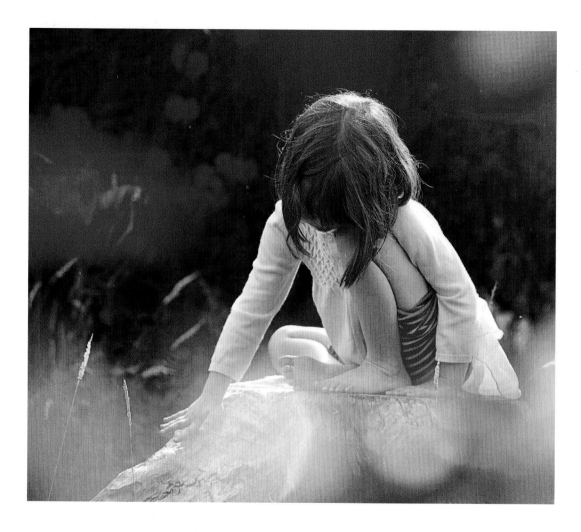

used to the movement and presence of others around her in these public places and I started to see her interact more not only with the new environments but with people too. It didn't always work, though. Sometimes we would see how she used to be: nervous and disturbed by the busyness that seemed to cave in on her. Very often those times happened when she was tired and we would take a step back and let her just be for a few days, and give her some more time in the garden or on bike rides. It was a constant balancing act between pushing the boundaries and letting her rest.

• •

In the winter we went to another zoo after the success of Iris's first visit but this time it wasn't car-based, so it was more challenging for her. She had to walk through crowds, stand in line, being close to others and passing groups of school children. She was fascinated by the elephants, spending a while observing them in their warm barn while they ate their hay. She loved the penguins and some of the other birds and said 'meow' to the meerkat. I was so proud of her and it was liberating for all of us to be able to go out as a family on trips like this. But you could never quite tell what was going to happen. The unpredictable nature of being in these public places meant that it didn't matter how much I planned ahead, an already challenging situation could easily turn into the impossible. I hadn't thought of it but winter is when parks and zoos do maintenance, so there was noise from builders and groundsmen making various repairs and upgrading parts of the zoo. That, coupled with the cold wind and showers, didn't exactly make it easy for her but Iris managed very well and enjoyed herself. Seeing her at times like that was incredible; she had come so far since starting the club. It had provided her with the confidence and experience she needed to be able to negotiate unfamiliar surroundings, noises, people and changing circumstances. At the end she was even confident enough to have a walk around the shop and pick out a present to take home. While it was tempting to stay warm at home, I was very pleased we made the effort to go out and the trip gave us our new topic: elephants.

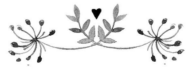

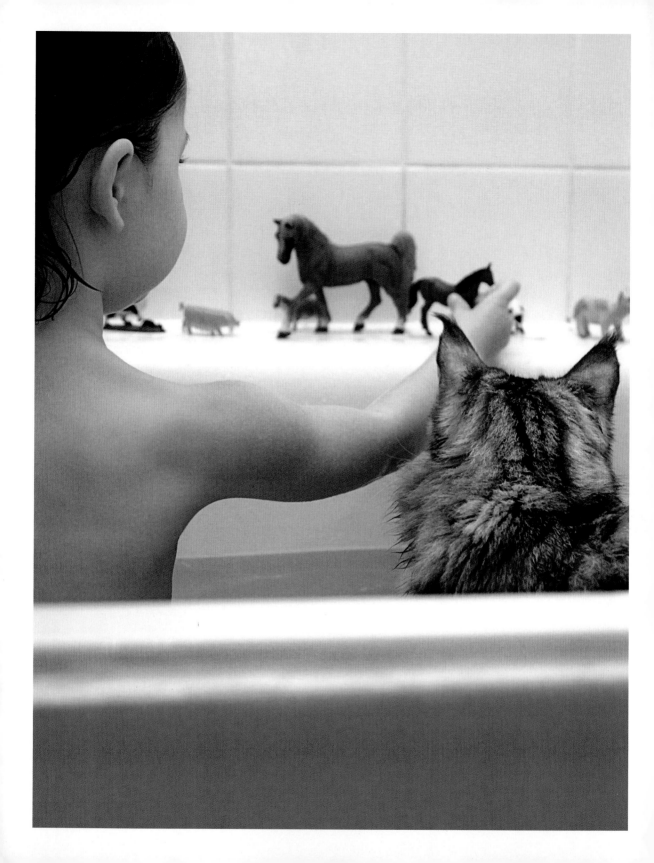

The three of us walk hand in hand along a grass track with small paddocks either side filled with an array of farm animals. Iris counts the chickens in their field but unfortunately they are too fast. I hear her trying and then, 'Oh no! One, two, three – uh-oh!'

Later in her bath she is determined to bring the animal theme with her and we are joined by a selection of animals including Thula. Iris looks at her and then back to the animals lined up on the edge. Thula looks so much smaller in the bath, half her body in miniature under the surface compared with the soft fluffy coat above. She learns about the 'sheepdog', 'pink pig', 'ram' and 'big horse'. Each in turn are presented for a sniff as Iris announces their name and gives a rendition of the sound they make. Then they are returned neatly to the line-up. She knows that Thula missed out on the farm visit and wants to share her knowledge and experiences.

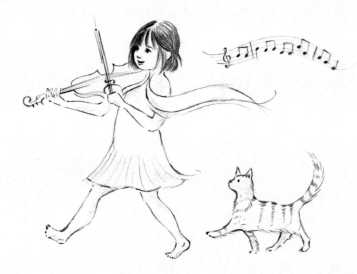

ten

Beethoven's Fifth echoed around the swimming pool and in between Iris's joyful 'da-da-da dums' we heard her say 'jellyfish, jellyfish'. She repeated the words over and over with hysterical giggles, apparently happy as a jellyfish in water. With her swimsuit and armbands on without a problem we were already on a high; after all, it wasn't so long ago that just getting a top on Iris had been a gold-medal-winning performance. The iPad apps and videos had done the trick, and she now understood the purpose of the armbands and welcomed them. We had paired swimming with Beethoven's famous symphony and it was working wonderfully; the energetic power from the music gave Iris so much confidence. Reaching out to P-J she held on to him and then ventured out on her own, propelling herself forward with little wriggles and frog-like movements with her legs.

We had known since Iris was a baby that music would always play an important role in her life, and lately orchestras and in particular the violin held Iris's attention above any other instrument. The meaning of it to Iris was still unclear to us. Her passion for violins was huge. They spoke to her. Sometimes when I looked around at home every surface would be covered in books all open on a page with a violin. I had been buying books one after the other and she loved them all. *My First Orchestra*, *The Story of the Orchestra*, *Instruments of the Orchestra*,

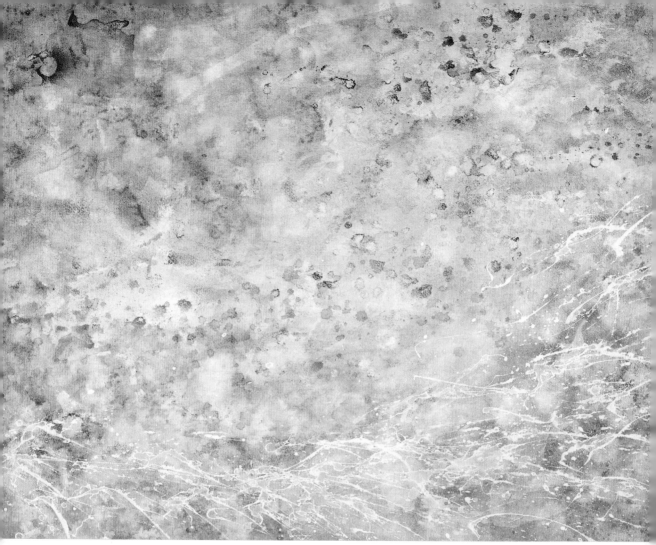

Magic Flute, acrylic, July 2013

Little Children's Music Book and *My First Classical Music Book*, they all surrounded her and she looked upon them like jewels glinting in the sunlight. The iPad would also be on with the Philharmonia Orchestra app running with a musician describing the main techniques of how to play the violin. The more I encouraged her interest in music, the more it developed.

One of the intriguing yet sometimes problematic behaviours of a child with autism is their ability to immerse themselves in a subject. It isn't always the case but very often their concentration levels and self-motivation can be outstanding for a topic that interests them. Sometimes they get interested to the point of obsession, but this does allow them to excel in certain areas, like with Iris's painting, and now I was seeing it with her interest in music. She was reading words from her music books and had already taught herself the names of all the instruments and what they sounded like so she could recognize each one. I believed that as long as she wasn't getting stuck and her behaviour was not too repetitive, where there was a continual flow of learning, then we should follow these interests and allow her to explore and learn at her own pace.

I spoke to a violin restorer who happened to have a violin that would fit Iris. I talked about her and he didn't brush off what I was saying about her intense interest in music at such a young age. He was intrigued to hear about her paintings and I felt like he understood what I wanted to do for her. I listened carefully as he told me that I should just let her enjoy the violin, to play with it, to have it around her as much as she wanted. Maybe try a few lessons, but if that didn't work, not to worry – it could just be too early. We agreed that I would drive over to his workshop in Stamford to see the violin and have another chat about how to proceed with Iris. It was a beautiful drive that I knew well from many weddings that I had photographed in the area but I did feel very tired. Iris had been up in the night and not even Thula had been able to settle her. She had been up at 2 a.m. and nothing would persuade her that it wasn't morning time. She had wanted to look at her books downstairs in the playroom and so I rested on the sofa while the pile of books on the floor grew. One after another she would go and collect one from the shelf, carefully going through it and then adding it to the pile. Rather like a quality-control stocktake, some were discarded and the loved ones were kept neatly beside her.

About halfway through the journey I passed under the Welland Viaduct. This staggering structure had always given me courage when I felt nervous before I got to a wedding I was photographing. As I drove under one out of the eighty-two arches I was in awe of it. When I felt tired and like I couldn't give any more I would sometimes think about places like this; they are true wonders of strength. The viaduct that I was driving under was constructed with over 30,000,000 bricks, all manufactured on site. It was completed at a pace that even I couldn't feel impatient with: the first brick being laid in March 1876, and all eighty-two arches completed two years later. Considering the basic tools used it was an inspiring achievement and there was no way I could feel tired after just one bad night's sleep thinking of that. I turned the radio on to Classic FM to get me in the mood but as I listened to the radio presenter talk I suddenly realized I had not got a clue what I was doing. I knew nothing about violins and nothing about music for that matter. I think Iris could actually say more about the instruments than I could. I was completely out of my depth. Did that matter? Thinking of all those places I had been, the adventures abroad with P-J, teaching myself about photography, I knew it didn't. Autism has a way of making you forget what came beforehand. It can be all-consuming. It pushed us to our limits time and again in so many different ways and sometimes you seemed to not only lose your child but yourself as well.

The restorer's workshop was small, like a galley kitchen, but instead of pots and pans on shelves and cupboards there were violins hanging everywhere and the surfaces were a carpenter's workstation. He stored his on the wall, so they were on display to see. I loved that idea. If you love something so much, why shut it away in a case every day? He went through the violins on display. Some were antiques and highly valuable, others were new intricate original designs. We stood side by side as there wasn't much room to move and I listened to him talk about all the beautiful instruments. It was like the Aladdin's cave of the music world and I felt excited to just have stepped through that door.

'Here she is.' He opened a tiny red violin case and delicately removed the violin, made a few adjustments and then played a tune. 'Sorry that's not the greatest. It's really difficult for me to play these smaller violins, but this one has a beautiful sound and I think it will do very nicely.'

It sounded heavenly to me and I went home with the little violin on the passenger seat beside me. He had told me not to say 'Iris can't play the violin' but instead 'Iris can't play the violin yet.' He was an incredibly positive open-minded character and the small word at the end changed the sentence dramatically, giving hope for the future. I reminded myself to add more 'yets' to my thoughts from then on. Each time I ventured into something new with Iris we were meeting people along the way, who were all playing their part in our lives. The loneliness had gone.

● ●

Iris's body was snuggled up against mine on the sofa: finally she was asleep. As she had drifted off her hand was still gripping her new violin, seemingly not wanting to ever let go. It had been a long day. A song called 'A Precious Place' by Patsy Reid played on a CD, a beautiful Scottish fiddle player who had cast a spell over Iris. She was mesmerized by her playing and wanted to hear her music again and again. Earlier on as the sun was going down she had taken her new friend to visit all her magical spots in the garden: the tree stump, the bench and down the path into the orchard banked with grasses. Rabbits scattered into the hedgerow and Iris stopped halfway down the path just before

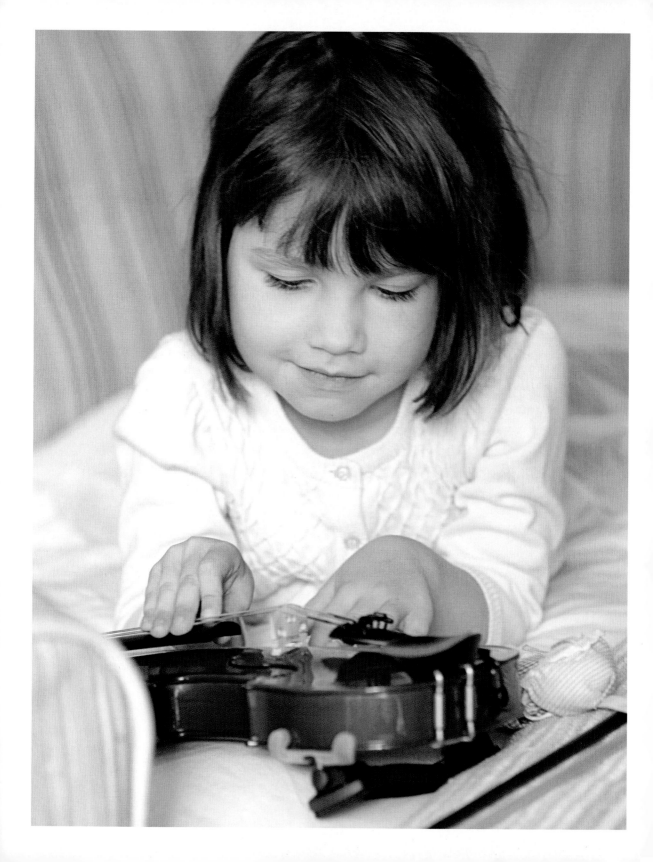

the old damson tree where the woodpeckers feed. She held the instrument high up in the air, looking at it in a beam of light and then bringing it down next to her cheek, and rested for a moment. She loved it with all of her heart.

Iris loved to play with a pop-up paper orchestra on the tree stump and we would say it was the 'Tree Stump Philharmonic', which she found hilarious. She pointed at each player, naming their instrument and then looked at Thula to make sure she was paying attention to her music lesson. I had been trying to find a suitable orchestra to take Iris to see for months, so I was delighted when I saw a listing for a local orchestra performing at the weekend. It was the perfect kind of concert: casual enough that nobody minded the fact we had a child in a cape walking with us and there were lots of violins. It started with Tchaikovsky's *Swan Lake*. I shall never forget the look on Iris's face during the applause at the end: pure happiness and joy, with her arms up in the air saying, 'Wow! Yeeeeeee!' In the quieter parts she wanted her orchestra book on her lap and went through the instruments one by one and then looked for them among the performing musicians. Her first experience of a live orchestra had been exhilarating and it spurred on a search for many more concerts to take her to.

There was something so powerful about live music that had an effect upon Iris. She would become more open socially and she would use her voice more, and seeing her in that state became a beautiful addiction. 'Where can we take her next?' P-J would say after a performance and I would do some more research. We took her to a wide variety of different concerts and music festivals. The ones in the open air were some of the most successful and I will never forget how free and happy she was listening to a local jazz band in the gardens of Kelmarsh Hall. When the heavens opened and it poured with rain the band and some of the crowd huddled under a small tent, and to my surprise instead of being upset by being so closely surrounded by others she was excited. The instruments and their players were all there so Iris felt confident. While they played it was as if she was transported into the music, connected; her fingers, mind and soul were with it almost as if she could see it. She was experiencing those musical sensations in a different way to how we felt them and afterwards those connections were open to us too as she talked to us, looking straight into our eyes and giving us a big hug.

The following Friday night wasn't following the normal bedtime routine but I didn't care; she was enjoying life and making great strides. I sang a song called 'Mellow Yellow' with a made-up story about Iris's painting that lay before us on the table. She laughed at me while she danced around her painting, adding more yellow with a wide brush.

'I'm going to record all your songs one day you know!' P-J called out from the garden room, teasing me.

'Don't you dare,' I said. I had made up little ditties for all sorts of activities and parts of Iris's daily routine: there was one for brushing teeth, another for using the bathroom and one for when we were leaving the park or saying goodbye to the bikes, iPad, music, books . . . Well, pretty much any situation. These improvised little songs helped Iris, guided her and encouraged interactions.

That evening Iris was in a great mood, and late into the night, after her bath, I had a very receptive little girl: happy to engage, talking and creating a beautiful painting. I knew that maybe I wasn't doing her or myself any favours by not keeping to a routine but for the first time Iris managed to say a clear 'painting' and 'paint' along with all sorts of other words she had used before. My excitement about this set her off running around the kitchen and to the hallway with her hands in the air as if she had scored a

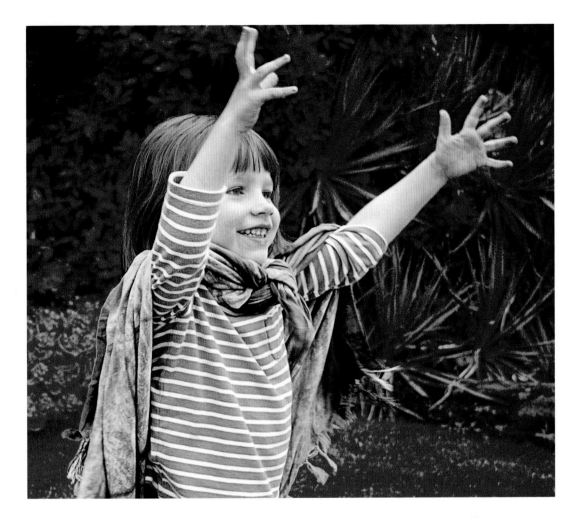

goal. Sometimes Iris could say words but the pronunciation was a little off, so only I would be able to tell what she was saying, but hearing her that night it was brilliantly clear. She returned and added some more paint to the paper and then rushed off again with the brush, over the carpeted floor, which made my heart leap, and then on to the sofa where Thula was. She lay on the sheet that I used to protect the furniture and dotted spots of the paint just in front of her paws. Iris wanted her to be

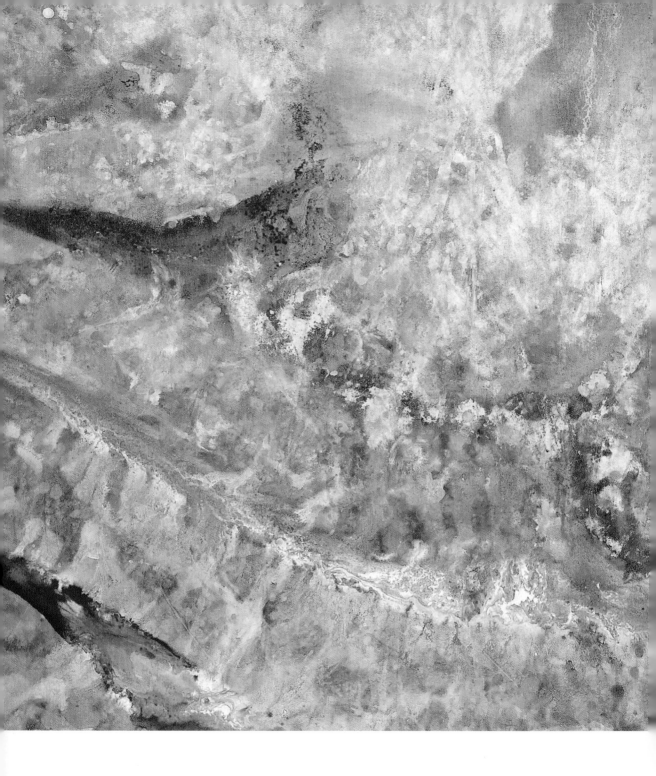

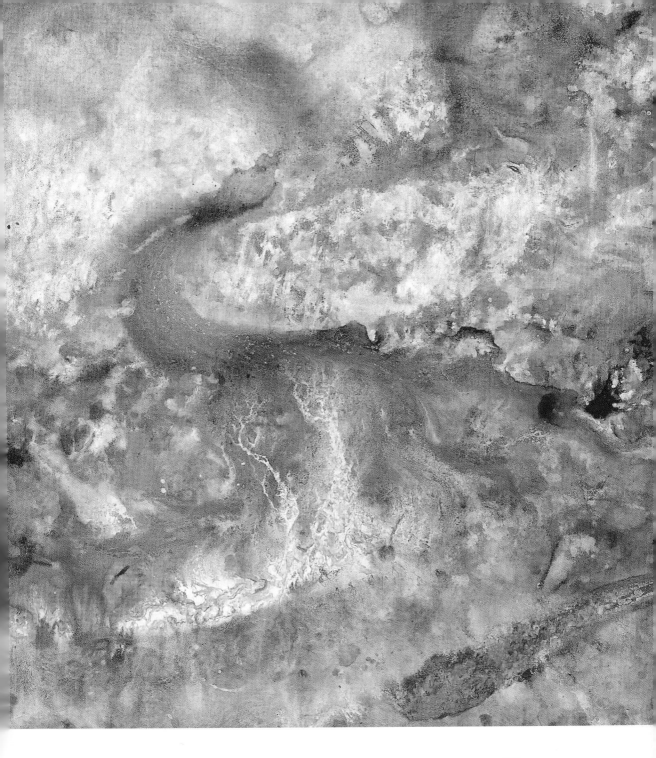

Painting a Lullaby, acrylic, Summer 2014

included in the activity too and enjoy the colours as she had. We laughed as Thula tried to catch the colour by putting her furry paws over the spots of paint. Soon after the games with Thula Iris went upstairs, climbed into bed and fell fast asleep within minutes, and so I named the piece *Painting a Lullaby*.

I would wake up in the mornings with Iris dancing around the house saying, 'Tuba, trombone, French horn, drum, oboe, bassoon, harp, violin . . .' Iris and Thula would then sit together on the sofa and Iris practised playing the violin, sometimes in the correct position, other times with the violin resting on her lap as she gently drew the bow across the strings. One morning as I tidied up the kitchen Iris started bringing in things from all over the house. First it was a CD she wanted on – *The Carnival of the Animals*, one of her favourites. Then she rushed off to get some music books, a chair and a great number of musical instruments. She carefully positioned the books round the edge of one of her paintings so they were standing upright and the instruments were at the end of the table. I had started to notice something; to her the arts were not separated into the neat categories that adults put them in – they were one. The music imitated a bird in the sky and Iris turned to a page with the flute and tried blowing against her fingers. I whistled and she giggled. Her attention was then on the painting itself; there was one area still not dry from the evening before and she scratched into the surface with a sculpting tool, moving in time to the music. A quick go on the xylophone and she was back to looking at the books and stirring some pale green paint while listening to more animals from Camille Saint-Saëns.

On another occasion Iris had a fantastic time at a concert that was especially for children in our local town. She heard the oboe playing Ravel and Dring. It started well. Iris was confident as we walked hand in hand from the car across a busy high street to the building. At first we sat with her on my lap listening to the music. She smiled at the musicians and then ventured further. When the oboe player asked if anyone had their dancing shoes on, she bounced up and down right in front of her with her pink shoes on and after the music had stopped she had a wonderful time dancing around the rest of the hall. Even when the other children were given their own drums and shakers, she coped by climbing on me and standing on my legs to get up high. She felt safer being able to see everyone from above and climbed back down when she could manage to join in; it was almost cat-like behaviour. When we arrived back home, paint flew all over a brand-new sheet of paper. Thula was, of course, relieved to have her girl back again and spent a long time inspecting this new painting; she was intrigued as the colour mixed on the paper: trails of green across red and a pale blue creating roots through the darker purple below.

Since Iris's confidence was at an all-time high and she seemed so much more receptive to social situations when paired with music, we felt the time was right for her first violin lesson. It didn't quite go as I had imagined. Ten minutes in, with wild eyes, ears back and tufty bits flying, Thula was swinging skilfully from the curtains way up high and then landing on the floor, running at speed in a cartoon-like motion. She leapt from the sofa, knocked over a lamp and ran across the room and out to the kitchen where Iris was sitting. Then she was up high again with legs dangling off the blind just above Iris's head, a mad look in her eyes, her mood feeding off Iris's anxiety. Cries could be heard from where we were sitting in the garden room. I walked over and grabbed Thula to put her away in the laundry, trying to regain some sort of calm in the mayhem.

It had all started so well: Thula was as she normally is, interested in the arrival of the violin teacher and settling in a magnificent pose on top of the piano ready to hear some music. Iris had been upset that morning but everything was fine when the teacher arrived. But her reaction to the intro lesson wasn't what I had expected. As soon as she heard the teacher's violin play she cried and ran out of the room and wouldn't return. It was a shock to me as the music was so beautiful and familiar to Iris, but her reaction was immediate. She didn't stay and inspect the new larger violin in the way I had envisaged. She was terribly upset and I couldn't figure out why. She did, however, stay in the kitchen for a while and enjoyed some of the music.

I was thankful that we had found such an understanding, lovely teacher. She was a recommendation from the violin restorer and had travelled a long way to come and see us. I'm sure most would have thought I had gone completely mad and that Iris obviously didn't like the instrument. Iris's communication skills had improved quite dramatically but not to the extent of being able to tell me why she reacted in this way. I couldn't help but feel sad; the violin had always brought her so much happiness. The absence of her usual music therapist, who had been on holiday, might have been the reason – perhaps she had been expecting her to be in the room and the change was a shock to the system. I will probably never know for sure, but we did try again and the next time I started to learn some basics on the violin in the hope that Iris would want to join us.

It wasn't to be. In the weeks afterwards Iris made it clear she didn't want me to play either by removing it from my hand, putting it down carefully and not letting anyone touch it. I did manage to have some lessons on the piano, though, so I could start to play for Iris myself. I realized then that maybe it was all too early for lessons, and like my attempts years earlier to introduce Iris to animals the timing wasn't right. The social aspects of a music lesson are intense and although Iris had come a long way she wasn't ready for that yet.

. . . .

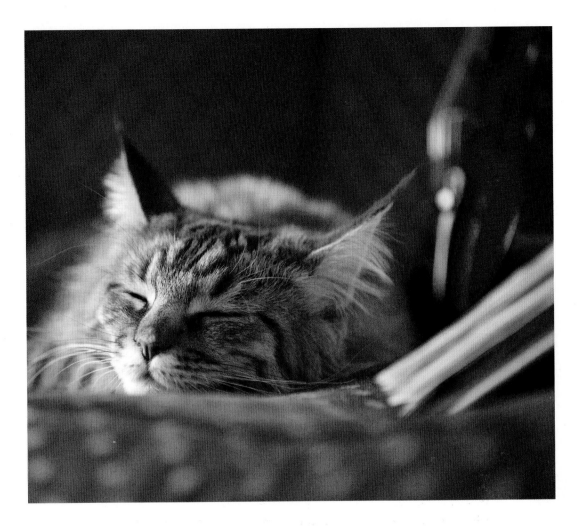

There was an arts centre in Leicester called Embrace Arts, now the Attenborough Arts Centre, that truly lived up to its name, making everyone welcome. Championed by Lord Attenborough, it is one of only two purpose-built spaces in the East Midlands for the promotion of arts and disability. With the deep resonant sound of the double bass playing, Iris relaxed as we made our way through the busy café area to the music hall, where we picked out a table on the front row facing the grand piano. I had

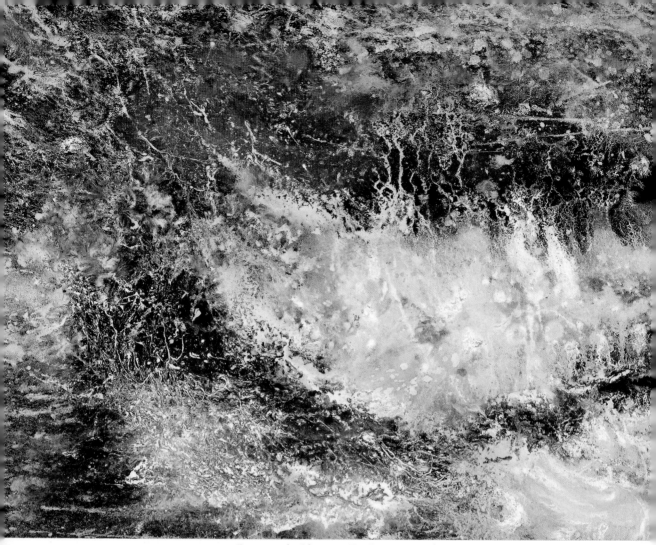

Dance to the Oboe, acrylic, Summer 2014

selected a range of small toys for her to play with and I passed them to her one by one. Iris looked over to the musicians with great interest as they warmed up. I was amazed at how calm she was, with me for a while on my lap and then happy to be on her own chair as she watched and listened to the skilful players. It was a jazz trio made up of the saxophone, the double bass and the piano. Not once throughout the whole performance did Iris look unnerved by the volume or the complexity of the tunes.

Then when the audience clapped, instead of being alarmed, she turned to see everyone's faces, smiling at them. I could hear her humming along to the music and occasionally doing that 'dooo-da-dadoo-da-dadoo' that people do when they are listening to jazz. It wasn't the case with all music; she didn't like children's tunes or many modern bands, but she loved classical, jazz and some music from around the world like African and folk songs. They all had a different effect upon her: invigorating, calming, relaxing, fun.

A few months later we returned for another concert. She listened to a small choir, a cello and a piano played by the Leicester University Musicians. The violinist, who must have been playing before we arrived, came to sit down in front of where we were. Iris couldn't take her eyes off the instrument, saying in her quiet voice, 'V, violin'. When it was packed away in its case I whispered to her that it would come out to play another day and I started to feel rather hot, worrying about an impending outburst of emotion, but she just smiled at me. She looked over instead to the student playing the piano so beautifully and she was content.

This time we had some seats at the back and she had more space to play with her toys while she listened. These 'Soundbites', as they were called, suited us perfectly. You were allowed to go in and out, move around if you needed to and eat your lunch from the café. It was all very relaxed and filled with acceptance and a love for music. It allowed us to help Iris practise her skills in areas that she found so hard, like the busyness of restaurants, unexpected social interactions and the movement of other people. She walked confidently holding our hands through the arts centre and out of the front doors with a big smile on her face, the blue cape dancing along with her.

But there was a problem that I had to face and that was people's reactions to us taking Iris out to these musical events. It was a

313

harsh reminder of my challenges ahead. Judgements, other people's opinions and thoughts would be catapulted at me whether I liked it or not. Up until that point I had been protected from this as we had mostly been based at home or with family. One time, away from the protection of home, the countryside and our bikes, we sat in a pew within a church – surely a place free from judgemental outbursts and a place we should feel safe. We were attending an afternoon concert, a Beethoven string quartet, and even though Iris was tired, she really enjoyed herself and occasionally hummed along to the music while playing with a few toys on the bench. She then climbed on to my knee and sat happily swaying to the violin while watching the movement carefully. The music was lovely and although I was enjoying it too, I dreaded every pause, every silence, due to the negativity I could feel behind me. I was willing Iris to keep as quiet as possible, but the music seemed to be making Iris very responsive and she whispered the names of her toys and even tried to replicate the violin's tune quietly after they had finished.

A couple in the audience were appalled at our presence, and felt the need to tell us so at the end of the concert. 'It's not appropriate for you to bring your child here. You have ruined it for us, for everyone else and insulted the musicians.'

'I'm sorry but my child has just as much right to be here as you. She's been very good. You could have moved somewhere else if she was bothering you,' said P-J.

I wished we had just hurried out. Why did P-J always have to say something back?

'You have ruined it for everyone,' the man repeated, furious with us.

Hearing those words nearly made me cry. Fighting the urge to burst into tears I held it in and walked as fast as I could with

Iris back to the car. I wanted to get home, to shut our gates on everyone and be in the garden. I realized how fragile my confidence was after many years of being isolated at home. We had been going out much more with Iris that year and I had been feeling free and happy, but I hadn't experienced judgement from others until then. Then I wished I had stood up to that couple and told them why we were there and backed up P-J. How could they be so quick to judge? It made me furious but I had said nothing and then disappeared as if I was in the wrong.

Of course they didn't know Iris's story. They didn't know how hard it had been, what courage it took to bring a

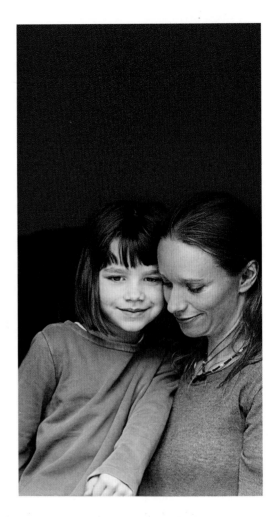

child with special needs to a concert. If they had known that Iris had watched the BBC Young Musician of the Year strings final over and over again, listened to countless recordings of violin players from around the world, seen YouTube videos of orchestras and read dozens of orchestra books and knew that music opened doors into her world, maybe they wouldn't have thought badly of us at all. If only they had known that these musicians who played so beautifully were like my heroes; they were giving Iris something I couldn't and in turn I was eternally grateful. It hurt deeply to think that they were insulted by our presence.

That day my confidence was knocked. I had to be brave and I wished people would be more understanding. Later that afternoon I emailed the musicians to apologize about any disturbance we had caused. What came next restored all that had been lost. They sent a message straight back saying how lovely it had been to see a child so connected to the music and enjoying herself, and that in no way at all were they offended. They then invited us to their rehearsals so that we could enjoy the music without feeling any pressure from others.

Later that month we accepted the musicians' very kind invitation. To have only Iris and the musicians with no audience to worry about, just the classical music, was a magical thought. As we entered the church, the last few people from a family service were leaving: there was lots of loud chatter and noise and Iris began to cry. We managed to find a quiet space upstairs, and immediately she was fine as we waited for the musicians to move into the church. At first we watched from the gallery. She was so excited she couldn't contain it. I could see she knew that she didn't have to with the whole place to herself. She bounced, danced, explored and found a brilliant viewing spot above where the musicians were playing. Then we made the move downstairs to be closer to the instruments. Here, Iris was very different to how she had been before. She didn't want to sit listening quietly, she wanted to dance to the saxophone, the cello and the violins. In the break she even turned the pages of one of the musician's music sheets, getting so close to all of them. She was interested in the electric piano and one of the violinists kindly offered to get it working for her. She played on it while we chatted to them about their performance. They were all intrigued by Iris, her interest in music and told me about how they all first started. It was wonderful listening to them. Music was never in my world as it was for them and they could see quite clearly how much it meant to Iris too. It was as if Iris was forging ahead beyond our knowledge and passions; it was inspiring and I admired her so much for that.

Music was not only helping with Iris's confidence and communication skills, it was also used in her education. I created a violin theme for her homeschooling and like all the other topics it all started with a motivator at its core, in this case the violin. The story of Peter and the Wolf by Sergei Prokofiev, a musical fairy tale in which each character is played by a different instrument of the orchestra, proved to be very effective, encouraging interaction, play, speech and reading. Peter is played by the violins and all the strings in the orchestra, the bird by the flute, the duck by the oboe, the cats by the clarinet, the grandfather by the bassoon, the wolf by the French horn and the hunters and their gunshots by the kettledrums and the big bass drum. Iris's reading had come on so well she was able to read many of the sentences out loud and it was a perfect starting point to launch from. As with 'The Owl and the Pussycat', I created many projects from one story. We then moved on to Vivaldi's *Four Seasons*, allowing me to focus on the weather and English seasons. We all went on adventures down to the stream. Thula would sit patiently beside Iris as she watched the water pass under the bridge. I would talk to them about the sounds we heard, and we played a game matching the different sounds and shapes in nature with instruments just like in *Peter and the Wolf*. A large tree in the wood became the double bass and the trickling water was the piccolo. I had bought Iris her own camera as she had been showing an interest in mine and she captured life from her point of view. She took an array of images, mostly close-up details of moss and water;

she loved the soft velvety texture and those tiny shoots that tickled her fingertips. So at the end of the day when I loaded the photographs on to my computer I learnt a lot about moss in all its glory through Iris's eyes.

•••

At the end of November I had a very exciting call from my brother who was away with his girlfriend Carolina.

'So tell me about Ireland. Where are you staying? What's it like?'

'It's great. It's been amazing. Listen, I have some news . . .'

'Tell me.'

'I've just proposed and Carolina said yes.'

'Oh, James, that's such wonderful news! Congratulations! We're thrilled for you. The whole family will be over the moon.'

I couldn't wait to see him over Christmas and celebrate. Since meeting Carolina something had changed about him; he was more relaxed and so happy.

We celebrated at my parents' party at Christmas, and in London that January with a beautiful engagement party at the Garden Museum. The ancient abandoned church had been rescued from demolition in the seventies and turned into a museum. Now it also serves as a gallery space and a magnificent venue for events. My mother's beautiful flowers and the dramatic lighting of the arches and windows created an air of excitement about their wedding. The plans were already coming together: a Swedish celebration in Stockholm where Carolina's parents lived. I couldn't help but get carried away hearing from the bridesmaids about all there was to see in their incredible country in the north.

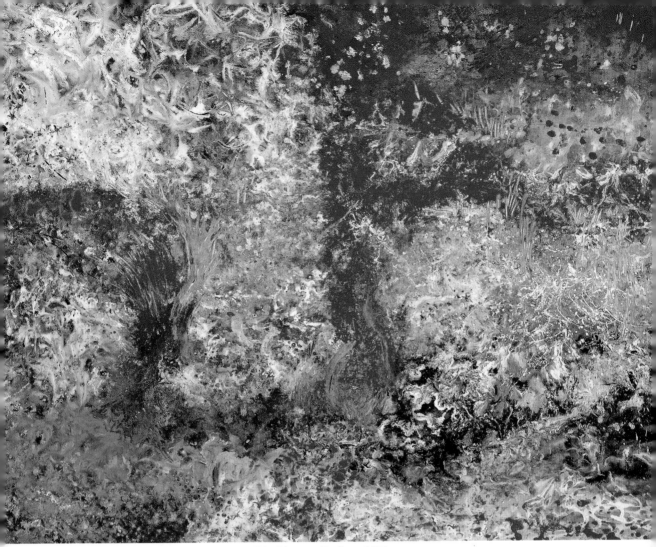

Zin Zin, acrylic, June 2015

The city sounded like a dream: magnificent architecture, parks, palaces, medieval cobbled streets – all surrounded by water.

Then I was torn. I would probably have to go alone as a trip like this would be too much for Iris. James and Carolina talked to me about it and wanted very much for Iris to be there, for us all to come as a family. Carolina's family had stayed in England before with my parents, and they hadn't batted an eyelid at Iris wandering around topless and shoeless or when she flapped her hands if she got excited or hummed at something that intrigued her. No judgements, just acceptance, and that gave me great comfort. Despite this there was still so much we had to overcome.

The date was set for the end of August, which meant I had about six months to work with Iris on certain issues. As I broke down the trip in my mind it was a daunting task. Iris hadn't been on any public transport yet: not a bus, train or plane. The holidays that we had tried to take in the past had ended with us returning home early. Our Cornwall trip when Iris was one and half years old had hardly been a success and nor was another attempt to enjoy ourselves in Wales the year after. That only lasted a couple of days before we had made our way back home. Iris was only just gaining confidence in public places and the thought of the massive Heathrow Airport in London and a plane packed full of people for two and half hours, strange noises, sensations and then arriving in a different country made me nervous. Then there was the wedding day itself, Iris would need to sit quietly through the ceremony, ride on a bus and a boat and handle a busy reception.

In all the celebrations and excitement I had been pushing away the reality of what was to come, what I would need to do to prepare Iris for this. I suddenly felt overwhelmed by the prospect and nervous about how I could possibly make it all work. Then I thought about how I had started the Little Explorers Activity Club because Iris found being around others so hard. That had changed over time. Could I really manage to do the same for this trip? Were we crazy to even think this was possible, let alone that we might have a great time?

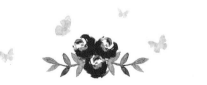

I don't want to disturb the magic. Iris is sitting cross-legged next to P-J on the sofa with Thula on the other side. She finishes the last line of the book so beautifully and I hold in my urge to rush over and hug her. In the story of Zin! Zin! Zin! A Violin the lonely trombone is joined by its musical friends to make up a chamber group of ten. Iris shouts out 'Encore, Encore!' to get them to come out and play once more.

Iris and P-J are working so well together, and a tear of happiness runs down my cheek. Then the worries return once again about the trip to come and the massive steps we are trying to take. But Iris, like the trombone, is no longer alone, and nor am I.

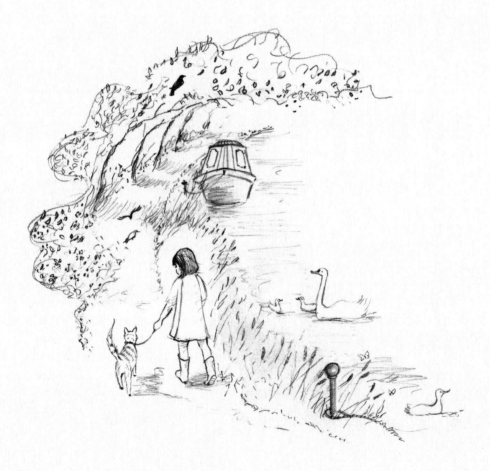

eleven

Thula stretched as far as she could on her back legs to reach the door handle.

'OK, I get it. You want to go out,' I said.

As I walked over she greeted me with a chirping trill, and I opened the door and she bounded out into the snow. It was the end of January 2015, the first snow was still falling and Thula couldn't wait to get out there. She was built for this kind of weather; her coat, sometimes silky and flat, was all puffed out with a regal mane of thick luxurious fur like a beautiful collar. Her rather oversized paws with their long tufts were perfect for making her way through the garden. When Iris had finished her breakfast she went to the window and saw Thula playing, pouncing down hard on something she had heard under the frozen layer. Her stripy black-and-white tail, bushy like a fox's, made Iris laugh. Then she watched Thula as she lay calmly in the sun upon her frozen blanket. The foliage, hedges and branches were all covered in a white frosting that glowed in the golden morning light.

'Shall we go out and play with Thula?' I asked.

'Snow, more snow,' Iris said, and then did a little jig, which I took as a yes. By the time I had her all dressed in her snowsuit and boots the snow had stopped falling and although we had music therapy soon I knew this was our chance. I could already hear it starting to melt; if we didn't go out now, it would be too late.

I was expecting Iris to react as she had done before, and be nervous of the crunching under foot. I thought she would probably need to be in my arms again, but this time she had her loyal friend at her side, so it was a different story. It took a while for Iris to acclimatize to her garden all in white: she just stood still, listening from the decking and watching everything with Thula beside her. She was intrigued by the sounds, and her fingers moved as if they were playing an instrument and she was connected to the water that melted from the branches. I could see she was calming, her breathing slowing down, her breath warm in the cold air as she studied the landscape in great detail. Thula made her move, bouncing through the snow and leaping up on to the tree stump. Iris walked over to join her and soon they were both happily exploring. I opened the gate and off they went down the hill into the orchard.

Something had caught Thula's attention and then Iris's too. I followed their gaze and saw a pair of muntjac making their way through the wood and up the track to the fields beyond. I loved that even in the winter our garden attracted so much wildlife. We were very relaxed gardeners; we certainly weren't going for the neat, well-groomed look. Any fruit on the trees that didn't get eaten was left for the animals. Our flower beds and hedges were left to grow wild for them to seed, providing many opportunities for the animals that lived around us. After the winter, just before the spring, we would clear everything and make way for the new growth, then the whole cycle would start again.

It was nearly time for Iris's music therapy session. She turned as soon as I said 'music' and made her way back up to the house with Thula trotting along behind. By lunchtime most of the snow had melted. It had been a beautiful but brief encounter.

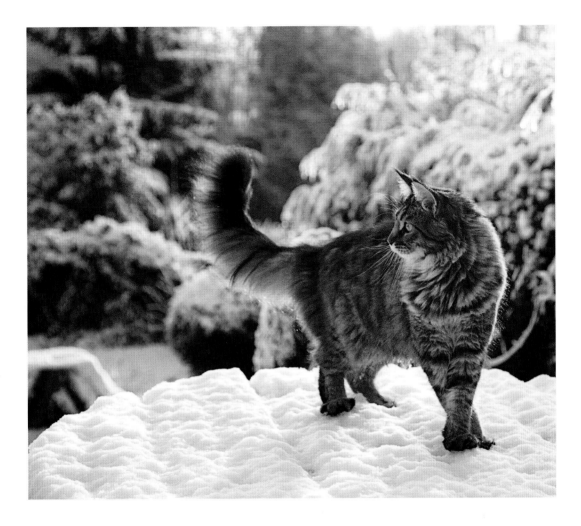

I heard Iris say in a sad voice, 'No more snow!'

'There'll be more. We have the snowdrops coming soon too.'

It was the snow that calmed my worries about how Iris would manage abroad. How far she had come since the first time she had seen snow, how she had adapted. I owed it to her to trust in her resilience.

• •

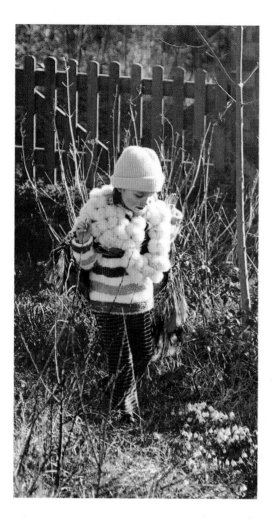

'So, what's the new plan?' P-J asked me.

I started to wonder when our conversations weren't going to be about problems and solutions . . . Sometimes I got so tired of it all, just wanting life to be 'normal', but I always came to the conclusion that this was our normal.

'I thought we should work on the first part of the trip, so that means the airport. Iris hasn't been to any big buildings yet with all the noises of people, trolleys, cafés, restaurants and shops. So my idea was to build up slowly, carry on as we were, taking her to places, pairing it up with things she likes but go bigger – much bigger.'

'Like where?'

'The theatre would be good. Maybe there's an orchestra we can go to that's held there.'

'I've been there before. It's very big in the entrance hall, loads of different floors, restaurants and bars, lots of people hanging around. It'll be a massive step, though. I'm not sure if she's ready for that.'

I agreed; she wasn't quite there yet. We needed to spend the next month building up to that sort of outing.

'How about some tourist places?'

'Yes, anywhere where we can get her used to crowds and queues. Then there's the issue of her not liking to eat in public places or use the bathroom. We need to figure all that out too and practise them.'

'List! Where's your list?' P-J said, laughing at me as I ran through yet more issues.

Much to his amusement I rushed off to get a pen and paper. Then for the next few days I researched and made bookings for various performances, found places where we could take Iris: more trips and fun adventures to go on. There was also her schooling to think about, so I thought we could potentially get two items ticked off my list at once with an outing to a bookshop. It would be busier than most of the shops she had been going to, but filled with something she loved and it might even help me find another topic for her schooling. Hopefully she would be so happy at the sight of a whole room filled with books that she wouldn't mind the crowds of people and children.

••

We made our way across the busy high street with Iris holding our hands. She was a little unnerved by a noisy lorry trundling through the town centre but we managed to get to the bookshop without a problem. It was as if we were taking her to a sweet shop: as soon as she was in, her eyes lit up and we made our way over to the brightly coloured children's section. She picked out a book all about a princess and wouldn't let go. She loved the colours and sparkly details, and where the glitter was stuck to the paper she felt the texture carefully with the tip of her index finger. She sat down at the table in the centre of the room and went through the book over and over again. She didn't seem to mind the other people or the noise: she was focused and nothing would take her eyes away from the princess. We bought the book and with it came a new topic for Iris's education – castles.

I had a call from my brother the following week. He was involved in a project to make a series of films using the new Sony Action camera. They wanted to tell Iris's story using one of these cameras and thought it would be a brilliant way to raise some more positive awareness for autism. We didn't like the idea at first; we had always protected Iris from the outside world and the media. The thought of a film crew at our house was worrying, but the more James explained about the project the more I saw the potential benefits for others. It was another way I could express how different was brilliant, changing the perceptions about living with autism. More tragic stories were hitting the headlines about the problems with bullying and autism in schools, and I wanted people to understand the potential hidden within a child on the spectrum. For Iris the project would potentially be very challenging. It would be intensely social as a film crew made up of a cameraman, director, sound technician and her uncle would be with us for three or four days. It would be action-packed and demanding for all of us, as they wanted to capture the key elements of her story. I had no doubts that Thula would relish the experience, but for Iris it might be a step too far. For many nights I thought about it, and the pros and cons in my mind shifted all the time, but in light of our goal for the summer we decided to go for it.

We agreed that we would carefully monitor Iris and I made it clear to the director that if she needed to have some time out then we would all need to give that to her. Filming was due to start at the end of March. The team first came up to meet Iris and to see the locations. Then they sent the tiny video camera to us the week before so that Iris could get used to it and could have a go at using it herself to record life from her perspective.

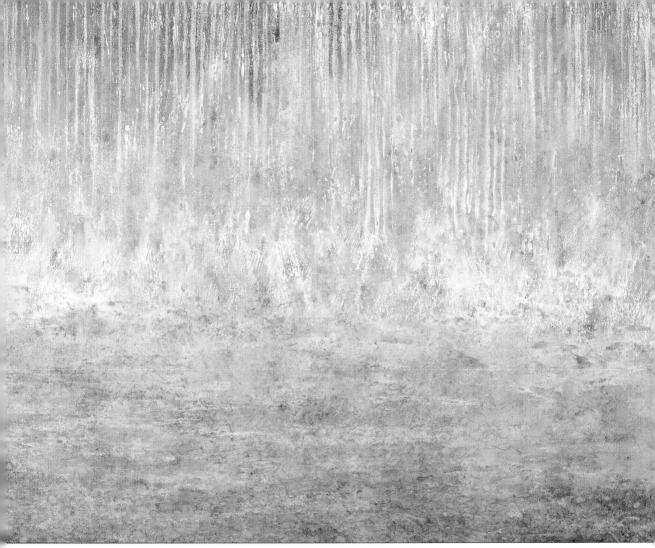

Waterfall Bounce, acrylic, April 2013

One of Iris's favourite places to film seemed to be in the bath with Thula. The footage made me laugh so much: Thula's thin legs under the water and then close-ups of her drinking or the depths of her soft coat and those long whiskers.

From start to finish I was astounded at Iris's progress. She allowed me to put a harness round her body so we could fix the camera on to her. She would wait patiently in the car or on the bikes as the team worked to set things up. Following instructions wasn't easy

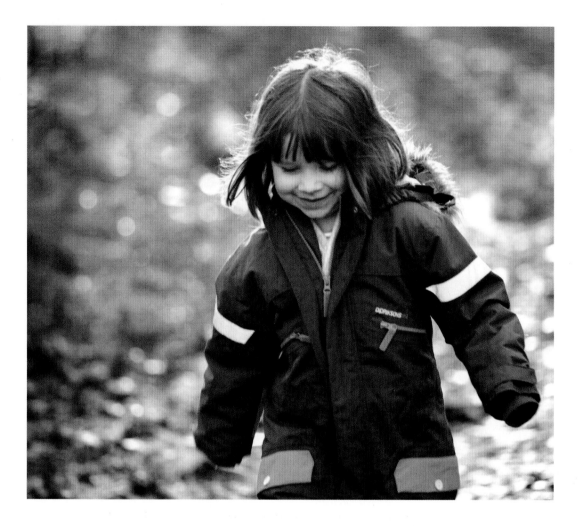

for her so we took a more go-with-the-flow approach and Thula
made us all proud as she took baths, went on the bikes, played
with bubbles and even had a swim in the swimming pool. The
house was full of people and at lunchtime the kitchen was packed
with equipment, laptops, screens, batteries charging, sound boom,
cameras and lenses . . . It felt exciting but exhausting at the same
time, but Iris was loving it. A whole week's worth of activities
were crammed into just one day and although tired at the end of
each day she was very happy.

There were times when I needed help with Iris and James would step in. He carried her up to the house on his shoulders when she needed a break, or gave her a snack and she would reply with a 'thank you'. He even swam with her in the pool using the underwater camera. He didn't put any pressure on her, but equally he didn't seem worried about just getting on with things. I loved watching Iris interact with him and the others at lunchtime as we all ate our food at the picnic table. She wanted to be included and to be with everyone, which was an incredible change as for so long social mealtimes had been such a challenge.

The project had started off as a way to help others but it turned into a fabulous way for Iris to practise her social skills with people who understood her. It gave me so much hope for the summer, inspiring us to keep going with our plan. There were downsides, but not in the way I had predicted; it was nothing to do with Iris and all to do with me. The process of creating a film and seeing the vision come to life from another's perspective about our life was hard. I had previously captured Iris's life through my own lens, and my romantic photography had a soft gentleness to it. The film ended up being more modern, attracting a younger crowd to go with the adventurous new action camera.

It was just over two minutes long, telling Iris's story from a unique perspective. The inclusion of old footage from when Iris was a baby brought it all back. Iris playing with her toys and not even looking up if we came into the room or said her name. Standing in the garden as a toddler with her arms out, her fingers feeling the wind. Our child, so removed from us but connected to nature, was there before me on the screen. During the filming I recorded a voiceover; the director asked me to think about that time, to think of how I felt back then, how Iris had been with us and our relationships. Doing that unearthed all those feelings from the early years and then seeing it all together in a film made me feel vulnerable. The feelings were raw and it opened

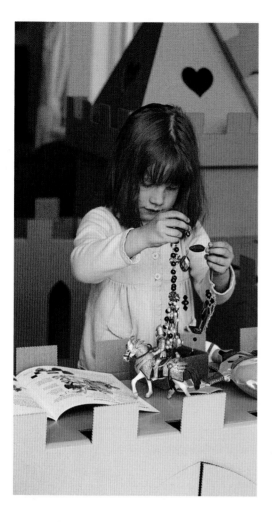

up that part of our lives once again. But we had moved on and Iris had overcome so much. It was upsetting but also empowering and helped give me the strength to move forward.

Preparations were underway for our 'castle' theme and in the spring we all worked on a new project together, building our very own castle in the garden room made out of pink cardboard. Thula and I were on turret duty while P-J and Iris worked on the walls together. Iris would say the odd word – 'Princess, prince, king, queen . . .' – as she held one side, while P-J bent it into the right shape. It took all morning but once it was finished our hard labour was rewarded. Thula prowled the internal corridors of the castle, then was on lookout, sitting majestically on one of the outer walls. Iris was in the inner courtyard inspecting her crown jewels and then playing with the knights, dragon and princess puppets. She had the grand idea of putting her trampoline in the centre and she bounced for hours within the walls of her castle. Over the next few days the castle was decorated with all sorts of stickers and paintings. The scene was set for an ambitious trip to Warwick Castle.

The back of the car was full, there were books propped up against Iris's bike seat and the puppets were stored away in Thula's basket. A whole range of knights, kings, queens and horse toys were scattered all over.

'Are you sure you've got enough stuff?' P-J said. Missing his sarcasm through my tiredness, I ran through the toys I had wanted Iris to have with her for the journey.

'Oh, I forgot the archer toy. Let me just go –'

'She's fine, look.'

I looked into the back and Iris said, 'Rag 'n' roll!'

My car seemed to be a mobile classroom on trips like this, but the long journey had its benefits as we made sure Iris

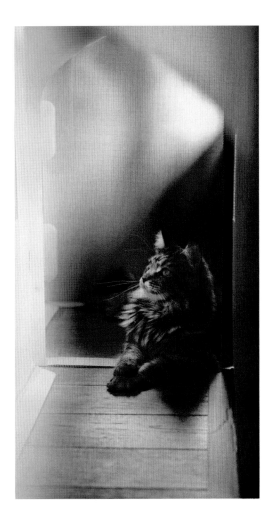

understood what we were about to see. I don't think anything could have prepared her for what was to come. The beauty and splendour of Warwick Castle, with its river running through the blossom-filled valley, was exhilarating, at times overpowering, but above all a wonderful place for her to explore. My concerns about the queues for tickets were unfounded; our early arrival meant there was only one other couple in front of us. We made our way into the interior of the castle, Iris admiring the armour on display in the Great Hall and the knights on their horses and then she was off. She made her way confidently past other visitors, P-J and I following as she went from room to room, stopping at objects or paintings that caught her attention and then hurrying down corridors, upstairs, downstairs, along more corridors, settling at a window seat for just a moment before setting off again. As we walked behind her I could hear lots of words, one after the other. She saw a portrait with a pair of lions in the State Dining Room and I heard her say, 'Lion. Lion says roar!' Then when she spotted an eagle on a fireplace: 'Eagle, wow!' She described and labelled everything she saw. She pronounced the famous portrait of King Charles I on horseback by Van Dyck a 'big knight, white horse'. She was a little confused by the lifesize waxwork models; she wanted to understand what they were all about, including their long dresses. I could see her thinking 'Mummy doesn't wear these' as she bent down and had a look under their skirts. At that moments like that I would point out something in the next room and she would hurry on so I could try to avoid being told off about her touching the fabrics.

Once Iris had explored the castle it was time for a walk on to the mound. She stopped in front of P-J and lifted her arms up: her signal to be carried.

'OK, Beanie, up on my shoulders you go,' he said, and she tucked her knees up as he lifted her, then as she got into position her hands flapped excitedly and we made our way up to the top.

But suddenly I could tell by her noises that something was bothering her. The hums were intensifying and she was getting frustrated. Maybe we'd done enough and it was time to go home.

My own legs began to ache. I was tired and the extra pressure to prepare Iris had taken its toll. I realized that I needed to pace myself as well as Iris. I had been so busy over that past week, with hardly a chance to stop and breathe. Even in the good times looking after a child on the spectrum comes with extra layers of thought, preparation, listening, watching, research and reading her non-verbal language to understand how she perceives the world. I needed to do this to help her avoid the meltdowns. Iris hadn't experienced any for ages but we needed to observe her carefully and rein things in if needed.

Back at the car P-J kissed Iris. 'That was amazing, Beanie, well done!' He turned to look at me; he was so happy, and even though I was tired his enthusiasm spread to me.

• •

A few weeks later we had our next trip upon us, one that made me more nervous than the others – the orchestra at the Northampton Theatre. I wished I could take on more of P-J's character in those times, his confident facade would come in handy in facing situations like that. It was the reaction from the audience to us bringing Iris that worried me. I tried my best to put that out of my mind and to stay positive. Iris walked confidently into the massive atrium, holding our hands, up the staircases, passing by the bars and cafés. The chatter echoed around her and yet she didn't mind. She was focused; she was going to see the orchestra and in her mind that was all that mattered.

Every silence in the performance still made me sweat and as she said 'bye-bye' to the opera singer my fears were mounting. Iris was becoming very vocal. She was connected to the powerful music and it was clear for everyone to see. I had to hold on to her sitting on my lap. Iris and the music were one, soaring high. In her heart she was on the kettledrums as they boomed, floating above the flutes and dancing along the xylophone. She whizzed along the coiled brass of the French horn and flew out of the flared bell. She sang with the violins and hummed to the double basses.

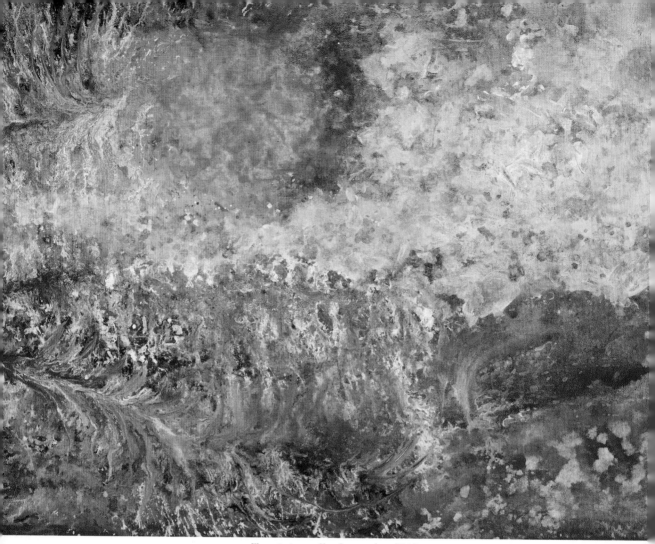

Trumpet, acrylic, September 2015

She adored every instrument and the musicians that played them, even the humble triangle was a delight to her senses. We left feeling elated, knowing that Iris could manage a large building like that if there was something that held her interest. In my mind I was making a plan, how to make the airport a place that Iris would connect with. I would find some apps for the iPad, games, books and toys on the airport theme and when we were finally there a visit to a bookshop would be a good start.

The actual journey to Stockholm was the main hurdle in our minds but other parts of the trip needed some preparation too. My brother had told me that after the ceremony we were all going to take a boat trip around the archipelago and so boats were also in focus. We decided that over the next month we would hire a boat and take it along the canal. Then both of us forgot about the idea until one day I opened up the garage to find that P-J's bike tyre was completely flat. The weather was beautiful and it seemed a shame not to go out, so a spontaneous trip along the canal came together and within the hour we were making our way to the wharf with Thula in tow. She had jumped into the car and waited patiently, making it quite clear there was no way she was going to miss out on another outing. There was a kind of childish thrill about stowing away our extra cargo and Iris was very excited to be bringing Thula. To keep her safe on the transfer from car to boat I coaxed her into a cat carrier that also doubled up as rucksack, perfect for such an occasion.

Our boat for the day wasn't a long canal boat but a shorter eight-and-a-half-metre one, still engine-powered but with the added bonus of a superb viewing area with benches and a table. The sides were open, making it light and airy. I settled Iris at the table with her books and a duvet and then let Thula out. She immediately jumped up on to the bench and curled up beside Iris on a cushion. The roles were reversed: instead of Thula comforting Iris it was Iris taking care of her nervous cat. Iris started to recognize where we were as we followed the tracks we had so often travelled along by bike. Within a few minutes they were both happy and we went on our way along the canal lined with trees, the fields beyond. The pace was slow; like anything related to the canal, a boat trip has its own time. You can't rush anywhere and that was good for me; I needed to slow down for a while. We passed ducks and their ducklings, swans, moorhens, and saw the brilliant turquoise blue of kingfishers swooping low over the water and then back into the reeds; and Iris chatted about what she could see. P-J was at the back of the boat steering, so we all joined him and Iris had a go.

Thula sat in the seat by the controls and then put her feet up on to the top of the boat and stood on her back legs, which brought many smiles from passers-by. I had started to become used to how she took things in her stride and always wanted to be involved: biker cat, nanny cat, bathtime cat, artist's assistant, educational assistant and now a boating cat. It was like she was one of us going off on all these adventures. We weren't just bringing our pet along for the ride; Thula was really enjoying these outings too. Whenever we got back home after a trip with her she would be so much more affectionate to all of us, the bonds had been strengthened by being somewhere new and experiencing something different together, and in parallel Iris behaved in the same way.

After lunch at Foxton Locks we turned the boat to make the journey back home. But about a mile from the wharf there was a terrible clunk and the engine stopped. We drifted to the far side of the canal and into thick bushes. P-J tried the engine again.

Beep, beep, beep . . . The intolerably loud beeping pierced Iris's mind. She couldn't bear it and leapt on to my lap, starting to pull at my clothes.

'Stop, P-J! Stop!'

He stopped trying to get the boat started and came over to me.

It was the noise, she couldn't stand it. 'Can you ring the boat company? Maybe they will know what to do?'

P-J went back to the controls and eventually got through to the manager who gave him some instructions. But when he turned over the engine and the beeping started all over again it was

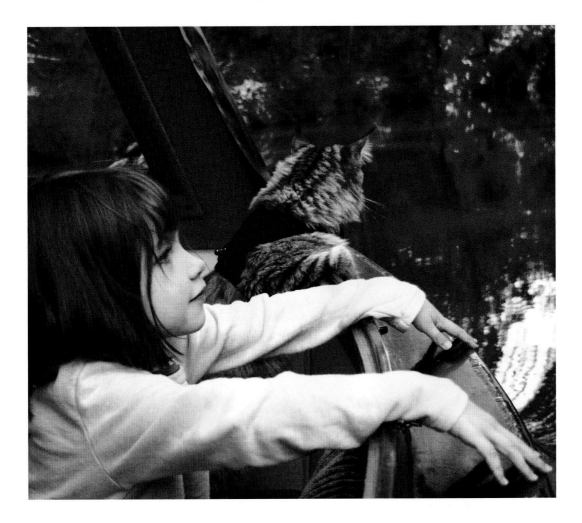

clear that Iris couldn't handle it. She grabbed at my face, taking my lips and squishing them shut very hard. It was the only way she could think of to say 'be quiet' but it hurt terribly and her pain was now mine. I hugged her close for a long while as she cried, gently rocking from side to side, not saying a word until she calmed down. Iris was normally so gentle, the sweetest-natured girl, but I was seeing our child under pressures that I could only imagine. That sound was obviously painful and she would do anything she could to stop it.

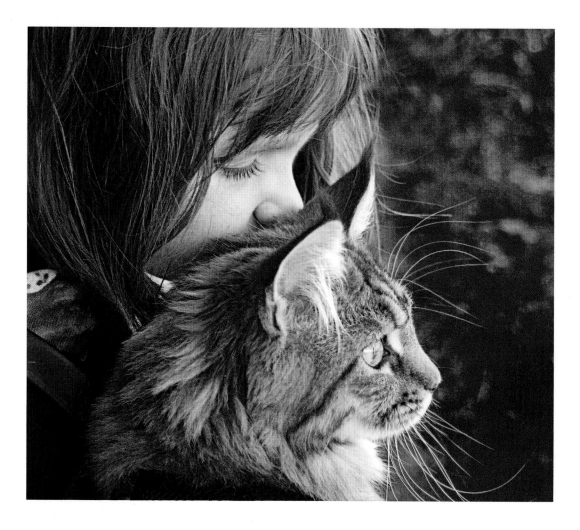

All four of us sat on the bench together and mulled over our situation. The bank on the other side was where we needed to get to and the track back to the car. But how to get there? We searched the boat. There was no pole to push us over, no rope long enough to throw to a passer-by. One of us could have got in the water to swim over and then pulled the boat across. But the walk home would have been horrible, soaking wet in dirty canal water – and I didn't even want to think about what lay at the bottom.

Luckily two policemen happened to walk by and offered to help. P-J found some rope from the buoys that hung down at the side of the boat to protect it. He tied them all together and after several attempts the rope was finally in the hands of the policemen on the other side and they pulled us over to the bank.

After securing the boat there was a rather embarrassing moment of offloading all my kit: food, drinks, toys, bags of books, duvet, my camera and Thula. We were like a pair of packhorses walking along hand in hand with Iris, Thula looking out at the view from the rucksack on my back. Before we left I had told Iris she needed to be brave for me, that this was all part of the adventure and that we had to walk to get back to the car. She was a little unsure at first but looked at Thula on my back and there seemed to be a moment of 'Well, if you're going.' And so we abandoned the boat and started the long walk home.

Our misfortune with the boat turned out to have an upside. We had not only practised going on a boat but also regaining our composure when things were not going to plan, coming back from the edge of a meltdown. Best of all, Iris had managed to deal with the change of circumstances and change of plan, all things that had been so challenging for her in the past and all potential components of our trip abroad.

On the transport theme there was another aspect of our journey that was worrying me. We might be taking a train from the airport to the centre of Stockholm. A trip was forming in my mind, an adventure to the capital: a train ride to London and then staying the night at a friend's flat. We could tackle a few issues in this one trip if all went well and maybe even go to a museum. I had fond memories of the Natural History Museum and since the dinosaurs had gone down so well at the club I felt sure that Iris would enjoy it. It was strange planning a trip like this. If someone had suggested taking Iris to London a year earlier I would have laughed – we all would. The concept of

Iris out and about in a city was inconceivable. But so much had changed. This would be another trip away from Thula but we needed to practise that too. Thula would stay at home while we were in Sweden and we needed to know Iris could manage without her before we left.

We were early. I, of course, was always prepared and Iris was following in my footsteps. She wanted to leave the house too soon but with so much eagerness to get to the train and her saying 'Train, rag 'n' roll', I could hardly say no. So we sat in the car park until it was time to go on to the platform. I was like a walking library, my overnight bag was stuffed full of books and my shoulder bag was so bursting at the seams I started to tilt to one side from the weight. Iris was excited and very happy. I protected her ears as our train pulled into the station. Iris's elation from the experience came with new abilities: she was talking more and using expressions we had never heard. When we went through a tunnel she said 'Into the dark' and started laughing hysterically, which set us off too.

She was particularly interested in one book I had brought along for the ride: a book called *The Water Hole* by Graeme Base, an extraordinary combination of wildlife, counting, narration and puzzles. There were animals hidden within the pictures, camouflaged cleverly. Amusement, education and delight was found on those beautifully illustrated pages. For the full hour, in between looking at the view, Iris wanted to hear the names of every detail she saw in that book. She practised her words and phrases, reading the sentences along with us and I couldn't believe that with so much going on in the train we were also having a very productive lesson. The new stimulus and environment seemed to be spurring her on. The book was the anchor and with us at her side she was as confident as I had ever seen her.

St Pancras station made her gasp in delight; the massive volume of space with its awe-inspiring Victorian Gothic architecture was a wondrous sight and Iris held my hand as we walked to the taxi. Feeling her hand in mine as we walked through the busy station was incredible. She walked quickly beside me looking up and around with an enchanted look in her eyes. It turned out that taxis were her new favourite thing: better viewing than from a car and more space. She sat bolt upright with her legs crossed like a little Buddha. The owners of the flat were away so we had the place to ourselves and there was a piano there that Iris immediately started to play; I had forgotten about the piano and it was very much appreciated as it gave Iris something familiar. She settled in well, even managing to use the bathroom – another item ticked off my list.

That night P-J went out to find some food for our supper. There was a restaurant just over the road and he explained about Iris and that it was her first trip to London and they let us take our plates over to the flat to eat in the sitting room so Iris could relax. The restaurant owners' refreshingly relaxed attitude made me smile; they understood that for her having a meal in a restaurant would be too much – she needed peace and space to move.

The following morning we all left the flat in high spirits. The plan seemed to be working and we were off to visit the Natural History Museum. We asked the taxi driver to put Classic FM on and the theme tune to *Jurassic Park* by John Williams started to play. It was as if it was a sign and everything was slotting into place. The music was inspiring, so when we arrived I wasn't nervous at all about Iris and how she would react to the museum. But the crowds were already starting to gather even though it had only just opened and as we waited a rep from the museum started to hype up the crowd.

'Are you excited?'

'Yes' everyone shouted.

Iris leapt at me, terrified. The sudden burst of noise was too much.

And then as we came into the entrance our bags were checked. Iris's favourite child loo seat and books were unearthed, and P-J struggled to get them all back into the rucksack. Tourists crowded around us and flashes of lights from their cameras were going off by the second as they saw the ginormous dinosaur in the central hall. Iris started to cry and we walked quickly away from the crowd up the stairs to try to escape the chaos echoing around us. But the problem was that the higher we climbed the more intense the noises seemed to become and Iris became inconsolable in P-J's arms. After many wrong turns we found our way to the big blue whale, a highlight in my mind that I thought Iris would love. But it was game over — another few flashes from a tourist camera and a meltdown began.

I could tell she was way past seeing, hearing or understanding her surroundings. She needed quiet, to be away from all those stuffed animals, that seemed to suddenly be everywhere, surrounding us. We walked frantically to try to find our way out, the voiceovers describing various animals and their habitats blaring out as our movement set them off. The voices reverberating around us, we kept going until we found the exit to the garden.

I tried to talk to P-J through the cries, suggesting he played some music on the iPhone, but he could hardly hear. Eventually we got it on, and after a while Iris settled with the trees and greenery surrounding her.

I didn't want it to end like this; I wanted to make good memories not bad, and we couldn't leave London now. I felt like the goal of Sweden was slipping away and it made me question if what we were doing was asking too much of Iris at this point. We decided that if Iris calmed down in the taxi we would try London Zoo. She had always adored going to the zoo. It was something familiar, surely a perfect day out in London. Why I thought dead animals behind glass would be fun was beyond me. I had fallen into the same old trap, recreating childhood memories of my own.

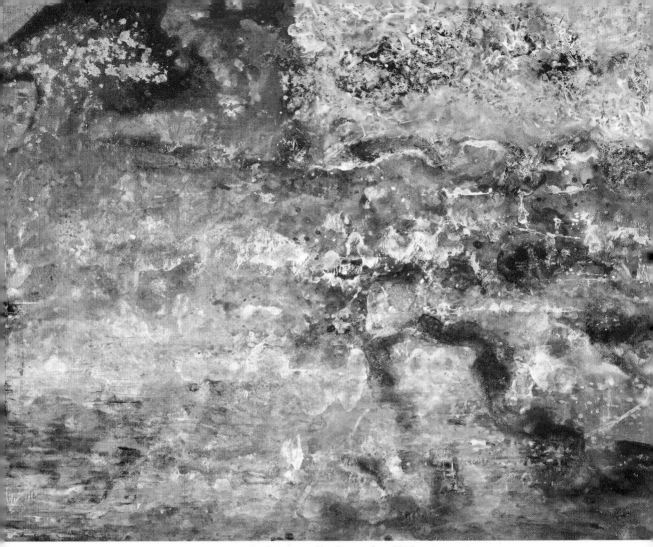

Story, acrylic, September 2015

But it turned out the zoo was no better. Work was being done in the grounds and we walked by crowds of school children. Once we overtook one lot, another would be on our tail. I felt as though it was a scene from *Tom and Jerry*: we were being chased and there were obstacles continually in our way. Angle grinders and cement mixers made way for agricultural-sized lawn mowers, then on to the penguin show with squeals and screams from masses of children. One after another our decisions were terrible

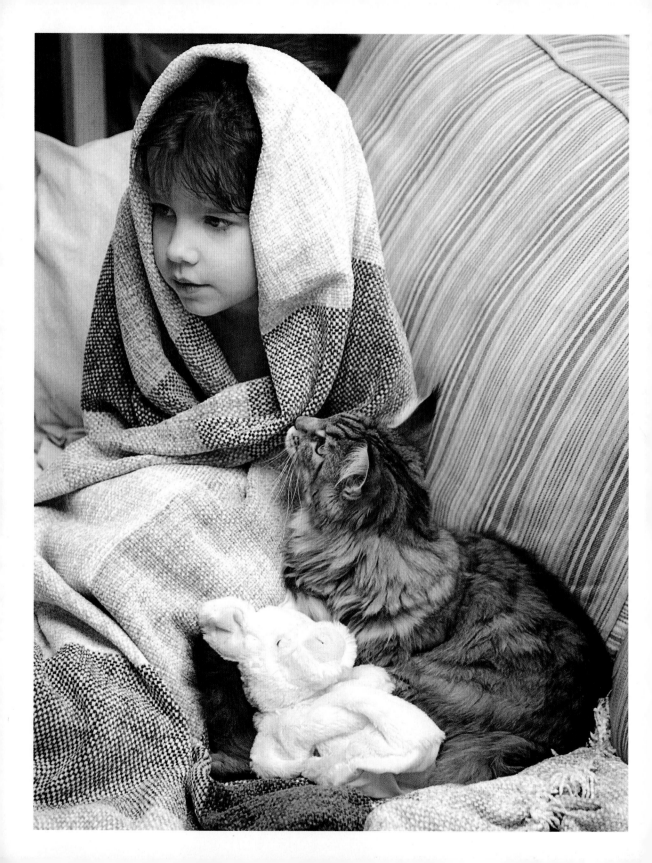

so we made our escape, leaping into the next available taxi and heading straight back to the flat.

P-J and I looked at each other. It was time to return to the Shire. Iris felt it too and was suddenly remarkably content on the ride back. She observed the city from the cool safety of her big black taxi cab and after a pizza we were heading home on the train through green fields, woods and rolling hills.

On our way home I had many regrets and started to once again question our motives. I had promised to follow, to be patient and kind. Was I losing that in this mission to experience a moment in time out in Stockholm? Then I thought of all our successes and decided that we were indeed making wonderful progress. I understood where we had gone wrong: taking her to busy museums, her senses had been overwhelmed. We were thinking of our childhoods and not focusing on Iris. If Stockholm was to be a success, we would need to follow Iris more carefully, to stop trying to do so much and to enjoy the simple pleasures. If Iris wanted to spend the days renting bikes and exploring the parks, looking at fountains, then that is what we would do. No more traipsing around museums; we would watch the water, the reflections, the boats and trees, and experience the city through Iris's eyes. We were asking a great deal from Iris so in return we would need to allow her to enjoy the trip in her own way.

Although Iris had come so far nothing would change the fact that she still experiences and feels the world differently; she will always be on the spectrum. She slides along that spectrum from moment to moment, and what we see on the surface is a fraction of what she is experiencing and feeling. Her communication skills have improved immensely but when under pressure those advances can fall away.

• •

▶

472–473 Lexicology

Scope: synonyms, antonyms, homonyms [*all formerly* 474]

472   Etymology

Phonetic, graphic, semantic development of words and morphemes

Including foreign elements

For notation, pronunciation, intonation, spelling, see 471

473   *Dictionaries

[474]   Synonyms, antonyms, homonyms

Class lexicology in 472–473, standard usage in 478

475   Structural system

Former heading: Grammar

Morphology and syntax

476   Prosody

477   Old, Postclassical, Vulgar Latin

478   *Standard Latin usage (Applied linguistics)

Classical Latin; classical revival (medieval and modern) Latin [*formerly* 479]; synonyms, antonyms, homonyms [*all formerly* 474]

479   Romance and other Italic languages

Including Osco-Umbrian languages

Class description and analysis of classical revival (medieval and modern) Latin in 471–476, standard usage in 478 [*both formerly* 479]

For Etruscan, see 499

.1   Romance languages

Class specific Romance languages in 440–460

* Divide as instructed under 430–490

480   Classical languages [*formerly* 489.1] and modern Greek

Class Latin in 471–478

.01–.09   Standard subdivisions of classical languages

.1–.9   Standard subdivisions of classical Greek

Class dictionaries of the language in 483

▶   481–486 Description and analysis of standard classical Greek

Class standard classical Greek usage in 488

481   Written and spoken codes

Abbreviations, acronyms, punctuation, intonation, capitalization, spelling, pronunciation, paleography

Including Minoan Linear B

▶   482–483 Lexicology

Scope: synonyms, antonyms, homonyms [*all formerly* 484]

482   Etymology

Phonetic, graphic, semantic development of words and morphemes

Including foreign elements

For notation, pronunciation, intonation, spelling, see 481

483   *Dictionaries

[484]   Synonyms, antonyms, homonyms

Class lexicology in 482–483, standard usage in 488

485   Structural system

Former heading: Grammar

Morphology and syntax

486   Prosody

* Divide as instructed under 430–490

487	Postclassical Greek

Hellenistic and Byzantine Greek

Including Biblical Greek

488	*Standard classical Greek usage (Applied linguistics)

Synonyms, antonyms, homonyms [*all formerly* 484]

489	Other Greek languages
[.1]	Classical languages

Class in 480

.3	*Modern Greek

Katharevusa and Demotic

490 Other languages

491	East Indo-European and Celtic languages

Do not use standard subdivisions

Class comprehensive works on Indo-European languages [*formerly* 491] in 411–418

.01–.09	Standard subdivisions of East Indo-European languages

.1	Indo-Iranian (Aryan) languages

For Indo-Aryan (Indic) languages, see **491.2–491.4**; *Iranian languages,* **491.5**

▶ 491.2–491.4 Indo-Aryan (Indic) languages

.2	Sanskrit

Vedic (Old Indic) and classical

* Divide as instructed under 430–490

► **491.3–491.4 Prakrits**

Class nonstandard Sanskrit (Primary Prakrits) in **491.2**

491.3   Middle Indic languages (Secondary Prakrits)

         Including Pali

.4   Modern Indic languages (Teritiary Prakrits)

         Sindhi, Punjabi, Hindi, Urdu, Bengali, Assamese, Bihari, Oriya, Marathi, Gujarati-Rajasthani, Sinhalese, Dard, Pahari, Romany

.5   Iranian languages

         Old and Modern Persian, Avestan (East Iranian), Pahlavi (Middle Persian), Ossetic, Kurdish, Pashto, Baluchi, Pamir, Tajiki

         Class Armenian [*formerly* **491.5**] in **491.9**

.6   Celtic languages

         Gaelic, Cornish, Welsh, Breton, Manx

.7   East Slavic languages

         Do not use standard subdivisions

.701–.709   Standard subdivisions of Russian

         Class dictionaries of the language in **491.73**

.71–.76   *Description and analysis of standard Russian

         Class standard Russian usage in **491.78**

.77   Nonstandard Russian

         Description, analysis, usage of Old Russian, Middle Russian, regional and nonregional variations

.78   *Standard Russian usage (Applied linguistics)

.79   Ukrainian and Belorussian

         Do not use standard subdivisions

* Divide as instructed under **430–490**

491.8	Balto-Slavic languages

Common Slavic, Bulgarian, Macedonian, Serbo-Croatian, Slovenian, Polish, Czech, Slovak, Wendish

Do not use standard subdivisions

> *For East Slavic languages, see* **491.7**; *Baltic languages,* **491.9**

.9 Baltic and other East Indo-European languages

Armenian [*formerly* **491.5**], Albanian, Old Prussian, Lithuanian, Latvian (Lettish), Anatolian, Tocharian, Thraco-Phrygian, Illyrian, Indo-Hittite

---

► ### 492–493 Afro-Asian languages

492 Semitic languages

Including Akkadian, Aramaic, Ethiopic, Samaritan, South Arabic, Canaanite-Phoenician, Minoan Linear A

.4 Hebraic languages

Do not use standard subdivisions

.401–.409 Standard subdivisions of Hebrew

Class dictionaries of the language in **492.43**

.41–.48 *Principles of Hebrew

.49 *Yiddish

.7 Arabic (North Arabic)

493 Hamitic and other languages

Old Egyptian, Coptic, Berber, Cushitic (Hamitic Ethiopian), Chad

> *For Hausa, see* **496**

* Divide as instructed under **430–490**

▶ ### 494–495 Asian and related languages

For East Indo-European languages, see **491**; *Afro-Asian languages,* **492–493**

494   ## Ural-Altaic, Paleosiberian, Dravidian languages

Altaic languages (Tungusic, Mongolic, Turkish); Uralic languages (Samoyedic, Hungarian, Finnish, Estonian, Lapp); Paleosiberian languages (Luorawetlin, Ainu, Gilyak, Ket); Dravidian languages (Tamil, Malayalam, Kanarese, Gondi, Khond, Telugu, Brahui)

495   ## Languages of East and Southeast Asia

Including Tibeto-Burman, Burmese, Thai, Vietnamese, Cambodian languages

.1   ### Chinese

Do not use standard subdivisions

.6   ### Japanese

.7   ### Korean

496   ## African languages

Including Hottentot, Bushman, Bantu, Hausa, Swahili

For Afro-Asian languages, see **492–493**

497   ## North American Indian languages

498   ## South American Indian languages

499   ## Austronesian and other languages

Including Negrito, Papuan, Malayan, Polynesian, Melanesian, Micronesian, Australian, Basque, Elamitic, Etruscan, Sumerian, Caucasian languages

.9   ### Artificial languages [*formerly* 408.9]

Esperanto, Interlingua, Volapük

Do not use standard subdivisions

500 Pure sciences

   .1   Natural sciences

   .2   Physical sciences

   .9   Natural history

501   Philosophy and theory

502   Miscellany

503   Dictionaries, encyclopedias, concordances

505   Serial publications

506   Organizations

507   Study and teaching

508   Collections, anthologies, travels, surveys

   .3   Travels and surveys

           For geographical treatment of travels and surveys, see **508.4–508.9**

   .4–.9   Geographical treatment of travels and surveys

           Add area notations **4–9** to **508**

509   Historical and geographical treatment

510 Mathematics

        Use **510.01–510.09** for standard subdivisions

   .78   Computation instruments and machines

           Mathematical principles of mechanical, electromechanical, electronic calculating devices

           Including analog instruments and digital machines

511   Arithmetic

   .021   Tabulated and related materials

           Class tables in **511.9**

511.024	Works for specific types of users
	Class business arithmetic in **511.8**
.07	Study and teaching
	Class problems in **511.9**
.8	Business arithmetic
	Including mensuration, mercantile rules, calculation of interest
.9	Problems and tables
512	Algebra
.021	Tabulated and related materials
	Class tables in **512.9**
.07	Study and teaching
	Class problems in **512.9**
.9	Problems and tables

▶ 513–516 Geometries

513	Synthetic geometry
	For trigonometry, see **514**; *descriptive geometry,* **515**
.07	Study and teaching
	Class problems in **513.9**
.9	Problems
514	Trigonometry
.07	Study and teaching
	Class problems in **514.9**
.9	Problems
515	Descriptive geometry

516   Analytic (Coordinate) geometry

  .07   Study and teaching

           Class problems in **516.9**

  .9   Problems

517   Calculus

  .07   Study and teaching

           Class problems in **517.9**

  .9   Problems

519   Probabilities and statistical calculations

520   **Astronomy and allied sciences**

         Do not use standard subdivisions

▶   520.1–520.9 Standard subdivisions of astronomy

  .1   Philosophy and theory

           Class natural astrology, ancient and medieval astronomy [*all formerly* **520.1**] in **520.9**

  .2–.8   Miscellany, dictionaries, serial publications, organizations, study and teaching, collections

  .9   Historical and geographical treatment

           Including natural astrology, ancient and medieval astronomy [*all formerly* **520.1**]

521   Theoretical astronomy and celestial mechanics

         Specific theories and their application to celestial bodies

522   Practical and spherical astronomy

         Observatories, telescopes and other astronomical instruments, observational techniques, corrections

523   Descriptive astronomy
           Use **523.001–523.009** for standard subdivisions

.01   Physical and chemical aspects
           Astrophysics, radio and radar astronomy
           Class spectroscopical methods in **522**

.1   Physical universe (Cosmology)
           Origin, development, structure, destiny of universe
           Including astrobiology, Milky Way

.2   Solar system
.207   Study and teaching
           Do not use for planetariums
           _____

►   523.3–523.8 Specific celestial bodies
           Physical features and constitutions, phases, orbits, distances,
           motions, eclipses, spectroscopy
           For transits, satellites, occultations, see **523.9**

.3   Moon
[.302 1]   Tabulated and related materials
                Do not use; class in **523.39**

[.302 2]   Illustrations
                Do not use; class in **523.39**

.39   Charts, photographs, tables

.4   Planets
           For earth, see **525**

[.402 1]   Tabulated and related materials
                Do not use; class in **523.49**

[.402 2]   Illustrations
                Do not use; class in **523.49**

.49   Charts, photographs, tables

166

523.5		Meteors and zodiacal light
.6		Comets
[.602 1]		Tabulated and related materials

Do not use; class in **523.69**

[.602 2]		Illustrations

Do not use; class in **523.69**

.69		Charts, photographs, tables

.7	Sun	
[.702 1]		Tabulated and related materials

Do not use; class in **525**

[.702 2]		Illustrations

Do not use; class in **523.79**

.79		Charts and photographs

.8	Stars	

For Milky Way, see **523.1**; sun, **523.7**

[.802 1]		Tabulated and related materials

Do not use; class in **523.89**

[.802 2]		Illustrations

Do not use; class in **523.89**

.89		Charts, photographs, tables

Including observers' atlases, star catalogs

.9		Transits, satellites, occultations

For moon, see **523.3**

525   Earth (Astronomical geography)

Constants, dimensions, heat, light, radiation, orbit and motions, seasons, tides, astronomical twilight and twilight tables, sun tables

For geodesy, see **526**; physical and dynamic geology, **551**

526 **Mathematical geography**

Including geodesy

.3 **Geodetic surveying**

Surveys in which curvature of the earth is considered in measurement and computation

.8 **Map projections**

Networks of parallel lines and meridians for map drawing

Class printing maps [*formerly* **526.8**] in **655.3**

.9 **Surveying**

Boundary, topographic, hydrographic surveying

Including aerial and terrestrial photogrammetry

Class engineering surveys in **622–628**

For geodetic surveying, see **526.3**; *snow surveys,* **551.5**

527 **Celestial navigation**

Determination of geographic position and direction from observation of celestial bodies

Class practical navigation with the subject

For finding time, see **529**

528 **Ephemerides (Nautical almanacs)**

Class tables of specific celestial bodies in **523**

529 **Chronology**

Intervals of time, calendars, horology (finding and measuring time)

Class extrameridional instruments, sidereal clocks and chronometers in **522**

530   Physics

.01   Philosophy and logic

Class theories in **530.1**

.02–.09   Other standard subdivisions

.1   Theories

.11   Relativity theory

.12   Quantum theory

Matrix, quantum, wave mechanics

Class classical mechanics in **531–533**

.13   Statistical and kinetic theories

Statistical mechanics and quantum statistics

Class classical mechanics in **531–533**

.14   Field theories

Unified and quantum field theories, problem of many bodies

.15   Mathematical physics

.16   Measurement theory

.4   States of matter

Solids (solid-state physics), liquids, gases

Class plasma in **537.1**

▶   **531–538 Classical physics**

531   Mechanics

Energetics, kinematics, dynamics, statics of solids and particles

Including simple machines

For mechanics of fluids, see **532**

.01–.09   Standard subdivisions

Class tables, review, exercise in **531.9**

.9   Tables, review, exercise

532   Mechanics of fluids

> Hydrostatics, hydrodynamics, surface and transport phenomena, other mechanical properties of liquids
>
> *For mechanics of gases, see* **533**

.001–.009   Standard subdivisions

> Class tables, review, exercise in **532.9**

.9   Tables, review, exercise

533   Mechanics of gases

> Statics, dynamics, surface and transport phenomena, other mechanical properties of gases
>
> Including vacuum and vacuum production

.01–.09   Standard subdivisions

> Class tables, review, exercise in **533.9**

.6   Aeromechanics (Aerostatics and aerodynamics)

.9   Tables, review, exercise

534   Sound and related vibrations

> Including generation thru vibration, propagation (transmission), characteristics, measurement, analysis, synthesis of sound waves

.01–.09   Standard subdivisions

> Class tables, review, exercise in **534.9**

.5   Related vibrations

> Subsonic and ultrasonic vibrations

.9   Tables, review, exercise

535   Visible light and paraphotic phenomena

> Former heading: Optics
>
> Including theories, physical and geometrical optics, spectral regions, spectroscopy

     .01–.09   Standard subdivisions

> Do not use for theories
>
> Class tables, review, exercise in **535.9**

     .5   Beams and their modification

> Polarization and amplification
>
> Including amplification by stimulated emission of radiation (lasers)

     .6   Color

     .9   Tables, review, exercise

536   Heat

> Theories, transmission (heat transfer), heat effects, temperature, cryogenics, calorimetry, thermodynamics

     .01–.09   Standard subdivisions

> Do not use for theories
>
> Class tables, review, exercise in **536.9**

     .9   Tables, review, exercise

537   Electricity and electronics

> *For magnetism, see* **538**

     .01–.09   Standard subdivisions

> Class theories in **537.1**; tables, review, exercise in **537.9**

     .1   Theories

> Electromagnetic and corpuscular theories, plasma and plasma dynamics

     .2   Electrostatics

> Charge and potentials, generators, dielectrics

537.5   Electronics

Emission, behavior and effects of electrons in gas and vacuum tubes, photoelectric cells and similiar mediums; spectroscopy, tubes, circuitry of radio waves, microwaves, X rays, gamma rays; electron and ion optics

For semiconductors, see **537.6**

.6   Electric currents

Direct and alternating currents, semiconductors, conductivity, thermoelectricity

For dielectrics, see **537.2**

.9   Tables, review, exercise

538   Magnetism

Magnets, magnetic materials and phenomena, magnetohydrodynamics, geomagnetism and allied phenomena

For atmospheric electricity, see **551.5**

.01–.09   Standard subdivisions

Do not use for theories

Class tables, review, exercise in **537.9**

.9   Tables, review, exercise

539   Modern physics

Molecular, atomic, nuclear physics

Scope: interpretation of structure thru spectroscopy

For electronics, see **537.5**

.01–.09   Standard subdivisions

Class tables, review, exercise in **539.9**

.7   Nuclear physics

Including fundamental radiations, subatomic particles, their acceleration, detection, measurement

---

►   539.75–539.76 Nuclear reactions

539.75   Transmutations

              Natural (radioactive decay) and artificial transmutations

    .76   High-energy reactions

    .762   Fission

    .764   Fusion

    .9   Tables, review, exercise

540   Chemistry and allied sciences

             Do not use standard subdivisions

►   540.1–540.9 Standard subdivisions of chemistry

    .1   Early theories

             Alchemy, phlogiston theory, philosopher's stone, other
             ancient and medieval philosophies

             Class theoretical chemistry in **541**

    .2–.9   Other

             Class apparatus and equipment in **542**

►   541–547 Chemistry

541   Physical and theoretical chemistry

             Systematic application of physical concepts and methods to
             chemical systems

             Class physical and theoretical organic chemistry in **547**

542   Laboratories, apparatus, equipment

             Including general procedures and manipulation of equipment

             Class a specific application with the subject

►   543–545 Analytical chemistry

             Class organic analytical chemistry in **547**

543   General analysis

       Use **543.001–543.009** for standard subdivisions

       For qualitative analysis, see **544**; *quantitative analysis,* **545**

544   Qualitative analysis

       Systematic macro and semiquantitative methods and procedures for detecting and identifying constituents of a substance

       Use **544.001–544.009** for standard subdivisions

545   Quantitative analysis

       Determination of the amount of a constituent in a substance

       Use **545.001–545.009** for standard subdivisions

546   Inorganic chemistry

       Elements and their inorganic compounds

547   Organic chemistry

       General, physical, analytical chemistry of nonpolar compounds

548   Crystallography

       Geometrical, chemical, mathematical, physical, structural, optical

549   Mineralogy

       Occurrence, description, classification, identification of naturally-occurring elements and compounds formed by inorganic processes

       For economic geology, see **553**

     .09   Historical and geographical treatment

       Class geographical distribution of minerals in **549.9**

     .1   Determinative mineralogy

       Determination by location, associations, and physical, chemical, crystallographic properties

       Class determinative mineralogy of specific minerals in **549.2–549.7**

▶ ────────── 549.2–549.7 Specific minerals

549.2 Native elements

   Metals, semimetals, nonmetals

.3 Sulfides, selenides, tellurides, antimonides, sulfosalts

.4 Halides

.5 Oxides

.6 Silicates

.7 Other minerals

   Phosphates, vanadates, arsenates, nitrates, borates, tungstates, molybdates, chromates, sulfates, carbonates

.9 Geographical distribution of minerals

   Add area notations 1–9 to 549.9

550 Earth sciences

551 Physical and dynamic geology

   Scope: geophysics and geochemistry of lithosphere, hydrosphere, atmosphere

   For astronomical geography, see **525**

.1 Gross structure and properties of the earth

   Structure and properties of earth's interior and crust

   For geomagnetism, see **538**

.2 Plutonic phenomena

   Volcanoes, earthquakes, fumaroles, hot springs, geysers

.3 Exogenous processes and their agents

   Erosion, weathering, deposition, sedimentation, transport thru action of ice, water, wind, frost

551.4 **Geomorphology**

Origin, development, transformations of topographic features, e.g., continents, islands, mountains, valleys, caves, plains, oceans, inland waters

Class physical geography [*formerly* **551.4**] in **910**

───────────

► **551.5–551.6 Meteorology, climatology, weather**

.5 **Descriptive and dynamic meteorology**

Physics of atmospheric circulation, temperature, pressure, electricity, moisture

Including snow surveys

[.59] **Climatology and weather**

Class in **551.6**

.6 **Climatology and weather** [*formerly* 551.59]

Weather belts, forecasting, reports, artificial modification and control, microclimatology

.7 **Historical geology (Stratigraphy)**

Do not use standard subdivisions

For paleontology, see **560**

.8 **Structural geology (Tectonophysics)**

Forms, position, deformation of rocks, e.g., stratifications, joints, cleavages, synclines, antisynclines, faults, folds, veins, dikes, necks, bosses, laccoliths, sills

.9 **Geochemistry**

Class chemical analysis of rocks and ores in **543**

552 **Petrology**

Origin, occurrence, constitution, classification of rocks

Use **552.001–552.009** for standard subdivisions

For mineralogy, see **549**; *economic geology,* **553**

553   Economic geology

Quantitative occurrence and distribution of rocks, minerals, other geological materials of economic importance

For a specific aspect of specific geological materials, see the subject, e.g., prospecting 622

▶
554–559 Regional geology

Geology of specific continents, countries, localities

Class a specific geological aspect of a region with the subject

554   Europe

Add area notation 4 to 55, e.g., geology of England **554.2**

555   Asia

Add area notation 5 to 55, e.g., geology of Japan **555.2**

556   Africa

Add area notation 6 to 55, e.g., geology of South Africa **556.8**

557   North America

Add area notation 7 to 55, e.g., geology of Ohio **557.71**

558   South America

Add area notation 8 to 55, e.g., geology of Brazil **558.1**

559   Other parts of world

Add area notation 9 to 55, e.g., geology of Australia **559.4**

560   Paleontology

.1   Philosophy and theory

.17   Stratigraphic paleobotany and paleozoology

Class specific fossils or groups of fossils in **561–569**

.9   Regional and geographical treatment

Divide like **574.9**, e.g., hydrographic paleontology **560.92**

561   Paleobotany

         Descriptive and taxonomic

.09   Historical treatment

         Do not use for regional and geographical treatment

▶   562–569 Taxonomic paleozoology

562   Invertebrate paleozoology

         For Protozoa, Parazoa, Metazoa, see **563**; *Mollusca and molluscoidea,* **564**; *other invertebrates,* **565**

563   Protozoa, Parazoa, Metazoa

         Unicellular animals, sponges, corals, starfishes

564   Mollusca and molluscoidea

         Clams, mussels, oysters, chitons, toothshells, snails, slugs, whelks, octopuses, squids, devilfishes, moss animals, lamp shells

565   Other invertebrates

         Worms, cyclops, fish lice, barnacles, sand fleas, sow bugs, wood lice, sea mantles, squillas, sea onions, lobsters, crabs, shrimps, mites, ticks, spiders, harvestmen, scorpions, millipedes, centipedes, insects

566   Vertebrate paleozoology (Chordata)

         For Anamnia, see **567**; *Sauropsida,* **568**; *Mammalia,* **569**

567   Anamnia (Cyclostomes, fishes, amphibians)

568   Sauropsida (Reptiles and birds)

569   Mammalia (Mammals)

570   **Anthropological and biological sciences**

[571]   Prehistoric archeology

         Class in **913**

572   Human races (Ethnology)

> Origin, distribution, physical characteristics of races
>
> Including causes of racial differences
>
> Class cultural anthropology [*formerly* 572] in 390
>
> > *For ethnopsychology, see* 155.8

.8   Specific races

> Divide like 420–490, e.g., Semitic races 572.892

.9   Races in specific countries

> Add area notations 3–9 to 572.9

573   Somatology (Physical anthropology)

> Including prehistoric man, environmental effects on physique, pigmentation, anthropometry
>
> > *For ethnology, see* 572

.021   Tabulated and related materials

> Class statistical tables in 312

.2   Organic evolution of man

> Heredity and environment (genetics), variation as factors in evolution

574   Biology

> *For botanical sciences, see* 580; *zoological sciences,* **590**; *special biological fields and techniques,* **575–579**

.09   Historical treatment

> Class regional and geographical treatment in 574.9

.1   Physiology

> Circulation, respiration, nutrition, metabolism, secretion, excretion, reproduction, histogenesis, movements, biophysics, biochemistry

.2   Pathology

> Anomalies, malformations, deformations, diseases

574.3	Maturation

Embryology and gametogenesis

For histogenesis, see **574.1**

.4 Morphology and descriptive anatomy

.5 Ecology

Interrelation of organisms to environment and to each other

.6 Economic biology

.8 Histology and cytology

Study of minute structure of tissues, and structure and physiology of cells

For histogenesis, see **574.1**

.9 Regional and geographical treatment

.909 Zonal and physiographic treatment

Class insular biology in **574.91**, hydrographic biology in **574.92**

.91 Insular biology

.92 Hydrographic biology

Including marine biology

.929 Fresh-water biology (Limnetic biology)

.93–.99 Geographical treatment

Add area notations **3–9** to **574.9**

▶ 575–579 Special biological fields and techniques

575 Organic evolution

Origin of species thru historic descent with modification

Including evolution thru sexual selection, evolutionary cycles, origin and evolution of sexes

Class organic evolution of man in **573.2**, of plants in **581**, of animals in **591**

.001–.009 Standard subdivisions

Class theories in **575.01**

575.01   Theories

> Darwinian, neo-Darwinian, orthogenetic, mutation, Lamarckian, neo-Lamarckian theories

.1   Genetics

> Heredity and variation as factors in evolution
>
> *For variation, see* **575.2**

.2   Variation

> Physiological and environmental aspects, hybrids, mutations, sports

576   Microbiology

> Including ultramicrobes (rickettsiae, viruses), microorganisms in relation to immunity and pathogenicity
>
> *For Thallophyta, see* **589**; *Protozoa,* **593**

.1   General principles

> Divide like **574**, e.g., fresh-water microorganisms **576.192 9**

577   General properties of living matter

> Origin and beginnings of life, spontaneous generation, comparison of living and nonliving substances and processes, conditions necessary for life, vitalism versus mechanism, degeneration and death, sex in nature
>
> *For biophysics and biochemistry, see* **574.1**

578   Microscopes and microscopy

> Slide preparation, description and use of microscopes
>
> Class a specific application with the subject

579   Collection and preservation of biological specimens

> Preparation and preservation of skeletons and total specimens, taxidermy, techniques of collecting and transporting, arrangement and maintenance in museums

580   Botanical sciences

For paleobotany, see 561; arrangement in museums, 579

581   Botany

Class specific classes, orders, families in **582–589**

.09   Historical treatment

Class regional and geographical treatment in **581.9**

.1–.9   General principles

Divide like **574.1–574.9**, e.g., plants of United States **581.973**

►   582–589 Taxonomic botany

582   Spermatophyta (Seed-bearing plants)

Use **582.001–582.008** for standard subdivisions

For Angiospermae, see 583–584; Gymnospermae, 585

.1   Special groupings

Class specific classes, orders, families in **583–585**

►   582.13–582.14 Herbaceous plants

Seed plants without persistent woody tissue

.13   Flowering plants

Class here comprehensive works on herbaceous and woody flowering plants

For woody flowering plants, see 582.16–582.18

.14   Shrubs and vines

Succulent, carpet, mat, cushion, bush herbals

▶ 582.16–582.18 Woody plants

Flowering and nonflowering woody plants

582.16 Trees (Dendrology)

.17 Shrubs

.18 Vines

▶ 583–584 Angiospermae (Flowering plants)

Class comprehensive works in **582.13**

583 Dicotyledones (Dicotyledons)

584 Monocotyledones (Monocotyledons)

585 Gymnospermae (Naked-seed plants)

586 Cryptogamia (Seedless plants)

Use **586.001–586.008** for standard subdivisions

For Pteridophyta, see **587**; *Bryophyta,* **588**; *Thallophyta,* **589**

587 Pteridophyta (Vascular cryptogams)

Quillworts, ferns, club mosses, horsetail family

588 Bryophyta

Mosses, liverworts, hornworts

589 Thallophyta

Including lichens, fungi, molds, algae, diatoms, fission plants other than bacteria

.9 Schizomycetes (Bacteriology)

Use **589.900 1 – 589.900 8** for standard subdivisions

590   Zoological sciences

For taxonomic paleozoology, see **562–569**; *arrangement in museums,* **579**

591   Zoology

Class specific classes, orders, families in **592–599**

.09   Historical treatment

Class regional and geographical treatment in **591.9**

.1–.9   General principles

Divide like **574.1–574.9**, e.g., animals of United States **591.973**

For human physiology, see **612**; *human anatomy,* **611**

▶   592–599 Taxonomic zoology

592   Invertebrates

Use **592.001–592.008** for standard subdivisions

For Protozoa, Parazoa, Metazoa, see **593**; *Mollusca and molluscoidea,* **594**; *other invertebrates,* **595**

593   Protozoa, Parazoa, Metazoa

Unicellular animals, sponges, corals, starfishes, hydras, medusas, jellyfishes, sea urchins, sea walnuts, comb jellies, sea cucumbers

594   Mollusca and molluscoidea

Clams, mussels, oysters, shipworms, chitons, tooth shells, snails, slugs, whelks, octopuses, squids, devilfishes, moss animals, lamp shells

595   Other invertebrates

Including worms, cyclops, fish lice, barnacles, sand fleas, sow bugs, wood lice, sea mantles, squillas, sea onions, lobsters, crabs, shrimps, mites, ticks, spiders, harvestmen, scorpions, millipedes, centipedes

595.7	Insecta (Insects)

Use **595.700 1 – 595.700 8** for standard subdivisions

.76	Coleoptera (Beetles)
.77	Diptera and related orders

Midges, gnats, mosquitoes, flies, fleas

.78	Lepidoptera

Moths and butterflies

.79	Hymenoptera

Ants, wasps, bees

596	Chordata (Vertebrates)

Including Tunicata (sea squirts and sea grapes)

Use **596.001–596.008** for standard subdivisions

For Anamnia, see **597**; *reptiles and birds,* **598**; *Mammalia,* **599**

597	Anamnia (Cyclostomes, fishes, amphibians)

Including caecilians, frogs, toads, salamanders, newts, mud puppies

Use **597.001–597.009** for standard subdivisions

.2	Cyclostomata (Lampreys)
.3	Chondrichthyes

Sharks, skates, rays, torpedoes, guitarfishes, sawfishes, chimeras

► 597.4–597.5 Osteichthyes

.4	Actinopterygii and related orders

Bowfins, river dogfishes, ganoids, sturgeons, paddlefishes, spoonbills, lobe-finned fishes, gars, lung fishes

.5	Teleostei

Morays, carps, catfishes, top minnows, sea horses, herrings, salmon, trout, tarpons, snappers, basses, mackerels, pompanos, tunas, swordfishes, other bony fishes

598	Reptiles and birds
.1	Reptilia (Reptiles)

Scope: herpetology

For amphibians, see 597

.11	Lepidosauria

Lizards and tuataras

For Serpentes, see 598.12

.12	Serpentes (Snakes)
.13	Chelonia (Turtles, tortoises)
.14	Crocodilia (Crocodiles, alligators)

.2	Aves (Birds)

For specific orders of birds, see 598.3–598.9

.209	History of ornithology

Class regional and geographical treatment in 598.29

.29	Regional and geographical treatment
.291	Zonal and physiographic treatment
.293–.299	Geographical treatment

Add area notations 3–9 to 598.29

598.3–598.9 Specific orders of birds

.3	Gruiformes and related orders

Cranes, limpkins, rails, gallinules, coots, gulls, skimmers, terns, auks, oyster catchers, plovers, woodcock, sandpipers, curlews, phalaropes, herons, bitterns, egrets, storks, ibises, spoonbills, flamingos

.4	Anseriformes and related orders

Swans, geese, ducks, mergansers, screamers, albatrosses, shearwaters, fulmars, petrels, pelicans, gannets, cormorants, darters, penguins, loons, grebes

.5	Palaeognathae

Ostriches, rheas, cassowaries, emus, kiwis, tinamous

| 598.6 | Galliformes and Columbiformes |
| | Curassows, guans, grouse, quails, pheasants, turkeys, domestic chickens, hoatzins, sand grouse, pigeons, doves |

.7 Psittaciformes, Trogoniformes, Cuculiformes

Parrots, parakeets, macaws, lories, jacamars, puffbirds, honey guides, toucans, woodpeckers, flickers, piculets, trogons, plantain eaters, cuckoos, roadrunners, anis

.8 Passeriformes (Passerine, perching birds)

Flycatchers, larks, swallows, titmice, nuthatches, wrens, mockingbirds, thrushes, wagtails, waxwings, crows, magpies, jays, shrikes, starlings, vireos, blackbirds, tanagers, grosbeaks, finches, sparrows, buntings

.89 Coraciiformes and Apodiformes

Kingfishers, rollers, todies, motmots, bee eaters, hoopoes, hornbills, swifts, hummingbirds

.9 Falconiformes (Birds of prey)

Hawks, falcons, buzzards, vultures, ospreys, eagles, owls, oilbirds, frogmouths, potoos, goatsuckers

599 Mammalia (Mammals)

Use 599.001–599.008 for standard subdivisions

.1 Monotremata

Spiny anteaters, platypuses

.2 Marsupialia

Opossums, opossum rats, kangaroos, marsupial mice, wallabies, bandicoots, phalangers, koalas, wombats

.3 Unguiculata and Glires

Edentates, lagomorphs, rodents, insectivores, dermopterans
For Chiroptera, see **599.4**; *Primates,* **599.8**

.4 Chiroptera (Bats)

599.5   Cetacea and Sirenia

         Whales, dolphins, porpoises, sea cows

    .6   Paenungulata

         Elephants, conies, dassies, hyraxes

         For Sirenia, see **599.5**

    .7   Mesaxonia, Paraxonia, Ferungulata

         Perissodactyls (horses, asses, tapirs, rhinoceroses), artiodactyls (pigs, hippopotamuses, ruminants, camels), carnivores

    .8   Primates

         Lemurs, monkeys, marmosets, tamarins, apes

         For Hominidae, see **599.9**

    .9   Hominidae (Man)

600 Technology (Applied sciences)

601   Philosophy and theory

602   Miscellany

       Class patents and inventions in **608.7**

603   Dictionaries, encyclopedias, concordances

605   Serial publications

606   Organizations

   [.4]   Fairs, expositions, temporary exhibits, competitions

       Class in **607**

607   Study and teaching

       Including fairs, expositions, temporary exhibits, competitions [*all formerly* **606.4**]

   .4–.9   In specific continents, countries, localities

       Add area notations **4–9** to **607**

608   Collections, anthologies, patents, inventions

   .7   Patents and inventions

       Add area notations **1–9** to **608.7**

609   Historical and geographical treatment

610   Medical sciences

   .6   Organizations and professions

   .69   Medical professions

       Physicians, surgeons, medical technicians, physician-patient relationships

       For nursing profession, see **610.73**

610.7   Study, teaching, nursing practice

> Class experimental medicine in **619**

.73   Nursing profession

> Duties and practices of professional and practical nurses, attendants, aides, orderlies

> If preferred, class a specific kind of nursing with the subject, e.g., Red Cross and other public health nursing **614.073**

> *For home nursing, see* **649.8**

611   Human anatomy

> Abnormal, prenatal, microscopic, gross

> Use **611.001–611.009** for standard subdivisions

> *For pathology, see* **616.07**

612   Human physiology

> Functions, biophysics, biochemistry, innervation of human body, its specific systems and organs

> Use **612.001–612.009** for standard subdivisions

> *For pathology, see* **616.07**

.6   Reproductive system and developmental periods

> Use **612.600 1 – 612.600 9** for standard subdivisions

.61   Male reproductive system

.62   Female reproductive system

.63   Pregnancy

> *For embryology, see* **612.64**

.64   Embryology

> Use **612.640 01 – 612.640 09** for standard subdivisions

.65   Child development

.66   Adult development

> From adolescence thru climacteric

> *For aging, see* **612.67**

.67   Aging (Physical gerontology)

613	**General and personal hygiene**

Health and its preservation

For public health, see **614**

.07 **Study and teaching**

Including health education [*formerly also* 371.7]

.1 **Environment and health**

Effects of climate, air, light, temperatures, humidity, air conditioning on health

For housing and health, see **613.5**

.2 **Food and health**

Food programs for general well-being and improved appearance

For beverages and health, see **613.3**

.3 **Beverages and health**

For alcohol, see **613.8**

.4 **Care of person**

Cleanliness and comfort thru bathing and adequate clothing

.5 **Housing and health**

.6 **Health and well-being under unusual conditions**

Industrial hygiene [*formerly* 331.82], self-defense, military and camp hygiene, shipboard hygiene, survival instructions

.7 **Rest, exercise, physical fitness**

Including physical education [*formerly* 371.7]

.8 **Addictions and health**

Habit-forming stimulants and narcotics as factors deleterious to health, e.g., alcohol, opiates, tobacco

613.9   Factors relating to heredity, sex, age

> Including inherited mental and physical disorders

   .94   Eugenic practices

> Sterilization and birth control

   .95   Sex hygiene

   .97   Hygiene for specific age groups

> *For a specific aspect, see the subject, e.g., cleanliness* **613.4**

614   Public health

> Safeguarding public health by registering, certifying, reporting births, deaths, diseases; by inspecting, standardizing, certifying, labeling common commodities; by providing programs for disease control, sanitation and environmental comfort

> Class vital statistics in **312**, forensic medicine in **340**, medical social work in **362**, toxicology in **615.9**

> Class laws, regulations, legal aspects in **340**, public administration aspects in **350** [*both formerly* **614**]

   .07   Study, teaching, nursing practice

   .073   Red Cross and other public health nursing

> (Optional; prefer **610.73**)

   .4   Control of disease

> *For control of specific diseases, see* **614.5**

   .5   Control of specific diseases

> Including control of specific infectious diseases and noncommunicable diseases, e.g., heart diseases, cancer

   .58   Mental hygiene [*formerly* 131.3]

614.8	Accidents and their prevention

Safety thru regulation, inspection, other protective measures

Including first aid

.83	By machinery and hazardous materials

Flammable materials, explosives, fireworks, electrical equipment and appliances, radioactive materials

.84	By fire

.85	In industry [*formerly* 331.82]

615	Therapeutics and pharmacology

Class therapies applied to specific diseases in **616**

.9	Toxicology

Source, composition, physiological effects, tests, antidotes of poisons

Use **615.900 1 – 615.900 9** for standard subdivisions

616	Medicine

Use **610.1–610.9** for standard subdivisions

For specialized medicine, see **617–618**

.01	Medical microbiology

Pathogenic microorganisms and their relation to disease

.07	Pathology

Symptomatology and diagnoses

.08	Psychosomatic medicine

► **616.1–616.8 Diseases of specific systems and organs**

.1	Diseases of cardiovascular system

Diseases of heart, blood vessels, blood

616.2   Diseases of respiratory system

Otorhinolaryngology, diseases of trachea, bronchi, lungs, pleura, mediastinum

Use 616.200 1 – 616.200 9 for standard subdivisions

For otology, see 617

.3   Diseases of digestive tract

Nutritional and metabolic diseases; diseases of mouth, throat, pharynx, esophagus, stomach, intestines, rectum, anus, biliary tract, pancreas, peritoneum

Class laryngology in 616.2

For diseases of endocrine system, see 616.4; *dentistry,* 617

.4   Diseases of blood-forming, lymphatic, endocrine systems

Diseases of spleen, bone marrow, lymphatics, breast, pancreatic internal secretion; of thymus, thyroid, parathyroid, adrenal, pituitary, pineal glands

For diseases of blood, see 616.1; *of urogenital system,* 616.6; *nutritional and metabolic diseases,* 616.3

.5   Diseases of integument, hair, nails (Dermatology)

For allergies, see 616.9

.6   Diseases of urogenital system

Diseases of kidneys, ureters, bladder, urethra, prostate, penis, scrotum, testicles and accessory organs

For gynecology, see 618.1

.7   Diseases of musculoskeletal system

Diseases of bones, joints, muscles, tendons, fasciae, bursae, sheaths of tendons, connective tissue

For nutritional and metabolic diseases, see 616.3

616.8	Diseases of nervous system (Neurology and psychiatry)

Use **616.800 1 – 616.800 9** for standard subdivisions

.801–.809   Standard subdivisions of neurology

►   616.85–616.86 Psychoneuroses

Class comprehensive works in **616.85**

.85   General works

Chorea, hysterias, epilepsy, speech and language disorders, cutaneous sensory disorders, migraine, disorders of personality, character, intellect

.86   Psychoneurotic addictions and intoxications

Alcoholism, metallic intoxications, addictions to narcotics, stimulants, tobacco

.89   Psychiatry

Functional diseases (psychoses) of nervous system, e.g., general paresis, manic-depressive psychoses, paranoia and paranoid conditions, schizophrenia, senile dementias

Including psychoanalysis as therapy [*formerly* 131.34]

Class puerperal psychoses in **618.7**

For psychoneuroses, see **616.85–616.86**

.890 073   Psychiatric nursing

(Optional; prefer **610.73**)

.9   Other diseases

Communicable diseases, allergies and anaphylaxis, diseases due to physical and climatic conditions, rheumatic fever, neoplastic diseases

Use **616.900 1 – 616.900 9** for standard subdivisions

Class communicable diseases predominantly affecting a specific part of the body with the part affected

.907 3   Communicable disease nursing

(Optional; prefer **610.73**)

► ## 617–618 Specialized medicine

For neoplastic diseases, see **616.9**

617 **Surgery**

Orthopedic, systemic, regional, plastic surgery; dentistry, ophthalmology and optometry, otology and audiology

Use **617.001–617.008** for standard subdivisions

618 **Other branches of specialized medicine**

► ## 618.1–618.8 Gynecology and obstetrics

Medical and surgical treatment

.1 **Gynecology**

Class malignant neoplasms of genital tract in **616.9**

.107 3 **Gynecological nursing**

(Optional; prefer **610.73**)

.2 **Obstetrics**

Symptomatology, diagnosis, prenatal care, multiple pregnancy

.207 3 **Obstetrical nursing**

(Optional; prefer **610.73**)

► ## 618.3–618.8 Diseases, disorders, management of pregnancy, parturition, puerperium

.3 **Diseases of pregnancy**

Ectopic pregnancy, fetal abnormalities, abortion, prematurity

.4 **Normal labor (Parturition)**

Mechanism and management of normal labor and childbirth

.5 **Complicated labor (Dystocia)**

.6 **Normal puerperium**

Postpartum management and care

618.7	Puerperal diseases
.8	Obstetrical surgery
.9	Patients by age groups

Class surgical treatment in **617**

.92 Pediatrics

General and specific diseases of children and their treatment

Use **618.920 001 – 618.920 009** for standard subdivisions

.920 007 3 Pediatric nursing

(Optional; prefer **610.73**)

.97 Geriatrics

General and specific diseases of the aged and their treatment

.970 73 Geriatric nursing

(Optional; prefer **610.73**)

619 Comparative and experimental medicine

Study of diseases and their treatment in laboratory animals

For veterinary sciences, see **636.089**

620 Engineering, and allied operations and manufactures

Including fine particle technology, systems engineering

Use **620.001–620.009** for standard subdivisions

▶ 620.1–620.4 Applied mechanics (Engineering mechanics)

For principles of flight, see **629.132**; *automatic control engineering,* **629.8**; *air conditioning engineering,* **697.9**

.1 Engineering materials, properties, tests

Class sound and related vibrations in **620.2**, mechanical vibration in **620.3** [*both formerly* **620.1**]

620.2	Sound and related vibrations [*formerly* 620.1]
	Applied acoustics and ultrasonics
.3	Mechanical vibration [*formerly* 620.1]
	For sound and related vibrations, see **620.2**
.8	Human engineering (Biotechnology)
	Designing for optimum man-machine and man-equipment relationships

621   **Applied physics**

Mechanical, electrical, electronic, electromagnetic, heat, light, nuclear engineering

Use **621.001–621.009** for standard subdivisions

.01–.09   Standard subdivisions of mechanical engineering

Class thermodynamics [*formerly* **621.01**] in **621.4**

▶   621.1–621.2 Fluid-power engineering

For aerodynamics, see **629.132**; *air compression,* **621.5**

.1   Steam

Engines, boilers, locomotives, tractors, rollers, steam generation and transmission, boiler-house practices

.2   Power derived from liquids

Hydraulic-power and other liquid-pressure mechanisms

Use **621.200 1 – 621.200 9** for standard subdivisions

.201–.209   Standard subdivisions of hydraulic power

.3   Electrical, electronic, electromagnetic engineering

Use **621.300 01 – 621.300 09** for standard subdivisions

.301–.309   Standard subdivisions of electrical engineering

621.31	Generation, transmission, modification of electrical energy

Including transformers, condensers, details and parts of generators, control devices at central stations

Class electricity derived from nuclear power in **621.48**, by chemical methods in **621.35**, electric motors as prime movers in **621.4**

.312	Central stations

For dynamoelectric (generating) machinery, see **621.313**

.313	Dynamoelectric (Generating) machinery

Direct-current, alternating-current, synchronous, asynchronous machinery

.319	Transmission
.32	Light and illumination engineering

Illumination systems regardless of source, other branches of light engineering, e.g., lasers

Do not use standard subdivisions

For municipal lighting, see **628**

.320 01–.320 09	Standard subdivisions of illumination engineering
.320 1–.320 9	Standard subdivisions of electric lighting
.33	Traction

Electric-power transmission for railways

Including electrification of railway systems

.35	Applied electrochemistry

Primary and storage batteries, fuel cells

.36	Paraphotic engineering

Infrared and ultraviolet technology

Class heat radiation in **621.4**

.37	Electrical measurements

Meters, instruments, measurement of electric and nonelectric quantities by electrical means

621.38   Electronic and communication engineering

   .381   Electronic engineering

Including microwave, circuit, X-ray, gamma-ray
electronics

Class electroacoustical devices [*formerly* 621.381] in
621.389

For communication engineering, see
621.382–621.389

   .381 7   Miniaturization and microminiaturization

   .381 9   Special developments

Including computers

►   621.382–621.389 Communication engineering

Electrical, electroacoustical, electronic devices

►   621.382–621.383 Wire telegraphy

   .382   Codes, systems, types

Acoustic and automatic systems; printing, writing,
facsimile, submarine cable types

   .383   Specific instruments and apparatus

Keys, transmitters, receivers, calling apparatus, relays,
repeaters, switches, recorders

   .384   Radio- and microwave communication

►   621.384 1 – 621.384 6 Radio

   .384 1   General principles

Including wave propagation and transmission,
circuitry, instruments and apparatus, stations,
manufacture of receiving sets

   .384 19   Special developments

Radio beacons, radio compasses, loran,
telecontrol, space communication

►   621.384 2 – 621.384 3 Radiotelegraphy

621.384 2   Systems, stations, types

             Including radiofacsimile

.384 3   Specific instruments and apparatus

►   621.384 5 – 621.384 6 Radiotelephony

.384 5   Systems, stations, types

.384 6   Specific instruments and apparatus

.384 8   Radar

             General principles, specific instruments and apparatus, systems, stations, scanning patterns, special developments, e.g., racon, shoran

►   621.385–621.387 Wire telephony

.385   Analysis, systems, stations

►   621.386–621.387 Instruments, apparatus, transmission

.386   Terminal instruments and apparatus

.387   Central station equipment and transmission

.388   Television

             Black-and-white and color television

             Including relay and satellite systems; measurements and standardization of impedance, frequency, wavelength, modulation, signal intensity

             Use **621.388 001 – 621.388 009** for standard subdivisions

.388 1   General principles

             Wave propagation and transmission, circuitry, optics

.388 3   Instruments and apparatus

             Transmitters, valves, cameras, antennas, receivers, supplementary instrumentation

621.388 6		Stations
.388 8		Manufacturing and servicing of receiving sets
.388 9		Special developments

Including space communication

.389 Other communication devices

Including electroacoustical devices [*formerly* 621.381], sound recording and reproducing systems [*formerly* 681.8], public address systems, language translators, underwater devices, e.g., projectors, hydrophones, sonar

.39 Other branches of electrical engineering

Including thermoelectricity, rural and household electrification, conduction and induction heating

Class generation and transmission of electricity regardless of method or purpose in **621.31**

.4 Heat and prime movers

Including thermodynamics [*formerly* 621.01], electric motors, external-combustion engines (hot-air engines), air engines (air motors), wind engines

Do not use standard subdivisions

For steam, see **621.1**

.43 Internal-combustion engines

Gas-turbine, spark-ignition, jet, rocket, diesel, semidiesel engines

.47 Solar-energy engineering

Solar engines, batteries, furnaces

.48 Nuclear engineering

Fission and fusion technology, their by-products (radioactive isotopes), treatment and disposal of radioactive waste

621.5   Pneumatic and low-temperature technology

Including air compression, refrigeration, ice manufacture, cryogenic techniques

For fans, blowers, pumps, see **621.6**

.55   Vacuum technology

.6   Mechanical fans, blowers, pumps

Class hydraulic pumps in **621.2**

.7   Factory operations

Automatic factories, machine-shop practice

Class manufacture of a specific product with the subject, machine tools in **621.9**

.8   Mechanical power transmission and related equipment

Mechanisms, transmission elements, materials-handling equipment, fastenings, lubrication

For pneumatic technology, see **621.5**; *power derived from liquids,* **621.2**

.9   Tools

Design, maintenance, repair, operations of machine, pneumatic, hand tools

Use **621.900 1 – 621.900 9** for standard subdivisions

Class special-purpose machinery in **681**

.97   Fastening machinery

Hammers and riveting machinery

622   Mining engineering and operations

Prospecting, surface and underground mining, ancillary equipment and operations, ore dressing, hazards and accidents

623	Military and naval engineering

Planning, structural analysis and design, construction methods, operations; maintenance, repairs

Including fortifications, demolition and defensive operations

.4	Ordnance

Class armored vehicles in **623.7**

.5	Ballistics and gunnery
.6	Transportation facilities

For vehicles, see **623.7**

.7	Other operations

Topography, communication facilities, vehicles, sanitation, power and light systems, camouflage

.8	Naval engineering

Including naval architecture, shipyards

.82	Ships and boats

Construction, maintenance, repairs of sailing craft, small and medium power-driven craft, merchant ships, warships and other government vessels, hand-propelled and towed craft

Do not use standard subdivisions

For parts and details of ships and boats, see **623.84–623.87**

▶ 623.84–623.87 Parts and details of ships and boats

.84	Hull construction
.85	Special systems

Mechanical, electrical, electronic systems for lighting, air conditioning, temperature controls, water supply and sanitation, communication

.86	Equipment and outfit
.87	Power plants (Marine engineering)

Engines, fuels, engine auxiliaries

623.88 **Seamanship**

Art and science of handling ships

.89 **Navigation**

Selection and determination of course thru piloting, dead reckoning, use of electronic and other aids

For celestial navigation, see **527**

624 **Civil engineering**

Planning, structural analysis and design, construction methods, maintenance and repairs of foundations and other supporting structures, tunnels, bridges, roofs

For specific branches of civil engineering, see **625–628**

▶ **625–628 Specific branches of civil engineering**

For vehicles, see **629.1–629.4**

625 **Railroads and their rolling stock, roads and highways**

Planning, structural analysis and design, construction methods, maintenance, repairs

Including special-purpose railways, e.g., roadbeds, tracks and accessories, conveying apparatus, rolling stock of inclined, cable, ship, electric railways, and trolleybuses

.1 **Railroads**

Monorailroads, standard- and narrow-gage railroads

Including model railroads and trains

Do not use standard subdivisions

.2 **Railroad rolling stock**

Running gear, work cars, passenger cars, freight cars, accessory equipment, locomotives, mechanical operation of monorail rolling stock, standard- and narrow-gage railroads

For model trains, see **625.1**

.7 **Roads and highways**

For artificial road surfaces, see **625.8**

625.8   Artificial road surfaces

> Design, construction, materials of vehicular thorofare and pedestrian pavements
>
> Class maintenance and repairs in **625.7**

627   Hydraulic engineering and construction works

> Planning, structural analysis and design, construction methods, maintenance, repairs of inland waterways, harbors, ports, roadsteads, dams and reservoirs, other measures for flood control, land and water reclamation

628   Sanitary and municipal engineering and construction works

> Water supply, sewerage and sewage, garbage and refuse treatment and disposal, air pollution and countermeasures, fire-fighting technology, municipal lighting, insect and rodent extermination

629   Other branches

> Planning, structural analysis and design, construction methods, operations, maintenance, repairs

▶   ———————
629.1–629.4 Vehicles

> Self-propelled conveyances with directional independence
>
> *For ships and boats, see* **623.82**

.1   Flight vehicles and engineering

> *For astronautics, see* **629.4**

.13   Aeronautics

> Do not use standard subdivisions

.132   Principles of flight

> Aerostatics, aerodynamics, navigation, piloting, flight guides, wreckage studies, command systems for guided aircraft

629.133	**Aircraft**

Lighter-than-air and heavier-than-air aircraft, their models

For aircraft details, see **629.134**

.134 **Aircraft details**

For aircraft instruments and equipment, see **629.135**

.135 **Aircraft instruments and equipment**

Instruments for navigation, flight operations, power-plant monitoring; electrical, electronic, other equipment

.136 **Airports**

[.138] **Astronautics**

Class in **629.4**

.2 **Motor land vehicles**

Including design and construction of automobiles, trucks, tractors, trailers, bicycles, motorcycles, and their parts

.22 **Types**

Passenger automobiles, trucks, tractors, trailers, cycles, racing cars, their models

Do not use for specific details

.28 **Tests, operation, maintenance, repairs**

.282 **Tests and related topics**

Road tests, periodic inspection and roadability tests, wreckage studies

---

► **629.283–629.284 Operation**

Methods of driving, factors in safe driving

.283 **Of passenger cars**

.284 **Of other types of motor vehicles**

.3 **Ground-effect machines (Air-cushion vehicles)**

629.4	Astronautics [*formerly* 629.138]
.42	Propulsion systems

Power plants (rockets) and ancillary instrumentation and equipment

.43	Flight of unmanned vehicles
.44	Space stations
.45	Flight of manned vehicles

►

629.46–629.47 Spacecraft

Structural analysis and design, construction methods, maintenance, repairs

For propulsion systems, see **629.42**

.46	Unmanned vehicles

Including expandable space structures

.47	Manned vehicles

Including life-support and ground-support systems

.8	Automatic control engineering

Open-loop and closed-loop (feedback) systems

630 Agriculture and agricultural industries

.1	Philosophy and theory

Including agricultural life

Class scientific aspects in **630.21–630.29**

.2	Miscellany

Class here without further subdivision miscellany provided for in standard subdivisions **021–029**

.21–.29	Scientific aspects

Divide like **510–590**, e.g., agricultural chemistry **630.24**

► ## 631–632 General principles

Class general principles applied to specific crops in **633–635**

631   Farming

[.1]   Business management of farms

      Class in **658**

.2   Farm structures

      Description, maintenance, use and place in farming of farmhouses, barns, granaries, silos, elevators, sheds, fences, walls, hedges, roads, bridges

.3   Farm tools, machinery, appliances

      Description, maintenance (farm mechanics), use and place in farming

      Class uses in a specific operation with the operation

.4   Soil and soil conservation

      For soil improvement, see **631.6–631.8**

[.409]   Historical and geographical treatment

      Do not use

.5   Crop production

► ### 631.6–631.8 Soil improvement

.6   Reclamation and drainage

      For irrigation and water conservation, see **631.7**

.7   Irrigation and water conservation

.8   Fertilizers and soil conditioners

632   Plant injuries, diseases, pests, and their control

─────────────

► **633–635 Production of specific crops**

633   Field crops

> Large-scale production of crops, other than fruit, intended for agricultural purposes and industrial processing
>
> Do not use standard subdivisions

634   Orchards, small fruit, forestry

.9   Forestry

> Formation, maintenance, cultivation, exploitation of forests

635   Garden crops (Horticulture)

> Commercial and home gardening

─────────────

► **635.1–635.8 Vegetables**

> Crops grown primarily for human consumption without intermediate processing other than preservation

.1   Edible roots

> Beets, turnips, carrots, parsnips, radishes, salsify, related crops

.2   Edible tubers and bulbs

> Potatoes, sweet potatoes, yams, Jerusalem artichokes, onions and other alliaceous plants

.3   Asparagus, artichokes, cabbages

.4   Cooking greens and related vegetables

> Spinach, chard, rhubarb
>
> *For cabbages, see* **635.3**

.5   Salad greens

.6   Edible fruits and seeds

> Melons, squashes, pumpkins, cucumbers, tomatoes, green peppers, eggplants, okra, legumes, corn

635.9   Flowers and ornamental plants (Floriculture)

Class flower arrangement [*formerly* 635.9] in 745.92

.93   General and taxonomic groupings

Including annuals, biennials, perennials

.933–.939   By families, genera, species

Divide like 583–589, e.g., dicotyledons 635.933

Class families, genera, species of trees in 635.97

───────────

▶   635.96–635.97 Special groupings

Class specific families, genera, species, other than trees, in 635.933–635.939

.96   By purpose

For flower beds, borders, edgings, ground cover, houseplants, rock gardens, water gardens, wild flower gardens

.97   Other groupings

Everlastings, vines, foliage plants, shrubs, hedges, trees

Including families, genera, species of trees

───────────

▶   636–638 Animal husbandry

Class culture of cold-blooded animals other than insects in 639

636   Livestock and domestic animals

Do not use standard subdivisions

.08   Stock production, maintenance, training

Including fur farming [*formerly* 636.9]

.089   Veterinary sciences

Veterinary anatomy, physiology, hygiene, public health, pharmacology, therapeutics, diseases and their treatment

636.1	**Horses and other equines**
	Including asses, mules, zebras
	Do not use standard subdivisions
.2	**Cattle and other larger ruminants**
	Including zebus, bison, antelopes, water buffaloes, eland, bongos, kudus, gazelles, musk-oxen, deer, elk, moose, reindeer, caribous, giraffes, okapis, camels, llamas, alpacas, vicuñas
	Do not use standard subdivisions
.3	**Sheep and goats (Smaller ruminants)**
	Do not use standard subdivisions
.4	**Swine**
	Do not use standard subdivisions
.5	**Poultry**
	Do not use standard subdivisions
.59	**Other domestic birds**
	Turkeys, guinea fowl, pheasants, peafowl, pigeons, ducks, geese
.6	**Birds other than poultry**
	Plumage, song and ornamental birds
.7	**Dogs**
	Do not use standard subdivisions

► **636.72–636.76 Specific breeds**

Class the miniature of any breed in **636.76**

.72	**Nonsporting dogs**
	Boston terriers, English and French bulldogs, chow chows, Dalmatians, Keeshonden, poodles, schipperkes
	For working dogs, see **636.73**

636.73 **Working dogs**

Alaskan malamutes, boxers, collies, Doberman pinschers, Eskimo dogs, German shepherds, Great Danes, Great Pyrenees, mastiffs, Newfoundlands, Samoyeds, schnauzers, sheepdogs, Siberian huskies, Saint Bernards, Welsh corgis

.75 **Sporting dogs**

Gun dogs, hounds, terriers

For Boston terriers, see **636.72**

.76 **Toy and miniature dogs**

Affenpinschers, Chihuahuas, English toy spaniels, Italian greyhounds, Maltese, Mexican hairless, papillons, Pekingese, Pomeranians, toy poodles, pugs, toy Manchester and Yorkshire terriers

.8 **Cats**

Domestic cats, ocelots, margays, cheetahs

.9 **Other warm-blooded animals**

Monotremes, marsupials, other mammals

Class fur farming [*formerly* **636.9**] in **636.08**

637 **Dairy and related industries**

Milk, butter, cheese, frozen desserts, eggs

638 **Insect culture**

Class culture of invertebrates other than insects [*formerly* **638**] in **639**

639 **Nondomesticated animals**

Hunting, fishing, culture, conservation practices

Including culture of invertebrates other than insects [*formerly* **638**]

Class hunting and fishing as sport in **799**, fur farming in **636.08**, insect culture in **638**

640   Domestic arts and sciences (Home economics)

Care of household, family, person

Class personal hygiene in **613**

.73   Consumer education [*formerly* 339.4]

Selection of consumer goods, guides to quality

Including reports on named products

641   Food and drink

For food service, see **642**

.1   Applied nutrition

Occurrence in food of nutrients required to meet needs of human body

.3   Foods and foodstuffs

Comprehensive works on production, manufacture, preservation, preparation, use

Do not use standard subdivisions

Class food customs in **390**, food supply in **338.1** [*both formerly* **641.3**]

Class production in **630**, manufacture (commercial preparation and preservation) in **663–664**, home preservation and preparation in **641.4–641.8**

► 641.4–641.8 Preservation and preparation

.4   Preservation for later use

Canning, drying, dehydrating, cold storage, deep freezing, brining, pickling, smoking, use of additives

----

► 641.5–641.8 Preparation for proximate use (Cookery)

With and without use of heat

Scope: cookbooks, recipes

| 641.5 | General cookery |
| .59 | Characteristic of specific geographic environments |

Add area notations 3–9 to **641.59**

Class general cookery, noncharacteristic recipes from specific places in **541.5** without subdivision

---

► **641.6–641.8 Special cookery**

Limited by dish, material, process

Observe the following table of precedence, e.g., roasting meats **641.6**

Composite dishes
Specific materials
Specific processes and techniques

| .6 | Specific materials |

Cookery using preserved foods, wines, beers, spirits, fruits, vegetables, meats, dairy products

| .7 | Specific processes and techniques |

Baking, roasting, boiling, simmering, stewing, broiling, grilling, barbecuing, frying, sautéing, braising

| .8 | Composite dishes |

Sauces, relishes, appetizers, savories, stews, meat pies, casserole dishes, salads, sandwiches, sugar products, desserts, beverages

Including bartenders' manuals [*formerly* 663]

| 642 | Food and meal service |

Menus, food services at public and private places, table service and decor

| 643 | The home and its equipment |

Selection, purchase, rental, location, orientation, arrangement, improvement and remodeling

| 644 | Household utilities |

Description, selection, operation, care of systems, appliances, fittings, fixtures, accessories for heating, lighting, ventilation, air conditioning, water supply

645   Household furnishings

Description, selection, installation, use, care, repair of floor, wall, ceiling coverings, of furniture and outdoor furnishings

Class design and decorative treatment of interior furnishings in 747

646   Clothing and care of body

Including selection of clothing and materials

Do not use standard subdivisions

Class fashion [*formerly* 646] in 391

.01–.09   Standard subdivisions of clothing

Use 646.09 for Frigid Zones, cold weather, Tropics, hot weather clothing

.2   Plain sewing

Including mending, darning, reweaving, machine sewing

For clothing construction, see 646.4

.4   Clothing construction

Patternmaking, cutting, fitting, remodeling

Do not use standard subdivisions

For construction of headgear, see 646.5

.5   Construction of headgear

Do not use standard subdivisions

.6   Care of clothing

Including cleaning, dyeing

For mending, see 646.2; *laundering,* 648

.7   Care of body (Toilet)

Hairdressing, facial care, manicuring, pedicuring, barbering, reducing, slenderizing

647   Housekeeping

Private and public households of all types

Class a specific operation with the subject

648	**Household sanitation**

Laundering, housecleaning, control and eradication of pests, storage and preparation for storage

649	**Child rearing and home nursing**

Do not use standard subdivisions

.01–.09   Standard subdivisions of child rearing

▶   649.1–649.7 Child rearing

.1   Care, training, supervision

Including works for expectant parents, baby-sitters

For specific elements of care, training, supervision, see **649.3–649.7**

▶   649.3–649.7 Specific elements of care, training, supervision

.3   Feeding

.4   Clothing and care of body

.5   Supervised activities

Including play with dolls

.6   Manners and habits

Training in toilet, cleanliness, dressing and feeding self, good behavior

.7   Moral, religious, character training

.8   Home nursing

Care of sick and infirm

650   Business and related types of enterprise

Organization, activities, processes, techniques

Do not use standard subdivisions

651   Office services

Organization, equipment, supplies, personnel, operations, records management

Including parish office methods [*formerly* 254]

Class personnel management of office services [*formerly* 651] in 658.3

For accounting procedures, see 657

.7   Communication

Internal and external transmission of oral and written information thru messenger, postal, telecommunication, other systems

Class business writing [*formerly* 651.7] in 808.06

.8   Data processing

652   Writing

Including handwriting

For shorthand, see 653; *calligraphy* (*elegant handwriting*), 741

.3   Typewriting

Do not use standard subdivisions

[.4]   Duplicating

Class in 655.2–655.3

.8   Cryptography

653   Shorthand

655	**Printing and related activities**

Scope: bookmaking and book arts [*both formerly* 002]

Do not use standard subdivisions

.01–.08	**Standard subdivisions of printing**

Class historical and geographical treatment in **655.1**

───────────

▶ 655.1–655.3 Printing

.1	**Historical and geographical treatment**

───────────

▶ 655.2–655.3 Processes

Scope: duplicating [*formerly also* 652.4]

Class processes of specific establishments in **655.1**

.2	**Typography and composition**

For special printing, see **655.3**

.3	**Other**

Mechanical and photomechanical techniques, special printing, e.g., music, Braille and other raised characters

Including maps [*formerly* 526.8]

───────────

▶ 655.4–655.5 Publishing

Production of books, periodicals, newspapers

Class standard subdivisions in **655.4**

Class bookselling (book trade) [*formerly* 655.4–655.5] in **658.8**

For printing, see **655.1–655.3**; *bookbinding,* **655.7**

.4	**Standard subdivisions**
.401–.409	**Specific standard subdivisions**

Class geographical treatment in **655.4** without subdivision

655.5	**Specific elements**

Publishing processes, kinds of publications and publishers

Including music publishing [*formerly* 781]

Class specific establishments in **655.4**, editorial techniques in **808.02**

For journalism, see 070

[.6]	**Copyright**

Class in **340**

.7	**Bookbinding**

657	**Accounting principles and procedures**

Scope: description, use, maintenance of equipment

──────────

► 657.2–657.6 **General principles**

Class general principles applied to accounting for specific kinds of enterprises in **657.8**

.2	**Constructive (Recording, Bookkeeping)**
.3	**Financial (Reporting)**
.4	**Administrative (Analytical)**

Cost analysis and internal auditing

.6	**Public accounting and auditing**
.8	**Accounting for specific kinds of enterprises**

658	**Management**

The executive function of planning, organizing, coordinating, directing, controlling, supervising a project or activity with responsibility for results

Scope: management of real estate business [*formerly* 333.3], of public utility services [*formerly* 380], business management of newspapers and periodicals [*formerly* 070.3], of farms [*formerly* 631.1]

Do not use standard subdivisions

For public administration, see 350

► 658.1–658.8 Specific elements

658.1   Management by control of structure

Thru promotion and organization, legal counsel, financial direction and supervision, intercorporate relations, international operations

.2   Management of plants (Plant engineering)

Management of equipment and facilities

Do not use standard subdivisions

.3   Management of personnel (Personnel management)

Procedure by which employees are hired, managed, replaced

Scope: personnel management of office services [*formerly* 651]

Do not use standard subdivisions

Class managerial personnel policies [*formerly* 658.3] in 658.4

.31   Administration of employment policies

Selection, recruitment, placement, promotion, transfer, termination of service, employer-employee relationships, employee morale

Including in-service training, work schedules [*both formerly* 658.38]

.32   Wage and salary administration

Payroll administration, compensation plans, pensions

Including classification and pay plans, pensions, retirement for library personnel [*formerly also* 023]

.37   Personnel management in specific kinds of enterprises and occupations

For a specific element of personnel management, see the subject, e.g., wage and salary administration 658.32

658.38   Promotion of personnel welfare, satisfaction, efficiency

         Health and safety programs, welfare services, counseling services, educational programs

         Class work schedules, in-service training in **658.31**, internal organization in **658.4** [*all formerly* **658.38**]

.4   Management at executive levels (Executive management)

         Including managerial personnel policies [*formerly* **658.3**], internal organization [*formerly* **658.38**], communication, use of consultants, security

         Do not use standard subdivisions

         Class a specific activity of executive management with the subject

─────────

►   658.42–658.43 Specific levels

.42   Top management

         Direction and control of organization and functions, coordination of interdivisional relationships by senior officers

.43   Middle management

         Direction and control of operations by junior officers

.5   Management of production (Industrial engineering)

         Management of extraction, manufacture, transportation, storage, exchange (procurement and marketing) of goods and services

         Do not use standard subdivisions

         For plant engineering, see **658.2**; *materials control,* **658.7**; *marketing,* **658.8**

.7   Management of materials (Materials control)

         Control of goods used and commodities produced

         For marketing, see **658.8**

658.8		Management of distribution (Marketing)

Of goods and services

Including sales management and promotion techniques, channels of distribution

Scope: bookselling (book trade) [*formerly* **655.4–655.5**]

Do not use standard subdivisions

.83 Market research and analysis

[.830 9] Historical and geographical treatment

Do not use

.85 Personal selling (Salesmanship)

Class personal selling of specific kinds of goods and services in **658.89**

.86 Wholesale marketing

.87 Retail (Consumer) marketing

Do not use standard subdivisions

.88 Credit management

Mercantile and consumer (retail) credit

Including deferred payment plans

.89 Personal selling of specific goods and services

659 Other activities, processes, techniques

.1 Advertising

Promotion of organizations, products, services thru publicity

───────────────

► 659.11–659.17 Specific elements

.11 Organization

Policies, agencies, campaigns

659.13	Visual and audio-visual advertising

Thru newspapers, magazines, direct mail, signs, entertainment, specialty features, e.g., blotters, calendars, programs, novelties

> *For advertising by display of goods and services, see* **659.15**; *broadcast advertising,* **659.14**

.14   Broadcast advertising

.15   Advertising by display of goods and services

Including fashion modeling

.17   Contests and lotteries

.2   Public relations

Promotion of rapport and good will, assessment of public reaction

660   Chemical technology and related industries

Including chemical engineering, applied physical chemistry, industrial microbiology

Do not use standard subdivisions

> *For elastomers and elastomer products, see* **678**

.01–.09   Standard subdivisions of chemical technology

661   Industrial chemicals (Heavy chemicals)

Large-scale production of chemicals used as raw materials or reagents in the manufacture of other products

Including cyclic chemicals [*formerly* **668.7**]

Do not use standard subdivisions

> *For industrial gases, see* **665**

662   Explosives, fuels, and related products

Including fireworks, propellants, detonators, matches, nonfuel carbons

Class fluid fossil fuels in **665**

► ### 663–664 Food and drink

Manufacture (commercial preparation and preservation), packaging of edible products for human and animal consumption

Class comprehensive works in **664**

For dairy and related industries, see **637**

663 ## Drinks, stimulants, their substitutes

Alcoholic and nonalcoholic beverages, stimulants used in preparation of beverages, e.g., coffee, tea, herbals, cocoa, chocolate

Class bartenders' manuals [*formerly* 663] in **641.8**

664 ## Food technology

Do not use standard subdivisions

Class honey in **638**

665 ## Industrial oils, fats, waxes, gases

Nonvolatile, saponifying, lubricating oils, fats, waxes of organic and mineral origin; natural, derived, manufactured gases

Including petroleum

Class beeswax in **638**

666 ## Ceramic and allied industries

Glass, enameling and enamels, pottery, refractories, synthetic minerals, artificial stones, masonry adhesives

667 ## Cleaning, color and related industries

Cleaning and bleaching of textiles, furs, feathers, leather; dyes, pigments, process dyeing and printing, inks, paints, varnishes and allied products, surface finishing

Class a specific application of surface finishing with the subject

For nonfuel carbons, see **662**

668   Other organic products

      Soaps, detergents, wetting agents, glycerin, glues, crude
      gelatin, gums, resins, sealants, plastics, perfumes, cosmetics,
      fertilizers, soil conditioners, pesticides

      Class plastic fibers and fabrics in **677**

        For elastomers, see **678**

[.7]   Cyclic chemicals

      Class in **661**

669   Metallurgy

      Scope: comprehensive works on metals

      Including scrap metals [*formerly* **671.9**]

      Use **669.001–669.009** for standard subdivisions

        For a specific aspect of metals, see the subject, e.g., metal
        manufactures **671**

▶   669.1–669.7 Extractive metallurgy of specific
           metals and their alloys

.1   Ferrous metals

▶   669.2–669.7 Nonferrous metals

      Class comprehensive works in **669.7**

.2   Precious and rare-earth metals

      Gold, silver, platinum, radium, uranium, other rare-earth
      metals

.3   Copper

      Brass, bronze, Muntz metal, gun metal, copper-aluminum
      alloys, copper-beryllium alloys, aluminum bronze

.4   Lead

.5   Zinc and cadmium

.6   Tin

.7   Other

669.8   Metallurgical furnaces

    Operation, maintenance, supplies

  .9   Physical and chemical metallurgy

    Assay practices, physical metallurgy, metallography

▶   **670–680 Manufactures**

670   **Products based on processible materials**

    For chemical technology and related industries, see **660**

671   Metal manufactures

    Fabrication of metals and manufacture of primary products

    Class specific metals in **672–673**

  .2   Foundry practice (Hot-working operations)

  .3   Mechanical working and forming

    Cold-working operations, treatment and hardening, powder metallurgy

  .5   Joining and cutting

    Welding, flame and arc cutting, soldering, brazing, riveting

  .7   Finishing and surface treatment

    Buffing, polishing, coating

  .8   Primary products

    Sheet products, tubes, pipes, wires, cordage, cables, powder products

  [.9]   Scrap metals

    Class in **669**

▶   *672–673* Specific metals manufactures

    Fabrication of specific metals and manufacture of primary products

672   Ferrous metals

673   Nonferrous metals

227

674   Lumber, cork, wood-using industries

         Do not use standard subdivisions

675   Leather and fur industries

         Preliminary tanning, dressing, finishing operations

676   Pulp and paper industries

         Materials, machinery, manufacturing processes, properties, tests, recovery of waste products, primary and converted paper products, final paper and paperboard products

677   Textiles

         Production of fibers, and manufacture of fabrics and cordage

         Including primary products, e.g., carpets, rugs, felt hats, blankets, lap robes, coverlets

         Do not use standard subdivisions

678   Elastomers and elastomer products

         Natural and synthetic rubber and latexes, synthetic rubber and derivatives, elastoplastics

         Including primary products, e.g., tires, overshoes, heels, rubber bands, hose, sheeting

679   Other products

         Including ivory and feather products, brooms, brushes, mops, cigars, cigarettes, products derived from waste materials

         Class products manufactured from a specific waste material with the subject

680   **Handcrafted, assembled, final products**

         Class final paper and paperboard products in **676**, rubber products in **678**, other products based on processible materials in **679**

681   Precision mechanisms and related machines

         Measuring instruments, cameras, business machines, printing and duplicating machines, timepieces, optical devices, conventional and mechanical musical instruments and devices

         Class hand construction of musical instruments in **786–789**

[681.8] Sound recording and reproducing systems

Class in **621.389**

682 Small forge work (Blacksmithing)

Horseshoeing, production of hand-forged tools and ironwork

683 Hardware

Locksmithing, gunsmithing, manufacture of household appliances

Class refrigerators and freezers in **621.5**

For heating, ventilating, air conditioning equipment, see **697**

684 Furnishings and wheeled supports

Do not use standard subdivisions

▶ 684.08–684.09 Home (Amateur) workshops

.08 Woodworking
.09 Metalworking
.1 Furniture

Do not use standard subdivisions

.3 Fabric furnishings

Draperies, hangings, slip covers, curtains

For carpets and rugs, see **677**

.7 Carriages, wagons, carts, wheelbarrows

For motor land vehicles, see **629.2**

685 Leather goods and their substitutes

Saddlery, harness making, leather and fur clothing, footwear, gloves, mittens, travel and camping equipment

For overshoes, see **678**

687 Clothing

For leather and fur clothing, see **685**

688   Other final products

Including models, costume jewelry, smokers' supplies, accessories for personal grooming

Class engineering models in **620**

For brushes, see **679**; *cosmetics,* **668**

.7   Recreational equipment

Toys, equipment for games and sports

For leather goods and their substitutes, see **685**; *motor land vehicles,* **629.2**

690   **Buildings**

Planning, structural analysis and design, construction methods, maintenance, repairs of habitable structures and their interior accessories

Use **690.01–690.09** for standard subdivisions

Class creative design and construction in **721**

.5–.8   Specific types of habitable structures

Divide like **725–728**, e.g., ranch houses **690.86**

Class forts and fortresses in **623**, trailers in **629.22**

691   Materials

Selection, preservation, construction properties of timber, natural and artificial stones, ceramic and clay materials, masonry adhesives, glass, structural metals, plastics, insulating materials, prefabricated housing materials, adhesives and sealants

692   Construction practices

Interpretation and use of architects' drawings for construction purposes, construction specifications, contracting, estimates of materials and time

Class drawing of plans [*formerly* **692**] in **720**

Class building laws in **340**, local government regulation in **352**

693   Systems of construction
             For materials, see **691**

             ———————

             ▶   693.1–693.3 Solid block masonry

      .1   Stone

      .2   Stabilized earth
             Brick, adobe, pisé, cob, tapia, tabby

      .3   Tile and terra cotta

      .4   Hollow block masonry
             Concrete block, cinder block, hollow tile, hollow brick

      .5   Solid concrete construction
             Poured, precast, prestressed

      .6   Plaster-, stucco-, lathwork
             Internal and external application

      .7   Metal construction

      .8   Resistant construction
             To fire, shock, pests, lightning, water, moisture, heat, sound

      .9   Construction in other materials
             Including ice, snow, sandwich panels, glass, prefabricated
             materials
             For wood construction, see **694**

694   Wood construction (Structural woodworking)
             Including planning, structural analysis and design
             Do not use standard subdivisions

   .01–.09   Standard subdivisions of carpentry

▶ **694.2–694.6 Carpentry**
For roofs, see **624**

694.2   Rough carpentry (Framing)

.6   Finish carpentry (Joinery)
Construction of details

695   Roofing, auxiliary structures, and their materials
Covering, maintaining, repairing roofs; installing, maintaining, repairing gutters, flashings, other weatherings

▶ **696–697 Utilities**
For household electrification, see **621.39**

696   Plumbing, pipe fitting, heating, ventilating
Design, installation, maintenance, repairs
Do not use standard subdivisions
Class heating and ventilating in **697**

697   Heating, ventilating, air conditioning engineering
Principles, systems, equipment, installation, maintenance, repairs
Do not use standard subdivisions

▶ **697.1–697.2 Local heating**
For chimneys and flues, see **697.8**

.1   With open fires (Radiative heating)
Including fireplaces, braziers

.2   With space heaters (Convective heating)

▶ ## 697.3–697.7 Central heating

For chimneys and flues, see **697.8**

697.3   Warm-air heating

.4   Hot-water heating

.5   Steam heating

         Including district heating

         Do not use standard subdivisions

.7   Other methods

         Including radiant-panel, solar, nuclear heating

.8   Chimneys and flues

.9   Ventilation and air conditioning

698   Detail finishing

         Application and installation of decorative and protective coatings and coverings

.1   Painting

         Exteriors and interiors

         For painting woodwork, see **698.3**

.2   Calcimining and whitewashing

.3   Finishing woodwork

         By staining, polishing, varnishing, lackering, painting

.5   Glazing and leading windows

.6   Paperhanging

.9   Floor coverings

         Measuring, cutting, laying linoleum, tiles, carpeting

700   The arts

Description and critical appraisal, materials and techniques of the fine, decorative, graphic, performing, recreational arts

Use 700.1–700.9 for standard subdivisions

For literature, see 800

▶   701–709 Standard subdivisions of fine arts

701   Philosophy and theory

.1   Nature and character

.15   Psychology

Including fine arts as products of creative imagination

.17   Esthetics

.18   Criticism and appreciation

Theory and technique, history

Including criticism and appreciation thru use of audio-visual aids

Class works of critical appraisal in **709**, audio-visual treatment of art in **702**

.8   Techniques

Composition, color, decoration, perspective, use of models

Class research methodology in **701.9**

For description, critical appraisal of artists, see **709**

.9   Research methodology

Class psychological aspects in **701.15**

702   Miscellany

Class techniques in **701.8**

703   Dictionaries, encyclopedias, concordances

704   **Persons occupied with art, collections and anthologies, iconography**

> Class development, description, critical appraisal, collections of works, biographical treatment of artists in **709**; art dealers in **706**

.9   **Collections, anthologies, iconography**

.94   **Iconography**

> Development, description, critical appraisal, collections of works
>
> Including human figures and their parts, natural scenes, still life, architectural subjects, symbolism and allegory

.945   **Abstractions**

.947   **Mythology and legend**

.948   **Religion and religious symbolism**

> *For mythology, see* **704.947**

705   **Serial publications**

706   **Organizations**

707   **Study and teaching**

> Class museums and permanent exhibits in **708**

708   **Galleries, museums, private collections**

> Including museum economy
>
> Do not use standard subdivisions
>
> Class collections and anthologies of writings in **704.9**, temporary and traveling exhibits in **707.4**

▶   **708.1–708.9 Treatment by continent, country, locality**

> Scope: guidebooks, catalogs of specific galleries, museums, private collections

.1   **In North America**

> Class galleries, museums, private collections in Middle America in **708.972**

.11   **Canada**

708.13–.19   United States

> Divide like area notations **73–79**, e.g., galleries, museums, private collections in Pennsylvania **708.148**

.2–.8   In Europe

> Divide like area notations **42–48**, e.g., galleries, museums, private collections in England **708.2**
>
> Class galleries, museums, private collections in countries not provided for in area notations **42–48** in **708.94**

.9   In other countries

> Add area notations **3–9** to **708.9**

709   Historical and geographical treatment

> Development, description, critical appraisal, collections of works, biographical treatment of artists

▶   709.01–709.04 Periods of development

.01   Primitive peoples and ancient times

.02   500–1500

> Including art of 15th century [*formerly* **709.03**]

.03   1500–1900

> Class art of 15th century [*formerly* **709.03**] in **709.02**

.04   1900–

.3–.9   Geographical treatment

710   **Civic and landscape art**

711   Area planning (Civic art)

> Design of physical environment for public welfare, convenience, pleasure on international, national, regional, local level
>
> *For landscape design, see* **712**

712   Landscape design (Landscape architecture)

Landscaping public, private, semiprivate, institutional parks and grounds

For specific elements in landscape design, see 714–717; design of trafficways, 713; of cemeteries, 718

713   Landscape design of trafficways

▶   714–717 Specific elements in landscape design

714   Water features

Natural and artificial pools, fountains, cascades

715   Woody plants

Nonflowering and flowering

716   Herbaceous plants

Nonflowering and flowering

Class here comprehensive works on herbaceous and woody flowering plants

For woody flowering plants, see 715

717   Structures

Relationship of buildings, terraces, fences, gates, steps, ornamental accessories to other elements of landscape design

718   Landscape design of cemeteries

719   Natural landscapes

Including public parks and natural monuments, wildlife reserves, forest and water-supply reserves

720   **Architecture**

Including drawing of plans [*formerly also* 692]

.9   Historical and geographical treatment

[.901–.904]   Periods of development

Do not use; class in 722–724

[720.93]   In the ancient world

Do not use; class in 722

721   Architectural construction

Comprehensive works on design and construction of structural elements, e.g., foundations, walls, columns, arches, vaults, domes, roofs, floors, ceilings, doors, windows, stairs, balustrades

For design of structural elements, see 729; building construction, 690; specific types of structures, 725–728

▶   722–724 Periods of development

Chronological development of architectural styles

Class development of specific types of structures in 725–728

For architectual construction, see 721; design and decoration of structures, 729

722   Ancient period to ca. 300

Oriental, classical, pre-Columbian American architectures

723   Medieval period, ca. 300–1400

Early Christian, Byzantine, Saracenic, Romanesque, Norman, Gothic architectures, not limited geographically

724   Modern period, 1400–

Not limited geographically

Including Renaissance, classical revival, Gothic revival, Renaissance revival, neoclassical, Swiss timber and half timber, Romanesque revival architectures

.9   20th century architecture

▶   725–728 Specific types of structures

Comprehensive works on design and construction

Scope: specific structures

For building construction, see 690

725   Public structures

Government, military, commercial, transportation, storage, industrial, welfare, health, recreational, prison, reformatory, exhibition, memorial buildings; arches, gateways, walls, towers, bridges, tunnels, moats, vehicles

Including morgues and crematories [*both formerly* 726.8]

726   Buildings for religious purposes

Including temples, shrines, mosques, minarets, synagogues, parish houses, baptistries, churches, cathedrals, Sunday school buildings, monastic buildings, mortuary chapels, tombs, parsonages, missions

[.8]   Morgues and crematories

Class in 725

727   Buildings for educational and research purposes

Library, school, university, college, laboratory, botanical and zoological garden, observatory, museum, art gallery, community center, learned society buildings

728   Residential buildings

Not used primarily for public, religious, educational, research purposes

Including temporary buildings, multiple dwellings (other than hotels, motels, row houses), club houses, resort dwellings, accessory domestic structures, e.g., gatehouses, garages, conservatories, farm buildings

.3   Houses of urban type

Row and duplex houses, separate houses of two or more stories

For large and elaborate dwellings, see 728.8

.5   Hotels and motels

.6   Dwellings of suburban and rural types

Cottages, bungalows, ranch and split-level houses, farmhouses, solar houses

For large and elaborate dwellings, see 728.8

728.8   Large and elaborate dwellings

> Castles, palaces, chateaux, mansions, manor houses, villas

729   Design and decoration of structures and accessories

> Design in vertical and horizontal planes; design and decoration of structural elements, e.g., foundations, walls, columns, arches, vaults, domes, roofs, floors, ceilings, doors, windows, stairs, balustrades; decoration in specific mediums; built-in ecclesiastical furniture
>
> *For specific types of structures, see 725–728; interior decoration, 747*

730   Sculpture and the plastic arts

> Do not use standard subdivisions

> ▶   730.1–730.9 Standard subdivisions of sculpture

.1   Philosophy and theory

.2   Miscellany

> Class techniques, apparatus, equipment in 731.3–731.4

.3–.8   Dictionaries, serial publications, organizations, study and teaching, collections

.9   Historical and geographical treatment

> Class geographical treatment of sculpture of primitive peoples [*formerly* 730.9] in 732

[.901–.904]   Periods of development

> Do not use; class in 732–735

[.93]   In the ancient world

> Do not use; class in 732–733

▶

731–735 Sculpture

Fine art of producing figures and designs in relief or the round by fashioning in plastic and rigid materials

731 Processes and representations

Including composition, materials

Class individual sculptors in **730.9**

.3 Equipment

Tools, machines, accessories

For techniques, see **731.4**

.4 Techniques

Modeling, molding, casting, carving, firing and baking, restoration

▶

731.5–731.8 Representations

Development, description, critical appraisal, collections of works

.5 Styles and forms

Idealistic, naturalistic, realistic, grotesque styles; forms in relief, as mobiles and stabiles

For sculpture in the round, see **731.7**; *iconography,* **731.8**

.7 Sculpture in the round

Garden sculpture and fountains, vases, urns, busts, masks, monuments

For iconography, see **731.8**

.8 Iconography

Portrayal of specific subjects

▶ 732–735 **Periods of development**

Chronological development of sculptural styles

▶ 732–733 **Sculpture of primitive peoples and ancient world**

732 Nonclassical

Including geographical treatment of sculpture of primitive peoples [*formerly* 730.9]

733 Classical

Greek (Hellenic), Roman, Etruscan

Class sculpture of Greek Archipelago in 732

734 Medieval period, ca. 500–1400

Early Christian, Byzantine, Romanesque, Gothic styles not limited geographically

735 Modern period, 1400–

Not limited geographically

▶ 736–739 **Other plastic arts**

Processes and products

For decorative and minor arts, see **745–749**

736 Carving and carvings

Including paper cutting and folding

Class seals, stamps, signets [*all formerly* 736] in 737

737 Numismatics

Including seals, stamps, signets [*all formerly* 736], medals, talismans, amulets, counters, tokens, jettons

.4 Coins

.49 Of specific countries

Add area notations 3–9 to 937.49

738	Ceramic arts

Class ceramic sculpture in **731–735**

For glass, see **748**

738.1–738.3 Pottery

.1	Processes

Materials, equipment, techniques, decorative treatments

.2	Porcelain (China)
.3	Earthenware and stoneware
.4	Enameling and enamels

Cloisonné, champlevé, basse-taille, surface-painted enamels

Class a specific application of enameling with the subject, e.g., nielloing **739**

.5	Mosaic ornaments and jewelry
.6	Ornamental bricks and tiles
.8	Other products

Lighting fixtures, candlesticks, stoves, braziers, figurines

739	Art metalwork

Decorative metallic forms other than sculpture

Including work in iron, steel, copper, bronze, brass, tin, pewter, nickel, aluminum, chromium

For numismatics, see **737**

.02	Miscellany

Do not use for techniques, apparatus, equipment

.2	Work in precious metals

Including goldsmithing, silversmithing, platinumwork

For watch- and clockcases, see **739.3**

.27	Jewelry

For mosaic ornaments and jewelry, see **738.5**

.3	Watch- and clockcases
.7	Arms and armor

740 Drawing and decorative arts

Do not use standard subdivisions

.1–.9 Standard subdivisions of drawing and drawings

Class techniques in **741.4**

▶ **741–744 Drawing and drawings**

741 Freehand drawing and drawings

Scope: calligraphy (elegant handwriting), artistic lettering

For freehand drawing and drawings by subject, see **743**

.02 Miscellany

Class technique, apparatus, equipment in **741.2–741.4**

.09 Historical and geographical treatment

Class historical and geographical treatment of collections of drawings in **741.9**

.2 Drawing in specific mediums

Materials, equipment, processes

For drawing for specific purposes, see **741.5–741.7**

.4 Drawing processes

Composition, techniques

For perspective, see **742**; *drawing in specific mediums,* **741.2**; *for specific purposes,* **741.5–741.7**

▶ **741.5–741.7 Drawing and drawings for specific purposes**

Mediums and processes

.5 Cartoons, caricatures, comics

Including materials and methods of drawing animated cartoons

.59 Collections

.593–.599 Geographical treatment

Add area notations 3–9 to **741.59**

741.6	Illustration (Commercial art)

.64   Books

Including book jackets, children's books

.65   Magazines and newspapers

.67   Advertisements and posters

Including fashion drawing

.68   Calendars, greeting and postal cards

.7   Silhouettes

.9   Collections of drawings

Regardless of medium or process

For collections of cartoons, caricatures, comics, see **741.59**

742   Perspective

Theories, principles, methods

For techniques of drawing specific subjects, see **743**

743   Freehand drawing and drawings by subject

Including techniques of drawing specific subjects

744   Technical drawing

.4   Drafting procedures and conventions

Engineering, mechanical, architectural, map drawing; production illustration, lettering, titling, dimensioning, shades, shadows, projections

For perspective, see **742**

.5   Preparation and reading of copies

Blueprints, photostats

For blueprinting process, see **772**; *production of photostats,* **778.1**

► ## 745–749 Decorative and minor arts

Processes and products not provided for in **736–739**

Class comprehensive works in **745**

745   Design and crafts

Do not use standard subdivisions

.1   Antiques

Class a specific form of antiques with the subject

► ## 745.2–745.4 Design

.2   Industrial art and design

Creative design of mass-produced commodities

.4   Pure and applied design and decoration

For industrial design, see **745.2**; *design in a specific art form, the form, e.g., design in architecture* **729**

[.409]   Historical and geographical treatment

Do not use

► ## 745.5–745.9 Crafts

Scope: folk art

.5   Handicrafts

Creative work done by hand with aid of simple tools or machines

► ## 745.51–745.57 In specific materials

For textile handicrafts, see **746**

.51   Woods

Marquetry, inlay trim, ornamental woodwork

For ornamental woodwork in furniture, see **749**

.53   Leathers and furs

745.54	Papers

End papers, gift wrappings, wallpaper

.55	Shells
.56	Metals
.57	Rubber and plastics
.59	Making specific objects

Handicrafts in composite materials

Including decorations for special occasions, artificial flowers, lampshades, candlesticks, toys

.6	Lettering, illumination, heraldic design
.7	Decorative coloring

Painting, lackering, japanning, stenciling, decalcomania, tolecraft

For printing, painting, dyeing textiles, see **746.6**

.8	Panoramas, cycloramas, dioramas
.9	Other decorative arts and crafts
.92	Floral arts

Selection and arrangement of plant materials and appropriate accessories

Including flower arrangement [*formerly* **635.9**]

746	Textile handicrafts
1	Weaving

For tapestry making, see **746.3**; *rug- and carpetmaking,* **746.7**

.2	Making laces and related fabrics

Needlepoint, bobbin, darned laces; passementerie

For knitting, crocheting, tatting, see **746.4**

.3	Tapestry making
[.309]	Historical and geographical treatment

Do not use

746.4	Other textile crafts

Braiding, matting, basketry, knitting, crocheting, tatting, embroidery, patchwork, quilting

For rug- and carpetmaking, see **746.7**

.5	Beadwork
.6	Printing, painting, dyeing

Block and silk-screen printing, resist-dyeing, hand decoration, stenciling

.7	Rug- and carpetmaking
[.709]	Historical and geographical treatment

Do not use

.9	Costume [*formerly* 391]
747	Interior decoration

Design and decorative treatment of interior furnishings

Including decoration of specific elements, e.g., ceilings, walls, doors, windows, floors; draperies and upholstery; decoration of specific rooms of residential and other types of buildings, for specific occasions

For furniture and accessories, see **749**

[.09]	Historical and geographical treatment

Do not use; class in 747.2

.2	Historical and geographical treatment

▶ 747.201–747.204 Historical treatment

Periods of development not limited geographically

.201	Ancient period to ca. 500 A.D.
.202	Medieval period, ca. 500–1400
.203	Renaissance period, 1400–1800
.204	Modern period, 1800–
.21–.29	Geographical treatment

Divide like 708.1–708.9, e.g., interior decoration in Pennsylvania 747.214 8

748   Glass

Including methods of decoration, specific articles other than
glassware

.2   Glassware

Blown, prest, molded, cast, decorated products other than
stained glass

[.209]   Historical and geographical treatment

Do not use

.5   Stained, painted, leaded, mosaic glass

[.509]   Historical and geographical treatment

Do not use

749   Furniture and accessories

Including built-in furniture, specific kinds of furniture,
ornamental woodwork, heating and lighting fixtures, wall
decorations

For upholstery, see 747

[.09]   Historical and geographical treatment

Do not use; class in 749.2

.2   Historical and geographical treatment

Scope: antiques and reproductions

.201–.204   Historical treatment

Divide like 747.201–747.204, e.g., Renaissance period
749.203

.21–.29   Geographical treatment

Divide like 708.1–708.9, e.g., French furniture 749.24

750   Painting and paintings

For commercial art, see 741.6; painting in a specific decorative art, the subject, e.g., painting textiles 746.6

.2   Miscellany

Class techniques, apparatus, equipment in 751.3–751.4

[.9]   Historical and geographical treatment

Do not use; class in 759

751   Processes and forms

Class individual painters in 759.1–759.9

▶   751.2–751.6 Processes

.2   Materials

Surfaces, pigments, mediums, fixatives, coatings

For techniques, see 751.4

.3   Equipment

Models, tools, accessories

For techniques, see 751.4

.4   Techniques

Painting with specific mediums

Class pastel in 741.2

.5   Reproduction and copying

Including forgeries, alterations, expertizing, determination of authenticity

For print making and prints, see 761–769

.6   Care, preservation, restoration

.7   Specific forms

Easel paintings, murals, panoramas, cycloramas, dioramas, theatrical scenery, miniatures

For specific subjects, see 753–758

752   Color theory and practice
       Including color symbolism

▶   753–758 Specific subjects
           Class individual painters in **759.1–759.9**

753   Abstractions, symbolism, mythology
       For religious symbolism, see **755**

754   Subjects of everyday life (Genre paintings)

755   Religion and religious symbolism

756   Historical events
       Battles, coronations, disasters

757   Human figures and their parts
       Not provided for in **753–756, 758**

758   Other subjects
       Landscapes, still life, marine scenes, animal and plant life,
       industrial and technical subjects, architectural subjects

759   Historical and geographical treatment

▶   759.01–759.06 Periods of development
           Not limited geographically

.01   Primitive peoples and ancient times
       Including geographical treatment of paintings of primitive
       peoples [*formerly* **759.1–759.9**]

.02   Medieval period, ca. 500–1400
.03   1400–1600
.04   1600–1800
.05   1800–1900
.06   1900–

▶
759.1–759.9 Geographical treatment

Scope: individual painters regardless of process, form, subject

Class geographical treatment of paintings of primitive peoples [*formerly* 759.1–759.9] in 759.01

759.1 North America

Class painting and paintings of Middle America in 759.972

.11 Canada

.13 United States

Class comprehensive works on painting and paintings of specific states in 759.14–759.19

.14–.19 Specific states of United States

Divide like area notations 74–79, e.g., painting and paintings of California 759.194

Class individual painters in 759.13, painting and paintings of Hawaii in 759.996 9

.2–.8 Europe

Divide like area notations 42–48, e.g., painting and paintings of Wales [*formerly* 759.9] 759.29

Class painting and paintings of countries not provided for in area notations 42–48 in 759.94

.9 Other parts of world

Add area notations 3–9 to 759.9

Class painting and paintings of Wales [*formerly* 759.9] in 759.29

760 Graphic arts

Do not use standard subdivisions

For drawing and drawings, see 741–744; painting and paintings, 750; photography and photographs, 770

.1–.8 Standard subdivisions of print making and prints

[760.9] Historical and geographical treatment of print making and prints

> Do not use; class in **769**

▶ 761–769 Print making and prints

▶ 761–767 Print making

761 Relief processes (Block printing)

> Printing from raised surfaces

763 Lithographic (Planographic) processes

> Printing from flat surfaces
>
> *For chromolithography, see* **764**

764 Chromolithography and serigraphy

▶ 765–767 Intaglio processes

> Printing from incised surfaces

765 Metal engraving

> Class here comprehensive works on metal relief and metal intaglio processes
>
> Including line, stipple, criblé engraving
>
> *For relief processes, see* **761**; *mezzotinting and aquatinting,* **766**; *etching and drypoint,* **767**

766 Mezzotinting, aquatinting, related processes

> Including composite processes

767 Etching and drypoint

769 Prints

> Description, critical appraisal, collections regardless of process
>
> Including postage stamps (philately [*formerly* **383.2**]), paper money, other special forms

770 Photography and photographs

.1 Philosophy and theory

Class chemical aspects in **771**

.2 Miscellany

.28 Techniques

Including reversing negatives, recovery of waste materials, preservation of negatives, transparencies, positives

Class equipment in **771**

.282 Camera use

Loading, focusing, exposure, plate and film removal

────────────

► 770.283–770.284 Darkroom practice

.283 Preparation of negatives

Developing, desensitizing, reducing, intensifying, rinsing, fixing, washing, drying exposed plates, films, paper

.284 Preparation of positives (Contact printing)

Exposing, developing, rinsing, fixing, washing, drying, retouching, toning, coloring, mounting

771 Equipment, supplies, chemistry

Class here comprehensive works on use and manufacture

Including studios, laboratories, darkrooms, furniture, fittings, developing and printing apparatus, chemical supplies, sensitometry

Class equipment and supplies used in special processes in **772–773**, in specific fields of photography in **778**, manufacture of a specific kind of equipment or supplies with the subject, e.g., of cameras **681**

.3 Cameras and accessories

► ## 772–773 Special processes

Equipment, supplies, methods

For processing techniques in color photography, see 778.6; photomechanical printing techniques, 655.3

772 ## Metallic salt processes

Blueprinting (cyanotype), direct positive and printing-out, platinotype processes

773 ## Pigment processes of printing

Carbon, carbro, powder (dusting-on), imbibition, gumbichromate, diazotype, photoceramic, photoenamel, oil processes

778 ## Specific fields of photography

Methods; comprehensive works on use and manufacture of equipment and supplies

Class manufacture of a specific kind of equipment or supplies with the subject, e.g., of cameras **681**

.1 ### Photoduplication (Photocopying)

Of photographs, sketches, paintings, drawings, documents, other printed and written matter thru production of facsimiles, photostats, projected prints

*For microphotography, see **778.3**; blueprinting process, **772***

.2 ### Photographic projection

Filmstrips and filmslides

*For stereoscopic projection, see **778.4**; motion-picture projection, **778.5***

.3 ### Scientific and technological applications

Photomicrography and microphotography in black-and-white and color, telephotography, radiography (X-ray photography), infrared, close-up, panoramic, aerial and space, high-speed photography

Class a specific application with the subject

*For photogrammetry, see **526.9***

778.4	Stereoscopic photography and projection

Production of effects of binocular vision

For stereoscopic motion-picture photography, see **778.5**

.5 Motion pictures

Photography (cinematography), editing, projection, photomicrography, preservation and storage of films, stereoscopic motion pictures

.6 Color photography and photography of colors

Orthochromatic and panchromatic photography, direct and indirect processing techniques in color photography

Class color motion-picture photography in **778.5**, color photomicrography and microphotography in **778.3**

.7 Photography under specific conditions

Outdoors, indoors, under water, under extreme climatic conditions

.8 Trick photography

Including tabletop photography; photography of specters, distortions, multiple images; silhouette photography

.9 Photography of specific subjects

Class photography of specific subjects by specific methods in **778.1–778.8**

779 Collections of photographs

780 **Music**

If preferred, distinguish scores and parts by prefixing **M** to number for treatises, e.g., scores and parts for string instruments **M787**

▶ 780.07–781.9 General works

Scope: instrumental music

.07 Music and society

Musicians, critics, musicologists, amateurs, support and regulation

780.1	Philosophy and esthetics

Class general principles ("theory of music") in **781**

.15	Criticism and appreciation

Analytical guides and program notes

Class scientific aspects in **781.1**

.2	Miscellany

Class techniques, apparatus, equipment in **781**

.7	Study, teaching, performances
.73	Performances

Concerts and recitals

781	General principles ("Theory of music") and techniques

Class principles and techniques of dramatic music in **782**, of sacred music in **783**, of music for specific mediums in **784–789**

Class music publishing [*formerly* 781] in **655.5**

.1	Scientific aspects

Mathematical, physical, physiological, psychological aspects

For musical sound, see **781.2**

.2	Basic considerations

Musical sound, nomenclature and systems of terms, notation

For musical structure, see **781.3–781.4**

▶ 781.3–781.4 Musical structure

For musical forms, see **781.5**

.3	Harmony
.4	Melody and counterpoint

Including canon and fugue

.5	Musical forms

Sonata, dance music, program music, jazz and related forms

For canon and fugue, see **781.4**

781.6	Composition and performance

For musical structure, see **781.3–781.4**

.7	Music of ethnic and national orientation

Class geographical treatment of music in **780.93–780.99**

.9	Other topics

Musical instruments, words to be sung or recited with music, bibliographies and catalogs of scores and parts

Class bibliographies of treatises on music in **016.78**, catalogs and lists of recordings in **789.9**

782	Dramatic music and production of musical drama
.1	Opera

Grand, comic, satiric, chamber

.12	Librettos
.13	Stories, plots, analyses
.15	Scores and parts

.8	Theater music

Operettas, musical comedies, revues, secular cantatas and oratorios, incidental dramatic music; film, radio, television music

.9	Other forms of dramatic music

Including music for pantomimes, masks, pageants, ballets

783	Sacred music

Music composed for public and private worship or dedicated to a religious purpose

.1	Instrumental music

Treatises on instrumental music and instrumental accompaniment to vocal music

Class scores and parts in **785–789**

783.2	Liturgical and ritualistic music

Including works combining texts (librettos) with scores

Do not use standard subdivisions

Class texts used by a specific religion with the religion, e.g., liturgy and ritual of Christian church **264**

.3	Oratorios

Including Passions

.4	Nonliturgical choral pieces

Anthems, motets, choruses, cantatas

For oratorios, see **783.3**

.5	Nonliturgical chants

Gregorian, Ambrosian, Anglican, Jewish chants

.6	Songs

Including carols

.7	Evangelistic music

Treatises on mission, revival, Sunday school music

Class scores and parts in **783.6**, scores and parts for congregational singing in **783.9**

.8	Church choirs and vocal groups

Including training and conducting

Class scores and parts of music for choirs with the kind of music, e.g., anthems **783.4**

.9	Hymns

Songs for congregational singing

► ## 784–789 Individual mediums of musical expression

Scope: appreciation, composition, performance, concerts and recitals

Observe the following table of precedence for works combining two or more mediums, e.g., voice and piano **784**

> Voice
> String instruments
> Wind instruments
> Percussion instruments
> Accordion
> Organ
> Harpsichord
> Piano

For dramatic music, see **782**

784   Voice and vocal music

With or without instrumental accompaniment

Scope: comprehensive works on or combining words and music (texts and scores)

For sacred music, see **783**; *words to be sung or recited with music,* **781.9**; *music for orchestra with incidental vocal parts,* **785.2**

► ## 784.1–784.7 Specific kinds of vocal music

► ## 784.1–784.3 Vocal music according to number of voices

For vocal music according to origin, subject, special interest, see **784.4–784.7**

.1   **Choruses and part songs**

Madrigals, glees, rounds, catches, other choral pieces not originally composed for orchestral accompaniment

Do not use standard subdivisions

.2   **Complete choral works**

Originally composed for chorus and orchestra with or without solo voices

Do not use standard subdivisions

784.3   Songs for from one to nine parts

> Vocal chamber music, art songs, dance songs, ballads, ballades, canzonets
>
> Do not use standard subdivisions

▶   784.4–784.7 Vocal music according to origin, subject, special interest

.4   Folk songs

> Do not use standard subdivisions
>
> Class national airs, songs, hymns and songs of specific ethnic and cultural groups in 784.7

.6   Songs for specific groups and on specific subjects

> Topical songs, songs for home, community, students, children, societies, service clubs
>
> Do not use standard subdivisions

.7   Other kinds of songs

> National airs, songs, hymns; songs of specific ethnic and cultural groups
>
> Do not use standard subdivisions

.8   Collections of vocal music

> Too general to be provided for in 784.1–784.7

.9   The voice

> Training, performance, vocal ensemble

▶   785–789 Instruments and instrumental music

> *For treatises on sacred instrumental music, see* 783.1

785   Instrumental ensembles and their music

.06   Organizations

> Including bands [*formerly* 785.1], orchestras, chamber music ensembles

.1   Symphonies and band music

> Class bands [*formerly* 785.1] in 785.06

785.2   Music for orchestra with incidental vocal parts

  .3   Miscellaneous music for orchestra

> Serenades and other romantic music, symphonic poems and other program music, variations

  .4   Music for small ensembles

> Dance music, jazz, music for rhythm and percussion bands
>
> *For chamber music, see* **785.7**

  .5   Independent overtures for orchestra

  .6   Concertos

> Class music for organ, piano, orchestra in **786.8**

  .7   Chamber music

> Compositions for two or more different solo instruments

  .8   Suites for orchestra

►   786–789 Specific instruments and their music

> Scope: design, hand construction, care, tuning, repairing of instruments

786   Keyboard instruments and their music

> *For celesta, see* **789**

  .1   Keyboard string instruments and their music

> *For instruments, see* **786.2**; *training and performance,* **786.3**; *music,* **786.4**

  .2   Keyboard string instruments

> Pianoforte (piano) and its early forms, harpsichord, spinet, virginal, clavichord
>
> *For player pianos, see* **789.7**

  .3   Training and performance on keyboard string instruments

786.4	Music for keyboard string instruments

Class instructive editions in **786.3**

.5	Keyboard wind instruments and their music

For a specific instrument, see the subject, e.g., organ **786.6**; *training and performance,* **786.7**; *music,* **786.8**

.6	Organ

Class electronic organs and reed organs in **786.9**

.7	Training in and performance on keyboard wind instruments

For accordion and concertina, see **786.9**

.8	Music for keyboard wind instruments

Class instructive editions in **786.7**

For accordion and concertina, see **786.9**

.9	Other keyboard instruments

Electronic organs, reed organs (harmoniums, melodeons, cabinet organs), accordions and concertinas and their music

Class training and performance in electronic and reed organs in **786.7**, music in **786.8**

▶ 787–789 Other instruments and their music

787	String instruments and their music

Bowed and plectral instruments and their music, e.g., violin, viola, violoncello, viols, harp, guitar, mandolin, lute, banjo, zither, ukulele

788	Wind instruments and their music

Brass and woodwind instruments and their music, e.g., trumpet, cornet, bugle, trombone, horns, flute, piccolo, fife, clarinet, saxophone, oboe, basson, bagpipe, harmonica (mouth organ)

789	Percussion, mechanical, electrical instruments

Including membranophones, cymbals, triangle, bells, carillons, chimes, glockenspiel, marimba, xylophone, celesta, vibraphone

▶ 789.7–789.9 Mechanical and electrical
reproduction of music

789.7   Mechanical instruments and devices

Including barrel organ, reproducing and player pianos and orchestrion

.8   Music box

.9   Electronic musical instruments and music recording

790   Recreation (Recreational arts)

Materials, equipment, techniques

.01   Philosophy, theory, programs

.013   Value, influence, effect

Including psychological aspects of recreation, effective use of leisure

.019   Recreation for specific classes

Including recreational programs for families, children, senior citizens, invalids, persons with handicaps

.02   Miscellany

.023   Hobbies

Including collecting

.03–.09   Other standard subdivisions

.2   The performing arts

Including comprehensive works on stage, motion pictures, radio, television [*formerly* **791.4**]

For music, see **780**

791   Public entertainment

.06   Organizations

Including amusement parks

.1   Traveling shows

Including medicine shows, minstrel shows and skits

For circuses, see **791.3**

791.3	Circuses

.4	Motion pictures, radio, television

Class comprehensive works on stage, motion pictures, radio, television in **790.2**, script writing for motion pictures, radio, television in **808.06** [*all formerly* **791.4**]

.43	Motion-picture entertainment

Class comprehensive works on motion-picture communication [*formerly* **791.43**] in **384.8**

.44	Radio

Class comprehensive works on radiobroadcasting [*formerly* **791.44**] in **384.54**

.45	Television

Class comprehensive works on television broadcasting [*formerly* **791.45**] in **384.55**

.5	Miniature, toy, shadow theaters

.6	Pageantry

Processions, festivals, illuminations, parades, floats for parades

For water pageantry, see **797.2**; *circuses,* **791.3**

.8	Animal performances

Including bullfighting, rodeos, cockfighting

For circuses, see **791.3**; *equestrian sports and animal racing,* **798**

792	Theater (Stage presentations)

For miniature, toy, shadow theaters, see **791.5**

[.02]	Miscellany

Do not use

►   792.1–792.8 Specific kinds of dramatic
             performance
                     For specific productions, see **792.9**

792.1   Tragedy and serious drama
                     Including historical, Passion, morality, miracle plays

    .2   Comedy and melodrama

    .3   Pantomime

    .7   Vaudeville, music hall, variety, cabaret, night club
              presentations

    .8   Ballet

    .809   Historical and geographical treatment
                      Do not use for specific performances

    .82   Ballet dancing
                     Including choreography

    .9   Specific productions
                     Including production scripts (stage guides)
                     Class specific ballets in **792.8**

793   Indoor games and amusements
                     For indoor games of skill, see **794**; *games of chance,* **795**

    .2   Parties and entertainments
                     Charades, tableaux, children's and seasonal parties

    .3   Dancing
                     Including folk and national dances, theatrical dances, sword
                     dances, cotillions, germans, balls

    .33   Ballroom dancing (Round dances)

    .34   Square dancing

    .4   Games of action

    .5   Forfeit and trick games

795	**Games of chance**

Including dice games, wheel and top games, dominoes, mah-jongg, bingo, gambling and betting systems

.4	**Card games**

Including card tricks

796	**Athletic and outdoor sports and games**

Scope: intramural and interscholastic athletics and games [*both formerly 371.7*]

For aquatic and air sports, see 797; equestrian sports and animal racing, 798; fishing, hunting, shooting, 799

.1	**Miscellaneous games**

Singing and dancing games, leapfrog, hide and seek, puss in corner, prisoner's base, play with kites and similar toys

For active games requiring equipment, see 796.2

.2	**Active games requiring equipment**

Including roller skating, quoits, horseshoe pitching

For ball games, see 796.3

.3	**Ball games**
.31	**Ball thrown or hit by hand**

Handball, lawn bowling

.32	**Inflated ball thrown or hit by hand**

Net ball, basketball, volleyball

.33	**Inflated ball driven by foot**

Including pushball

.332	American football
.333	Rugby

Union and League

.334	Soccer (Association football)
.335	Canadian football

268

796.34	Racket games

Table tennis [*formerly* 794.7], court tennis, paddle tennis, lawn tennis, rackets and squash, badminton, lacrosse

.35	Ball driven by club, mallet, bat

Including polo, croquet, field hockey

.352	Golf
.357	Baseball
.357 2	Strategy and tactics

Defensive and offensive play

.357 3	Umpiring
.357 6	Specific types of baseball

Night, sandlot, precollege, college, professional, semiprofessional

For specific games, see **796.357 7**; *strategy and tactics,* **796.357 2**

.357 7	Specific games
.357 8	Variants

Softball, baseball for girls and women, indoor baseball, one old cat

.358	Cricket
.4	Athletic exercises and gymnastics

Calisthenics, track and field athletics, jumping, vaulting, throwing, use of horizontal and parallel bars, trapeze work, rope climbing, wire walking, acrobatics, tumbling, trampolining, contortion, the Olympic games

.5	Outdoor life

Including walking, mountaineering, spelunking

.54	Camping
.56	Dude ranching and farming

796.6   Cycling
> Use of wheeled vehicles driven by manpower
> Including bicycle, soapbox racing

.7   Driving motor vehicles
> For racing, for pleasure

.8   Combat sports
> Wrestling, jujitsus, boxing, fencing

.9   Ice and snow sports
> Ice skating, snowshoeing, skiing, tobogganing and coasting, curling, ice hockey, iceboating

797   Aquatic and air sports

.1   Boating
> Canoeing, rowboating, sailboating, motorboating, yachting, surf riding, water skiing, boat racing and regattas

.2   Swimming and diving
> Including water pageantry, water games
> Do not use standard subdivisions

.21   Swimming
> *For submarine swimming, see* **797.23**

.23   Submarine swimming
> Skin diving, scuba diving

.24   Springboard and precision diving

.5   Air sports
> Aircraft racing, flying for pleasure, stunt flying, gliding and soaring, parachuting (skydiving)

798   Equestrian sports and animal racing
> Horsemanship, horse racing, driving and coaching, racing other animals

799   Fishing, hunting, shooting

  .1   Fishing

         Fresh- and salt-water

  .17   Fishing for specific kinds of fish

         Divide like **597.2–597.5**, e.g., trout fishing **799.175**

  .2   Hunting

         Small and big game

         Including falconry

[.209]   Historical and geographical treatment

         Do not use; class in **799.29**

  .24   Birds

  .25   Small game other than birds

  .26   Big game other than birds

         For specific kinds, see **799.27**

  .27   Specific kinds of big game other than birds

  .29   Historical and geographical treatment

         Add area notations **1–9** to **799.29**

  .3   Shooting other than game

         With guns at stationary and moving targets, e.g., trapshooting, skeet shooting; with bows and arrows (archery)

800 Literature (Belles-lettres) and rhetoric

Scope: literature itself, works about literature

Observe the following table of precedence for works combining two or more literary forms, e.g., English poetic drama **822**

> Drama
> Poetry
> Fiction
> Essays
> Speeches
> Letters
> Satire and humor
> Miscellany

If preferred, give precedence to satire and humor over all other forms

▶ ## 801–807 Standard subdivisions of literature

Class collections and anthologies in **808.8**, history, description, critical appraisal, biographical treatment in **809**

801 Philosophy and theory

Including theory, technique, history of literary criticism

802 Miscellany about literature

Class techniques in **808.02–808.7**

803 Dictionaries, encyclopedias, concordances

[804] Essays and lectures

Class in **809**

805 Serial publications of and about literature

806 Organizations

807 Study and teaching

808	Rhetoric, collections, anthologies

Do not use standard subdivisions

▶ 808.02–808.06 Rhetoric (Composition)

Techniques of oral and written communication for clarity and esthetic pleasure

Class rhetoric in specific literary forms in **808.1–808.7**

.02 Authorship and editorial techniques [*formerly* 029.6]

Preparation of manuscripts

Including preparation of theses [*formerly* **378.2**], plagiarism, writing for publication

.04 Composition in specific languages

For composition for specific purposes and types of readers, see **808.06**

.06 Composition for specific purposes and types of readers

Professional, technical, expository writing; writing for children in specific literary forms

Including news writing [*formerly* **070.4**], business writing [*formerly* **651.7**], script writing for motion pictures, radio, television [*all formerly* **791.4**]

If preferred, class techniques of writing on specific subjects in standard subdivision **01**

▶ 808.1–808.7 Rhetoric in specific literary forms

Observe table of precedence under **800**

Class specific forms for children in **808.06**

.1 Poetry

.2 Drama

.3 Fiction

.31 Short stories

.4 Essays

273

808.5	Speech

Scope: voice, expression, gesture

.51	Public speaking (Oratory)

Platform, radio, after-dinner speaking

For debating and public discussion, see **808.53**; *preaching,* **251**

.53	Debating and public discussion
.54	Recitation

Storytelling, reading aloud

.55	Choral speaking
.56	Conversation
.6	Letters
.7	Satire and humor
.8	Collections and anthologies of literature

Scope: works emphasizing equally collections of literary texts and history, description, critical appraisal of literature

Class literatures of specific languages in 810–890

For history, description, critical appraisal of literature, see **809**

► 808.81–808.88 In specific forms

Observe table of precedence under **800**

.81–.87	In specific literary forms

Divide like **808.1–808.7**, e.g., collections of public speeches **808.851**

.88	Miscellany

Quotations, epigrams, diaries, journals, reminiscences, prose literature

Class a specific form of prose literature with the form, e.g., essays **808.84**

.89	For and by persons having common characteristics

For literature in specific forms, see **808.81–808.88**

[808.9]   Literatures of artificial languages

> Class in **899.9**

809   History, description, critical appraisal, biographical treatment of literature

> Scope: essays and lectures [*both formerly* 804]
>
> Class theory, technique, history of literary criticism in **801**, literatures of specific languages in **810–890**

.1–.7   In specific forms

> Divide like **808.1–808.7**, e.g., poetry **809.1**

.8   For and by persons having common characteristics

> *For literature in specific forms, see* **809.1–809.7**; *displaying specific features,* **809.9**

.9   Displaying specific features

> Including Bible as literature [*formerly* 220.88]
>
> *For literature in specific forms, see* **809.1–809.7**

► **810–890 Literatures of specific languages**

> By language in which originally written
>
> Scope: literature in dialect
>
> If preferred, class translations into a language requiring local emphasis with the literature of that language

810   **American literature in English**

> English-language literature of Western Hemisphere and Hawaii
>
> If desired, distinguish literature of a specific country by initial letter, e.g., literature of Canada **C810**, of United States **U810**; or, if preferred, class literatures not requiring local emphasis in **819**

.8   Collections and anthologies by more than one author

> Class collected works of single authors not limited to or chiefly identified with one specific form [*formerly* 810.81] in **818**

810.9　　　History, description, critical appraisal, biographical treatment

> Class description, critical appraisal, biographical treatment of single authors not limited to or chiefly identified with one specific form in **818**

▶　　　811–818 Specific forms

Observe table of precedence under **800**

Class under each form without further subdivision description, critical appraisal, biographical treatment, single and collected works of single authors; but, if preferred, class these regardless of form in **818**

Use **001–009** under each for standard subdivisions

811　　　Poetry

812　　　Drama

813　　　Fiction

> If preferred, do not class works of fiction

814　　　Essays

815　　　Speeches

816　　　Letters

817　　　Satire and humor

818　　　Miscellany

> Quotations, epigrams, diaries, journals, reminiscences, prose literature; collected works of single authors not limited to or chiefly identified with one specific form [*formerly* **810.81**]
>
> (Optional: class here description, critical appraisal, biographical treatment, single and collected works of single authors regardless of form; prefer **811–818**)
>
> *For a specific form of prose literature, see the form, e.g., essays* **814**

819　　　Literatures not requiring local emphasis

> In libraries emphasizing United States literature: Canadian and other; in libraries emphasizing Canadian literature: United States and other
>
> (Optional; prefer **810**)

▶ ## 820–890 Other literatures

820 Of English and Anglo-Saxon languages

Do not use standard subdivisions

If desired, distinguish English literature of a specific country by initial letter, e.g., literature of England **E820**, of Ireland **Ir820** (or of all British Isles **B820**), of Australia **A820**, of India **In820**; or, if preferred, class literatures not requiring local emphasis in **828.99**

For American literature in English, see **810**

.1–.7 Standard subdvisions of English literature

.8 Collections and anthologies of English literature by more than one author

> Class collected works of single authors not limited to or chiefly identified with one specific form [*formerly* **820.81**] in **828**

.9 History, description, critical appraisal, biographical treatment of English literature

> Class description, critical appraisal, biographical treatment of single authors not limited to or chiefly identified with one specific form in **828**

▶ ## 821–828 Specific forms of English literature

Observe table of precedence under **800**

Class under each form without further subdivision description, critical appraisal, biographical treatment, single and collected works of single authors; but, if preferred, class these regardless of form in **828**

Use **001–009** under each for standard subdivisions

821 Poetry

822 Drama

.3 William Shakespeare

823 Fiction

> If preferred, do not class works of fiction

824 Essays

825   Speeches

826   Letters

827   Satire and humor

828   Miscellany

> Quotations, epigrams, diaries, journals, reminiscences, prose literature; collected works of single authors not limited to or chiefly identified with one specific form [*formerly* 820.81]
>
> (Optional: class here description, critical appraisal, biographical treatment, single and collected works of single authors regardless of form; prefer 821–828)
>
> *For a specific form of prose literature, see the form, e.g., essays* 824

.99   English-language literatures not requiring local emphasis

> In libraries emphasizing British literature: Australian, Indian, other; in libraries emphasizing Australian literature: British, Indian, other
>
> (Optional; prefer 820)

829   Anglo-Saxon (Old English)

830   **Of Germanic languages**

> Do not use standard subdivisions

.1–.7   Standard subdivisions of German literature

.8   Collections and anthologies of German literature by more than one author

> Class collected works of single authors not limited to or chiefly identified with one specific form [*formerly* 830.81] in 838

.9   History, description, critical appraisal, biographical treatment of German literature

> Class description, critical appraisal, biographical treatment of single authors not limited to or chiefly identified with one specific form in 838

► ## 831–838 Specific forms of German literature

Observe table of precedence under **800**

Class under each form without further subdivision description, critical appraisal, biographical treatment, single and collected works of single authors; but, if preferred, class these regardless of form in **838**

Use **001–009** under each for standard subdivisions

831   Poetry

832   Drama

833   Fiction

    If preferred, do not class works of fiction

834   Essays

835   Speeches

836   Letters

837   Satire and humor

838   Miscellany

    Quotations, epigrams, diaries, journals, reminiscences, prose literature; collected works of single authors not limited to or chiefly identified with one specific form [*formerly* **830.81**]

    (Optional: class here description, critical appraisal, biographical treatment, single and collected works of single authors regardless of form; prefer **831–838**)

      For a specific form of prose literature, see the form, e.g., essays **834**

839   Other Germanic languages

    Divide like **439**, e.g., Swedish **839.7**

▶ ## 840–860 Of Romance languages

Class comprehensive works in **879.9**

840   French, Provençal, Catalan

Do not use standard subdivisions

If desired, distinguish French literature of a specific country by initial letter, e.g., literature of Canada **C840**, of France **F840**; or, if preferred, class literature not requiring local emphasis in **848.99**

.1–.7   Standard subdivisions of French literature

.8   Collections and anthologies of French literature by more than one author

Class collected works of single authors not limited to or chiefly identified with one specific form [*formerly* 840.81] in **848**

.9   History, description, critical appraisal, biographical treatment of French literature

Class description, critical appraisal, biographical treatment of single authors not limited to or chiefly identified with one specific form in **848**

▶ ## 841–848 Specific forms of French literature

Observe table of precedence under **800**

Class under each form without further subdivision description, critical appraisal, biographical treatment, single and collected works of single authors; but, if preferred, class these regardless of form in **848**

Use **001–009** under each for standard subdivisions

841   Poetry

842   Drama

843   Fiction

If preferred, do not class works of fiction

844   Essays

845   Speeches

846   Letters

847   Satire and humor

848   Miscellany

> Quotations, epigrams, diaries, journals, reminiscences, prose literature; collected works of single authors not limited to or chiefly identified with one specific form [*formerly* 849.81]
>
> (Optional: class here description, critical appraisal, biographical treatment, single and collected works of single authors regardless of form; prefer 841–848)
>
> > *For a specific form of prose literature, see the form, e.g., essays* 844

.99   French-language literatures not requiring local emphasis

> In libraries emphasizing Canadian literature: literature of France, Belgium, other; in libraries emphasizing literature of France: literature of Canada, Belgium, other
>
> (Optional; prefer 840)

849   Provençal and Catalan

850   **Italian, Romanian, Rhaeto-Romanic**

> Do not use standard subdivisions

.1–.7   Standard subdivisions of Italian literature

.8   Collections and anthologies of Italian literature by more than one author

> Class collected works of single authors not limited to or chiefly identified with one specific form [*formerly* 850.81] in 858

.9   History, description, critical appraisal, biographical treatment of Italian literature

> Class description, critical appraisal, biographical treatment of single authors not limited to or chiefly identified with one specific form in 858

▶ 851–858 Specific forms of Italian literature

Observe table of precedence under **800**

Class under each form without further subdivision description, critical appraisal, biographical treatment, single and collected works of single authors; but, if preferred, class these regardless of form in **858**

Use **001–009** under each for standard subdivisions

851 Poetry

852 Drama

853 Fiction

If preferred, do not class works of fiction

854 Essays

855 Speeches

856 Letters

857 Satire and humor

858 Miscellany

Quotations, epigrams, diaries, journals, reminiscences, prose literature; collected works of single authors not limited to or chiefly identified with one specific form [*formerly* **850.81**]

(Optional: class here description, critical appraisal, biographical treatment, single and collected works of single authors regardless of form; prefer **851–858**)

For a specific form of prose literature, see the form, e.g., essays **854**

859 Romanian and Rhaeto-Romanic

860 **Spanish and Portuguese**

Do not use standard subdivisions

If desired, distinguish Spanish literature of a specific country by initial letter, e.g., literature of Chile **Ch860**, of Colombia **Co860** (or, of all American countries **A860**), of Spain **S860**; or, if preferred, class literature not requiring local emphasis in **868.99**

.1–.7 Standard subdivisions of Spanish literature

860.8	Collections and anthologies of Spanish literature by more than one author

Class collected works of single authors not limited to or chiefly identified with one specific form [*formerly* 860.81] in **868**

.9	History, description, critical appraisal, biographical treatment of Spanish literature

Class description, critical appraisal, biographical treatment of single authors not limited to or chiefly identified with one specific form in **868**

▶ 861–868 Specific forms of Spanish literature

Observe table of precedence under **800**

Class under each form without further subdivision description, critical appraisal, biographical treatment, single and collected works of single authors; but, if preferred, class these regardless of form in **868**

Use 001–009 under each for standard subdivisions

861	Poetry
862	Drama
863	Fiction

If preferred, do not class works of fiction

864	Essays
865	Speeches
866	Letters
867	Satire and humor
868	Miscellany

Quotations, epigrams, diaries, journals, reminiscences, prose literature; collected works of single authors not limited to or chiefly identified with one specific form [*formerly* 860.81]

(Optional: class here description, critical appraisal, biographical treatment, single and collected works of single authors regardless of form; prefer 861–868)

For a specific form of prose literature, see the form, e.g., essays **864**

868.99   Spanish-language literatures not requiring local emphasis

> In libraries emphasizing Mexican literature: literature of other Hispanic-American countries and of Spain, other; in libraries emphasizing literature of Spain: Hispanic-American and other
>
> (Optional; prefer **860**)

869   Portuguese

> Scope: literature in Galician (Gallegan) dialect
>
> If desired, distinguish literature of a specific country by initial letter, e.g., literature of Brazil **B869**, of Portugal **P869**; or, if preferred, class literatures not requiring local emphasis in **869.899**

.08   Collections and anthologies by more than one author

> Class collections of single authors not limited to or chiefly identified with one specific form [*formerly* **869.081**] in **869.8**

.09   History, description, critical appraisal, biographical treatment

> Class description, critical appraisal, biographical treatment of single authors not limited to or chiefly identified with one specific form in **869.8**

►   869.1–869.8 Specific forms

Observe table of precedence under **800**

Class under each form without further subdivision description, critical appraisal, biographical treatment, single and collected works of single authors; but, if preferred, class these regardless of form in **869.8**

.1–.7   Specific literary forms

> Divide like **811–817**, e.g., essays **869.4**
>
> Use **001–009** under each for standard subdivisions

869.8   Miscellany

Quotations, epigrams, diaries, journals, reminiscences, prose literature; collected works of single authors not limited to or chiefly identified with one specific form [*formerly* 869.081]

(Optional: class here description, critical appraisal, biographical treatment, single and collected works of single authors regardless of form; prefer 869.1–869.8)

Use **869.800 1 – 869.800 9** for standard subdivisions

For a specific form of prose literature, see the form, e.g., essays **869.4**

.899   Literatures not requiring local emphasis

In libraries emphasizing Brazilian literature: literature of Portugal and other; in libraries emphasizing literature of Portugal: Brazilian and other

(Optional; prefer **869**)

870   Of Italic languages

Do not use standard subdivisions

.1–.7   Standard subdivisions of Latin literature

.8   Collections and anthologies of Latin literature by more than one author

Class collected works of single authors not limited to or chiefly identified with one specific form [*formerly* 870.81] in **878**

.9   History, description, critical appraisal, biographical treatment of Latin literature

Class description, critical appraisal, biographical treatment of single authors not limited to or chiefly identified with one specific form in **878**

► ## 871–878 Specific forms of Latin literature

Classical Latin; classical revival (medieval and modern) Latin [*formerly* 879]

Observe table of precedence under 800

Class under each form without further subdivision description, critical appraisal, biographical treatment, single and collected works of single authors; but, if preferred, class these regardless of form in 878

Use 001–009 under each for standard subdivisions

871   Poetry

> *For dramatic poetry, see* 872; *epic poetry,* 873; *lyric poetry,* 874

872   Dramatic poetry and drama

873   Epic poetry and fiction

874   Lyric poetry

875   Speeches

876   Letters

877   Satire and humor

878   Miscellany

> Quotations, epigrams, diaries, journals, reminiscences, prose literature; collected works of single authors not limited to or chiefly identified with one specific form [*formerly* 870.81]
>
> (Optional: class here description, critical appraisal, biographical treatment, single and collected works of single authors regardless of form; prefer 871–878)
>
> > *For a specific form of prose literature, see the form, e.g., speeches* 875

879   Other Italic languages

> Class classical revival (medieval and modern) Latin literature [*formerly* 879] in 871–878

.9   Romance languages

> Including Osco-Umbrian languages
>
> Class literatures of other specific Romance languages in 840–860

880 Of classical languages and modern Greek

Do not use standard subdivisions

Class literature of Latin language in **870**

.1–.7 Standard subdivisions of classical Greek literature

.8 Collections and anthologies of classical Greek literature by more than one author

Class collected works of single authors not limited to or chiefly identified with one specific form [*formerly* **880.81**] in **888**

.9 History, description, critical appraisal, biographical treatment of classical Greek literature

Class description, critical appraisal, biographical treatment of single authors not limited to or chiefly identified with one specific form in **888**

▶ 881–888 Specific forms of classical Greek literature

Ancient Greek; medieval (Byzantine) Greek [*formerly* **889**]

Observe table of precedence under **800**

Class under each form without further subdivision description, critical appraisal, biographical treatment, single and collected works of single authors; but, if preferred, class these regardless of form in **888**

Use **001–009** under each for standard subdivisions

881 Poetry

For *dramatic poetry, see* **882**; *epic poetry*, **883**; *lyric poetry*, **884**

882 Dramatic poetry and drama

883 Epic poetry and fiction

884 Lyric poetry

885 Speeches

886 Letters

887   Satire and humor

888   Miscellany

> Quotations, epigrams, diaries, journals, reminiscences, prose literature; collected works of single authors not limited to or chiefly identified with one specific form [*formerly* 880.81]

> (Optional: class here description, critical appraisal, biographical treatment, single and collected works of single authors regardless of form; prefer 881–888)

>> *For a specific form of prose literature, see the form, e.g., speeches* 885

889   Modern Greek

> Katharevusa and Demotic

> Class medieval (Byzantine) Greek literature [*formerly* 889] in 881–888

890   **Of other languages**

891   East Indo-European and Celtic languages

> Divide like 491, e.g., literature of modern Persian language 891.5

892   Semitic languages

> Divide like 492, e.g., literature of Yiddish language 892.49

893   Hamitic and other languages

> Literatures of Old Egyptian, Coptic, Berber, Cushitic (Hamitic Ethiopian), Chad-family languages

>> *For Hausa, see* 896

894   Ural-Altaic, Paleosiberian, Dravidian languages

> Literatures of Altaic languages (Tungusic, Mongolic, Turkic families); Uralic languages (Samoyedic, Magyar, Permian, Finnish, Estonian, Lapp languages); Paleosiberian languages (Luorawetlin, Ainu, Gilyak, Ket); Dravidian languages (Kota, Toda, Kurukh, Tamil, Malayalam, Kanarese, Gondi, Khond, Telugu languages); Brahui

895   Languages of East and Southeast Asia

Literatures of Chinese, Japanese, Korean, Tibeto-Burman, Burmese, Thai, Vietnamese, Cambodian languages

Divide like **495**, e.g., literature of Chinese language **895.1**

896   African languages

Literatures of Hottentot, Bushman, Bantu, Hausa, Swahili languages and dialects

Class Afro-Asian literatures in **892–893**

897   North American Indian languages
898   South American Indian languages
899   Austronesian and other languages

Including literatures of Negrito, Papuan, Malayan, Polynesian, Melanesian, Micronesian, Australian, Basque, Elamitic, Etruscan, Sumerian, Caucasian languages

.9   Artificial languages [*formerly* 808.9]

Literatures in Esperanto, Interlingua, Volapük

900

900 General geography and history and related disciplines

Do not use standard subdivisions

Class historical and geographical treatment of a specific subject with the subject

▶ **901–908 Standard subdivisions of general history**

Class history of specific continents, countries, localities in 930–990

901 Philosophy and theory

Class civilization of ancient world [*formerly* 901] in 913.03

.9 Civilization

Man's spiritual, intellectual, social, material situation and progress

If preferred, class in **909**

Class areal treatment in **910**

.92 In the years 500–1500

.93 In the years 1500–1900

.94 In the years 1900–

902 Miscellany

Including chronologies

903 Dictionaries, encyclopedias, concordances

904 Collected accounts of specific events

Including adventure [*formerly* 910.4]

905 Serial publications

906 Organizations

907	Study and teaching
908	Collections and anthologies
909	World history

Use **909.001–909.009** for standard subdivisions
(Optional: civilization; prefer **901.9**)
Class history of ancient world to ca. 500 A.D. in **930**

.07   Medieval, to 1450/1500

       Comprehensive works only

.08   Modern, 1450/1500–

       Comprehensive works only
       Class history of 1700–1799 in **909.7**, of 1800– in **909.8**

.7	1700–1799
.8	1800–
.81	1800–1899
.82	1900–

       For World War I, see **940.3**

.824   1940–1949

       For World War II, see **940.53**

| .825 | 1950–1959 |
| .826 | 1960–1969 |

910   **General geography**

Areal differentiation and traveler's observation of the earth
(physical geography [*formerly* **551.4**]) and man's civilization upon
it

Use **910.001–910.008** for standard subdivisions; but class charts
and plans in **912**

.02   The earth (Physical geography)

.03   Man and his civilization

910.09   Historical and regional treatment

> Including geography of regions not limited by continent, country, locality; discovery, exploration, growth of geographic knowledge
>
> Class geography of specific continents, countries, localities in **913–919**

.1   Topical geography

> (Optional; prefer specific subject, e.g., economic geography **330.91–330.99**)
>
> Divide like **001–899**, e.g., economic geography **910.133**

.2–.3   Miscellany, dictionaries, encyclopedias, concordances of travel

.4   Accounts of travel

> Trips around the world, ocean travel, seafaring life, shipwrecks, mutinies, buried treasure, pirates' expeditions
>
> Class adventure [*formerly* **910.4**] in **904**
>
> Class discovery and exploration in **910.09**, collections and anthologies of travels in **910.8**, scientific travels in **508.3**

.5–.9   Other standard subdivisions of travel

> Class travel in specific continents, countries, localities in **913–919**

911   Historical geography

> Growth and changes in political divisions

912   Graphic representations of earth's surface

> Atlases, maps, charts, plans
>
> *For map projections, see* **526.8**

.1   Specific subjects

.3–.9   Specific continents, countries, localities

> Add area notations **3–9** to **912**

▶ ## 913–919 Geography of specific continents, countries, localities

Scope: comprehensive works on geography and history of specific continents, countries, localities

If preferred, class in **930–990**

Class history of specific continents, countries, localities in **930–990**, geography of regions in **910.09**

For historical geography, see **911**; *graphic representations of earth's surface,* **912**

913 ## Geography of ancient world

Including prehistoric archeology [*formerly* **571**]

Use **913.001–913.008** for standard subdivisions

.02 ### The earth (Physical geography)

.03 ### Man and his civilization [*formerly also* **901**]

Including archeology (study of man's past civilizations thru discovery, collection, interpretation of his material remains)

.04 ### Travel

.3 ### Continents, countries, localities

Add area notation 3 to **913**, e.g., geography of ancient Italian peninsula **913.37**

▶ ## 914–919 Geography of modern world

Class customs of specific continents, countries, localities [*formerly* **914–919**] in **390.09**

914 ## Europe

Add area notation **4** to **91**, e.g., geography of British Isles **914.2**; then add **001–008** for standard subdivisions

915 ## Asia

Add area notation **5** to **91**, e.g., geography of Japan **915.2**; then add **001–008** for standard subdivisions

916   Africa

        Add area notation **6** to **91**, e.g., geography of South Africa **916.8**; then add **001–008** for standard subdivisions

917   North America

        Add area notation **7** to **91**, e.g., geography of Ohio **917.71**; then add **001–008** for standard subdivisions

        Class Indians and their civilization in **970.1**

918   South America

        Add area notation **8** to **91**, e.g., geography of Brazil **918.1**; then add **001–008** for standard subdivisions

        Class Indians and their civilization in **980.1**

919   Other parts of world

        Add area notation **9** to **91**, e.g., geography of Australia **919.4**; then add **001–008** for standard subdivisions

920   General biography, genealogy, insignia

        Including biography of Indians of North America [*formerly* **970.2**], of South America [*formerly* **980.2**], of slaves [*formerly* **326**]

        Do not use standard subdivisions

        Class biography of persons associated with a specific subject with the subject

.001–.008   Standard subdivisions of biography

.009   Historical and geographical treatment of biography

        Class treatment by continent, country, locality in **920.03–920.09**

▶   920.02–920.09 General collections of biography

.02   Not limited geographically

.03–.09   By continent, country, locality

        Add area notations **3–9** to **920.0**, e.g., collections of biographies of Englishmen **920.042**

▶ 920.1–928 Biography of specific classes of persons

(Optional; prefer standard subdivision **092**)

920.1   *Bibliographers

.2   *Librarians and book collectors

.3   *Encyclopedists

.4   *Publishers and booksellers

.5   *Journalists and news commentators

.7   *Persons by sex

.71   *Men

.72   *Women

.9   *Persons associated with other subjects

Not provided for in **920.1–920.5, 921–928**

921   *Philosophers and psychologists

922   *Religious leaders, thinkers, workers

Including collected biographies of communicants of specific religions and sects

923   *Persons in social sciences

Heads of state, nobility, public administrators, politicians, statesmen, military persons, philanthropists, social reformers, educators, explorers, geographers, pioneers; persons in economics (including labor leaders), law (including criminals), commerce, communication, transportation

924   *Philologists and lexicographers

925   *Scientists

926   *Persons in technology

927   *Persons in the arts

928   *Persons in literature

Including historians

* Optional; prefer standard subdivision **092**

929   Genealogy, names, insignia

.1   Genealogy

For sources, see **929.3**; *family histories,* **929.2**

.2   Family histories

For royal houses, peerage, gentry, see **929.7**

.3   Genealogical sources

Registers, wills, tax lists, census records, court records compiled for genealogical purposes

For epitaphs, see **929.5**

.4   Personal names

.5   Epitaphs

.6   Heraldry

For armorial bearings, see **929.8**

.7   Royal houses, peerage, landed gentry

Rank, precedence, titles of honor

.8   Armorial bearings

Coats of arms, crests, seals

.9   Flags

National, state, ship, ownership flags

Class military use in **355.1**

▶   **930–990 Geographical treatment of general history**

History of specific continents, countries, localities

(Optional: geography of specific places; prefer **913–919**)

Add area notations 3–9 to 9, e.g., general history of British Isles **942**; then, unless otherwise specified, add further as follows:

001–008	Standard subdivisions
01–09	Historical periods
	As shown in the schedules that follow

930	**The ancient world to ca. 500 A.D.**

Use 930.01–930.08 for standard subdivisions

931	*China to 420 A.D.
932	*Egypt to 640 A.D.
933	*Palestine to 70 A.D.
934	*India to 647 A.D.
935	*Mesopotamia and Iranian Plateau to 642 A.D.
936	*Europe north and west of Italian peninsula
937	*Italian peninsula and adjacent territories to 476 A.D.
938	*Greece to 323 A.D.
939	Other parts of ancient world to ca. 640 A.D.

► **940–990 The modern world**

940   Europe

From fall of Rome, 476, to present

Use 940.01–940.08 for standard subdivisions

.1   Middle Ages, 476–1453

.2   Modern period, 1453–

For World War I, see **940.3**; *20th century, 1918–   ,* **940.5**

.3   World War I, 1914–1918

Social, political, economic, diplomatic history, causes, results

Including participation of specific countries and groups of countries

For military history, see **940.4**

.4   Military history of World War I (Conduct of the war)

Including celebrations, commemorations, memorials, prisons, health, social services, secret service and spies, propaganda

Use 940.400 1 – 940.400 8 for standard subdivisions

* Add as instructed under 930–990

940.5	20th century, 1918–
.53	World War II, 1939–1945

For military history, see **940.54**

.531	Social, political, economic history

Including diplomatic causes and results

For diplomatic history, see **940.532**

.532	Diplomatic history
.533	Participation of specific groups of countries

United Nations, Axis Powers, neutrals, occupied countries

For participation of specific countries, see **940.534–940.539**; *a specific activity, the subject, e.g., diplomatic history* **940.532**

.534–.539	Participation of specific countries

Scope: governments in exile, underground movements, anti-Axis and pro-Axis national groups, mobilization

Add area notations **4–9** to **940.53**

For a specific activity, see the subject, e.g., diplomatic history **940.532**

.54	Military history of World War II (Conduct of the war)

Including strategy, mobilization, racial minorities as troops, repressive measures and atrocities, military participation of specific countries

Use **940.540 01 – 940.540 08** for standard subdivisions

.541	Operations

For specific campaigns and battles, see **940.542**; *aerial operations,* **940.544**; *naval operations,* **940.545**

.542	Specific campaigns and battles
.544	Aerial operations
.545	Naval operations
.546	Celebrations, commemorations, memorials

940.547	Prisons, health, social services
.548	Other topics

> Military life and customs, intelligence, subversion, sabotage, infiltration, psychological warfare (propaganda)

.55	Later 20th century, 1945–

► ## 941–949 Specific parts of Europe

941	*Scotland and Ireland

> Do not use standard subdivisions

.001–.008	Standard subdivisions of Scotland
.5	*Ireland

> Use **941.501–941.508** for standard subdivisions

942	*British Isles
.01	Early history to 1066
.02	Norman period, 1066–1154
.03	House of Plantagenet, 1154–1399
.04	Houses of Lancaster and York, 1399–1485
.05	Tudor period, 1485–1603
.06	Stuart period, 1603–1714
.07	House of Hanover, 1714–1837
.08	Victoria and House of Windsor, 1837–
.081	Victoria, 1837–1901
.082	20th century, 1901–

> *For George V, see* **942.083**; *period of World War II,* **942.084**; *later 20th century,* **942.085**

.083	George V, 1910–1936
.084	Period of World War II, 1936–1945

> Reigns of Edward VIII, 1936 and George VI, 1936–1952

.085	Later 20th century, 1945–

> Reign of Elizabeth II, 1952–

* Add as instructed under **930–990**

943   *Central Europe

   Do not use standard subdivisions

.001–.008 Standard subdivisions of Germany

.08   Germany since 1866

.085   Weimar Republic, 1918–1933

.086   Third Reich, 1933–1945

.087   Later 20th century, 1945–

944   *France

.04   Revolution, 1789–1804

.05   First Empire, 1804–1815

.06   Restoration, 1815–1848

.07   Second Republic and Second Empire, 1848–1870

.08   Third, Fourth, Fifth Republics, 1870–

.081   Third Republic, 1870–1945

.082   Fourth Republic, 1945–1958

.083   Fifth Republic, 1958–

945   *Italy and adjacent territories

.09   Italy since 1870

.091   Fascist regime, 1918–1946

.092   Republic, 1946–

946   *Iberian Peninsula and adjacent islands

   Do not use standard subdivisions

.001–.008 Standard subdivisions of Spain

.08   Spain since 1868

.081   Second Republic, 1931–1939

.082   Regime of Francisco Franco, 1939–

* Add as instructed under **930–990**

947   *Eastern Europe

          Do not use standard subdivisions

.001–.008   Standard subdivisions of Russia

.08   Russia since 1855

.084   Communist regime, 1917–   (Union of Soviet
          Socialist Republics, 1923–   )

          For later 20th century, see **947.085**

.085   Later 20th century, 1953–

948   *Scandinavia

949   *Other parts of Europe

950   **Asia**

          Use **950.01–950.08** for standard subdivisions

.4   20th century, 1905–

.41   Early 20th century, 1905–1945

.42   Later 20th century, 1945–

951   *China and adjacent areas

          Do not use standard subdivisions

.001–.008   Standard subdivisions of China

▶   951.04–951.05 China since 1912

.04   Early 20th century, 1912–1949

.05   People's Republic, 1949–

952   *Japan and adjacent islands

          Do not use standard subdivisions

.001–.008   Standard subdivisions of Japan

▶   952.03–952.04 Japan since 1868

.03   Re-establishment of imperial power, 1868–1945

.04   Postwar period, 1945–

* Add as instructed under **930–990**

953	*Arabian Peninsula and adjacent areas
954	*South Asia
.03	British rule, 1774–1947
.04	Independence and partition, 1947–
955	*Iran (Persia)
956	*Middle East
957	*Siberia (Asiatic Russia)
958	*Central Asia
959	*Southeast Asia

960   Africa

Use **960.01–960.08** for standard subdivisions

961	*North Africa
962	*Egypt and Sudan

Do not use standard subdivisions

.001–.008   Standard subdivisions of Egypt

963	*Ethiopia
964	*Northwest African coast and offshore islands

Do not use standard subdivisions

.001–.008   Standard subdivisions of Morocco

965	*Algeria
966	*West Africa and offshore islands
967	*Central Africa and offshore islands
968	*South Africa
969	*South Indian Ocean islands

* Add as instructed under 930–990

970   North America

(Optional: discovery and exploration to ca. 1600; prefer **973.1**)

Use **970.001–970.008** for standard subdivisions

.1   Indians of North America

History and civilization

For specific tribes, see **970.3**; *Indians in specific places,* **970.4**; *government relations,* **970.5**

[.2]   Biography of Indians

Class biographies of persons associated with a specific subject in standard subdivision **092**, of persons not so related in **920**

.3   Specific Indian tribes

For government relations, see **970.5**

.4   Indians in specific places

For specific tribes, see **970.3**; *government relations,* **970.5**

.5   Government relations with Indians

History and policy

Class Indian wars of a specific place and period with history of the appropriate place and period

[.6]   Specific subjects in relation to Indians

Class with the subject

971   *Canada

.01   Early history to 1763

.02   Early British rule, 1763–1791

.03   Period of the separate colonies, 1791–1841

.04   Growth of responsible government, 1841–1867

.05   Dominion of Canada during period 1867–1914

.06   20th century, 1914–

* Add as instructed under **930–990**

972   *Middle America

Use **972.000 1 – 972.000 8** for standard subdivisions

.001–.008   Standard subdivisions of Mexico

.08   Mexico since 1867

973   United States

Use **973.01–973.08** for standard subdivisions

.1   Discovery and exploration to 1607

Scope: discovery and exploration of America; if preferred, class in **970**

Class discoveries and explorations in a specific country with history of the country

.2   Colonial period, 1607–1775

Class local history in **974–975**

.3   Revolution and confederation, 1775–1789

.31   Social, political, economic history

For diplomatic history, see **973.32**

.32   Diplomatic history

Relations of United States with other nations

.33   Operations

For naval operations, see **973.35**

.35   Naval operations

Including ships, privateering

.38   Treason, secret service, spies, propaganda

.4   Constitutional period, 1789–1809

Administrations of Washington, John Adams, Jefferson

* Add as instructed under **930–990**

973.5	Early 19th century, 1809–1845

Administrations of Madison, Monroe, John Quincy Adams, Jackson, Van Buren, William Henry Harrison, Tyler

Including War of 1812

.6	Middle 19th century, 1845–1861

Administrations of Polk, Taylor, Fillmore, Pierce, Buchanan

Including Mexican War

.7	Administration of Lincoln, 1861–1865 (Civil War)
.71	Social, political, economic history

For diplomatic history, see **973.72**

.72	Diplomatic history
.73	Operations

For naval operations, see **973.75**

.75	Naval operations

Including ships, privateering, blockade running

.77	Prisons, health, social services
.78	Military life and customs, secret service and spies
.8	Later 19th century, 1865–1901 (Period of reconstruction)

Administrations of Andrew Johnson, Grant, Hayes, Garfield, Arthur, Cleveland, Benjamin Harrison, McKinley

Including Spanish-American War

.9	20th century, 1901–
.91	Early 20th century, 1901–1953

Including administrations of Theodore Roosevelt, Taft, Wilson, Harding, Coolidge, Hoover

.917	Administration of Franklin D. Roosevelt, 1933–1945
.918	Administration of Truman, 1945–1953

973.92	Later 20th century, 1953–
.921	Administration of Eisenhower, 1953–1961
.922	Administration of Kennedy, 1961–1963
.923	Administration of Lyndon B. Johnson, 1963–

► 974–979 Specific states of United States

974 *Northeastern states

975 *Southeastern (South Atlantic) states

976 *South central states

977 *North central states

978 *Western states

979 *States of Great Basin and Pacific Slope

980 South America

Use **980.001–980.008** for standard subdivisions

.1–.5 Indians of South America

Divide like **970.1–970.5**, e.g., specific tribes **980.3**

Class biographies of persons associated with a specific subject in standard subdivision **092**, of persons not so related in **920** [*both formerly* **980.2**]

[.6] Specific subjects in relation to Indians

Class with the subject

981 *Brazil

982 *Argentina

983 *Chile

984 *Bolivia

985 *Peru

* Add as instructed under **930–990**

986   *Northwestern South America and Panama

987   *Venezuela

988   *Guiana

989   *Other parts of South America

990   **Other parts of world**

       Do not use standard subdivisions

▶   991–996 Pacific Ocean islands (Oceania)

▶   991–995 Southwest Pacific

991   *Malay Archipelago

       Use **991.000 1 – 991.000 8** for standard subdivisions

  .001–.008   Standard subdivisions of Indonesia

992   *Sunda Islands

993   *New Zealand and Melanesia

994   *Australia

995   *New Guinea (Papua)

996   *Other parts of Pacific

       Do not use standard subdivisions

997   *Atlantic Ocean islands

998   *Arctic islands

999   *Antarctica

* Add as instructed under **930–990**

Table of Standard Subdivisions

As fully explained in the introduction, section 3.37, and as shown by the dashes that precede them, the following standard subdivisions (formerly known as form divisions) are never used alone, but may be used as required with any number from the general tables, e.g., classification (01 in this table) of modern Indic languages (491.4): 491.401.

—01   **Philosophy and theory**

Classification, value, linguistic and scientific aspects, indexes, research methodology, psychological aspects

(Optional: techniques of writing, prefer **808.06**; bibliographies and catalogs, prefer **016**; professional and occupational ethics, prefer **174**)

For dictionaries, see standard subdivision 03

—02   **Miscellany**

Including synopses, outlines, manuals, humorous and audio-visual treatment, commercial miscellany

—021   **Tabulated and related materials**

Tables, formulas [*both formerly* standard subdivision **083**], specifications, lists, inventories, catalogs of articles

For catalogs of museums and exhibits, see standard subdivision **074**

—022   **Illustrations [*formerly* standard subdivision 084]**

Pictures, charts, designs, plans

—023   **The subject as a profession, occupation, hobby**

If preferred, class the subject as a profession or occupation in **331.7**

—024   **Works for specific types of users**

—025   Directories [*formerly* standard subdivision 058]

—026   Law

         (Optional; prefer **340**)

—027   Inventions and identification marks

         Patents, trademarks, service marks, ownership marks, artists' and craftsmen's marks

—028   Techniques, apparatus, equipment

—03   Dictionaries, encyclopedias, concordances

—[04]   Collected essays and lectures

         Class in standard subdivision **08**

—05   Serial publications

         Class administrative reports and proceedings of organizations in standard subdivision **06**

—[058]   Directories

         Class in standard subdivision **025**

—06   Organizations

         History, charters, regulations, membership lists, administrative reports and proceedings

---

►   —061–063 Professional

         International, national, state, provincial, local organizations not engaged in profit-motive activities

—061   Permanent government organizations

—062   Permanent nongovernment organizations

—063   Temporary organizations

—065   Business organizations

         Individual proprietorships, partnerships, companies, corporations, combinations

—[069]   Professional and occupational ethics

         Class in **174**

—07   Study and teaching
—071   Schools and courses
—072   Research
            Historical, descriptive, experimental

—074   Museums and exhibits
            Collections, guidebooks, catalogs

—075   Collecting and collections of objects
            For museums and exhibits, see standard subdivision 074

—076   Review and exercise
            Workbooks with problems, questions, answers
            Including civil service examinations [*formerly* 351.3]

—077   Programed teaching and learning
—078   Use of apparatus and equipment
            Including use of teaching machines

—079   Competitions and awards
            Prizes, scholarships, fellowships, honorary titles

—08   Collections and anthologies
            Collections not planned as composite works
            Including collected essays and lectures [*both formerly* standard
            subdivision 04]

—[081]   Critical appraisal of a person's work
            Class in standard subdivision 092

—[083]   Tables and formulas
            Class in standard subdivision 021

—[084]   Illustrations
            Class in standard subdivision 022

—09   Historical and geographical treatment

—091   Regional treatment

History and description by region, area, place, group in general, not limited by continent, country, locality

Add area notation 1 to 09, e.g., the subject in Torrid Zone **091 3**

—092   Persons

Critical appraisal [*formerly* standard subdivision **081**] and description of work, biography of persons associated with the subject

Scope: Indians of North America [*formerly* **970.2**], of South America [*formerly* **980.2**], slaves [*formerly* **326**]

If preferred, class biography in **920.1–928**

Class biography not clearly related to any specific subject in **920**

Observe exceptions under **180–190, 750, 809, 810–890**

—092 2   Collected

—092 4   Individual

If preferred, class in **92** or **B**

—093–099   Geographical treatment

History and description by continent, country, locality, specific instance of the subject

Add area notations **3–9** to 09, e.g., the subject in United States **097 3**

Class persons associated with the subject in standard subdivision **092**

Area Table

As fully explained in the introduction, section 3.353 1, and as shown by the dashes that precede them, the following area notations are never used alone, but may be used as required (either directly when so noted or thru the interposition of standard subdivision 09) with any number from the general tables, e.g., cultural processes (301.29) in Japan (52 in this table): 301.295 2.

SUMMARY

—1   Regions, areas, places, groups in general
—2   Persons
—3   The ancient world
        —4–9 The modern world
—4   Europe
—5   Asia
—6   Africa
—7   North America
—8   South America
—9   Other parts of world

—1   Regions, areas, places, groups in general

Not limited by continent, country, locality

▶ —11–13 Zonal regions

—11   Frigid Zones

—12   Temperate Zones (Middle Latitude Zones)

—13   Torrid Zone (Tropics)

▶ —14–16 Physiographic regions

—14   Land and land forms

Islands [*formerly* area 9], continents, mountains, caves, plains, coastal regions, soil

—15   Types of vegetation

Forests, grasslands, deserts

—16   Air and water

Including ocean and sea waters, fresh and brackish waters

—161   Atmosphere

—17   Socioeconomic regions and groups

—171   Political orientation

Empires and political unions [*both formerly* areas 3–9], blocs, nonself-governing territories

—172   Degree of economic development

Regions of high, medium, low development

—173   Concentration of population

Urban, suburban, rural regions

—174   Ethnic groups

Including ancient European tribes [*formerly* area 36], Arabs [*formerly* area 53], Jews [*formerly* area 569 3], Negroes [*formerly* area 67], Gipsies [*formerly* 397]

—175   Lingual regions
—176   Religious culture groups

—18   Other kinds of terrestrial regions

Including Western [*formerly* area 7], Eastern, Northern, Southern hemispheres; Mediterranean [*formerly* area 4], Atlantic, Pacific, Indian Ocean basins

Class here the Occident

—19   Space

—2   Persons
—22   Collected
—24   Individual

► —3–9 Specific continents, countries, localities

Class regions, areas, places, groups not limited by continent, country, locality in area **1**

Class empires and political unions [*formerly* areas **3–9**] in area **171**

—3 The ancient world

If preferred, class in areas **4–9**

—31 China

—32 Egypt

—33 Palestine [*formerly also* area **39**]

Including Judea

—34 India

—35 Mesopotamia and Iranian Plateau

Class region east of Caspian Sea in area **39**

—36 Europe north and west of Italian peninsula

Class ancient European tribes [*formerly* area **36**] in area **174**

—37 Italian peninsula and adjacent territories

—38 Greece

For Aegean Sea islands, see area **39**

—39 Other parts of ancient world

Aegean Sea islands, Asia Minor, Cyprus, Syria, Arabia, Black Sea and Caucasus regions, central Asia, north Africa, southeastern Europe

Class Palestine [*formerly* area **39**] in area **33**

►   —4–9 The modern world

(Optional: the ancient world; prefer area **3**)

—4   Europe

Class Mediterranean region [*formerly* area **4**] in area **18**

SUMMARY

—41	Scotland and Ireland
—42	British Isles
—43	Central Europe
—44	France
—45	Italy and adjacent territories
—46	Iberian Peninsula and adjacent islands
—47	Eastern Europe
—48	Scandinavia
—49	Other parts of Europe

—41   Scotland and Ireland

►   —411–414 Divisions of Scotland

—411   Northern Scotland

Shetland and Orkney Islands, Caithness, Sutherland, Ross and Cromarty

—412   North central Scotland

Inverness, Nairn, Moray, Banff, Aberdeen, Kincardine

—413   Central Scottish Lowlands

Angus, Perth, Fife, Kinross, Clackmannan, Stirling, Dunbarton, Argyll, Bute

—414   Southern Scotland

Renfrew, Ayr, Lanark, the Lothians, Berwick, Peebles, Selkirk, Roxburgh, Dumfries, Kirkcudbright, Wigtown

—415   Ireland

For divisions of Ireland, see areas **416–419**

▶ —416–419 Divisions of Ireland

—416   Ulster
        Class here Northern Ireland

—417   Connacht (Connaught)
—418   Leinster
—419   Munster
—42   British Isles
        Class here Great Britain, United Kingdom
        For Scotland and Ireland, see area 41

▶ —421–428 England

—421   Greater London
        Including Outer Ring, Middlesex
        *For a specific part of Outer Ring, see the county in
        which located, e.g., Surrey area* 422

—422   Southeastern England
        Surrey, Kent, Sussex, Hampshire, Berkshire, Isle of Wight
        For Greater London, see area 421

—423   Southwestern England and Channel Islands
        Wiltshire, Dorset, Devon, Cornwall, Somerset

—424   Midlands of England
        Gloucester, Monmouth, Hereford, Shropshire, Stafford,
        Worcester, Warwick
        For East Midlands, see area 425

—425   East Midlands of England
        Derby, Nottingham, Lincoln, Leicester, Rutland,
        Northampton, Huntingdon, Bedford, Oxford, Buckingham,
        Hertford, Cambridge, Soke of Peterborough, Isle of Ely;
        the Fens

—426   Eastern England
              Norfolk, Suffolk, Essex

—427   North central England
              Cheshire, Lancashire, York

—428   Northern England and Isle of Man
              Durham, Northumberland, Cumberland, Westmorland;
              Lake District

—429   Wales
              For Monmouth, see area 424

—43   Central Europe
              Class here Germany

—436   Austria and Liechtenstein
              Class Trieste in area **45**, Slovenia and Dalmatia in area
              497 [*all formerly* area **436**]

—437   Czechoslovakia
              Class Galicia in area **438**, Bukovina in area **498** [*both
              formerly* area **437**]

—438   Poland
              Including Galicia [*formerly* area **437**]

—439   Hungary
              Class Transylvania in area **498**, Slavonia, Croatia, Bosnia
              and Herzegovina in area **497** [*all formerly* area **439**]

—44   France
              For Corsica, see area **459**; *a specific department outside
              Metropolitan France, the subject, e.g., Martinique area* **729 8**

—443   Paris metropolitan area
—449   Riviera
              Including Monaco

—45	Italy and adjacent territories

Including Trieste [*formerly* area **436**], independent state of San Marino

—453	Venice
—455	Florence
—456	Rome and Vatican City
—458	Sicily and Malta
—459	Sardinia and Corsica

—46	Iberian Peninsula and adjacent islands

Including Spain (with Balearic Islands), Andorra, Gibraltar

For Canary Islands, see area **64**

—469	Portugal

Including Madeira and Azores

—47	Eastern Europe

Class here Union of Soviet Socialist Republics (Soviet Union)

For Asiatic Russia, see area **57**; *Soviet Republics of central Asia, area* **58**; *Balkan Peninsula, area* **496**

—471	Finland
—473	Moscow
—477	Moldavian [*formerly* area 498 5] and Ukrainian Soviet Socialist Republics

—479	Caucasus

Including Armenian Soviet Socialist Republic [*formerly* area 566 4]

—48	Scandinavia

Class here northern Europe

For Finland, see area **471**; *Iceland, area* **491**

—481	Norway

For divisions of Norway, see areas **482–484**

────────────

►   —482–484 Divisions of Norway

—482   Southeastern Norway

Vest-Agder, Aust-Agder, Telemark, Vestfold, Ostfold, Oslo, Akershus, Buskerud, Opland, Hedmark counties

—483   Southwestern Norway

Rogaland, Hordaland, Bergen, Sogn og Fjordane, More og Romsdal counties

—484   Central and northern Norway

Sor-Trondelag, Nord-Trondelag, Nordland, Troms, Finnmark counties

—485   Sweden

For divisions of Sweden, see areas **486–488**

────────────

►   —486–488 Divisions of Sweden

—486   Southern Sweden (Gotaland)

Malmohus, Kristianstad, Blekinge, Kalmar, Kronoberg, Halland, Jonkoping, Alvsborg, Goteborg och Bohus, Skaraborg, Ostergotland, Gotland counties

—487   Central Sweden (Svealand)

Sodermanland, Stockholm, Uppsala, Vastmanland, Orebro, Varmland, Kopparberg, Gavleborg counties; Stockholm city

—488   Northern Sweden (Norrland)

Jamtland, Vasternorrland, Vasterbotten, Norrbotten counties

For Gavleborg, see area **487**

—489   Denmark

For Faeroes, see area **491**; *Greenland, area* **98**

—49	Other parts of Europe
—491	Iceland and Faeroes
—492	Netherlands (Holland)
—493	Belgium and Luxembourg
—494	Switzerland
—495	Greece

For Aegean Sea islands, see area **499**

—496	Balkan Peninsula

Including Turkey in Europe, Albania

If preferred, class Turkey in Europe in area **563**

Class here Ottoman Empire

For a specific country of Balkan Peninsula, of Ottoman Empire, see the subject, e.g., Greece area **495**

—497	Yugoslavia and Bulgaria

Including Slovenia and Dalmatia [*both formerly* area **436**]; Slavonia, Croatia, Bosnia and Herzegovina [*all formerly* area **439**]

—498	Romania

Including Bukovina [*formerly* area **437**], Transylvania [*formerly* area **439**]

—[498 5]	Moldavian Soviet Socialist Republic

Class in area **477**

—499	Aegean Sea islands

—5   Asia

Class here the Orient, Eurasia

—————————

▶   —51–52 Far East

For Siberia, see area 57; *Southeast Asia, area* 59

SUMMARY

—51   China and adjacent areas
—52   Japan and adjacent islands
—53   Arabian Peninsula and adjacent areas
—54   South Asia
—55   Iran (Persia)
—56   Middle East
—57   Siberia (Asiatic Russia)
—58   Central Asia
—59   Southeast Asia

—51   China and adjacent areas

—512   Taiwan (Formosa), and Hong Kong and Macao colonies

—515   Tibet

—517   Outer Mongolia (Mongolian People's Republic)

—519   Korea

—52   Japan and adjacent islands

Class southern Sakhalin, Kurile Islands [*both formerly* area 52] in area 57

—521   Tokyo

—528   Ryukyu and Bonin Islands

—53   Arabian Peninsula and adjacent areas

Including Sinai Peninsula, Bahrein

Class Arabs [*formerly* area 53] in area 174

—54   South Asia

Class here India

For Southeast Asia, see area **59**

—[547]   Pakistan

Class in area **549**

—[548 9]   Ceylon and Maldive Islands

Class Ceylon in area **549 3**, Maldive Islands in area **549**

—549   Pakistan [*formerly* area 547] and other jurisdictions

Including eastern Baluchistan [*formerly* area **588**], Maldive Islands [*formerly* area **548 9**], Nepal, Sikkim, Bhutan

—549 3   Ceylon [*formerly* area 548 9]

—55   Iran (Persia)

Including western Baluchistan [*formerly* area **588**]

—56   Middle East

Class here Near East

For a specific country of Middle or of Near East, see the subject, e.g., Iran area **55**

—561   Asia Minor and adjacent islands

Class here Turkey

For divisions of Asia Minor and adjacent islands, see areas **562–566**; *Aegean Sea islands, area* **499**

▶   —562–566 Divisions of Asia Minor and adjacent islands

—562   Western Asia Minor

Canakkale, Balikesir, Manisa, Kutahya, Usak, Afyon, Denizli, Burdur, Mugla, Aydin, Izmir (Smyrna) provinces of Turkey

---

—563   North central Asia Minor

Bursa, Bilecik, Kocaeli, Bolu, Eskisehir, Ankara, Cankiri, Zonguldak, Kastamonu, Sinop, Samsun, Amasya, Corum, Yozgat, Sakarya provinces of Turkey

(Optional: Turkey in Europe; prefer area **496**)

—564   South central Asia Minor and Cyprus

Including Antakya, Isparta, Konya, Kirsehir, Kayseri, Nevsehir, Nygde, Icel, Seyhan (Adana), Hatay, Gaziantep provinces of Turkey

—564 5   Island of Cyprus

—565   East central Asia Minor

Trebizond (Trabzon), Gumusane, Giresun, Ordu, Tokat, Sivas, Maras, Malatya, Adiyaman, Urfa provinces of Turkey

—566   Eastern Asia Minor

Armenia (Rize, Coruh, Erzurum, Kars, Agri, Van, Hakari provinces of Turkey), Kurdistan (Erzincan, Elazig, Tunceli, Diyarbakir, Mus, Bingol, Bitlis, Sürt, Mardin provinces of Turkey)

—[566 4]   Armenian Soviet Socialist Republic

Class in area **479**

—567   Iraq

—569   Eastern Mediterranean

—569 1   Syria

—569 2   Lebanon

—[569 3]   Jews after dispersion

Class in area **174**

—569 4   Israel

Class here Palestine

For Jordan, see area **569 5**

—569 5   Jordan

—57	Siberia (Asiatic Russia)

Including southern Sakhalin, Kurile Islands [*both formerly* area 52]

Class here Soviet Union in Asia

For Soviet Republics of central Asia, see area 58

—58	Central Asia

Including Kirghiz, Kazakh, Turkmen, Tadzhik, Uzbek Soviet Socialist Republics

—581	Afghanistan
—[588]	Baluchistan

Class eastern Baluchistan in area 549, western Baluchistan in area 55

—59	Southeast Asia

For Malay Archipelago, see area 91

—591	Burma
—593	Thailand (Siam)
—594	Laos
—595	Malaysia

Class Malaysian Borneo in area 911

—596	Cambodia
—597	Vietnam
—6	Africa
—61	North Africa

Including Libya, Tunisia

For a specific part of North Africa, see the subject, e.g., Algeria area 65

—62   Egypt and Sudan

              For Sinai Peninsula, see area **53**

—624   Sudan

              For provinces of Sudan, see areas **625–629**

▶   —625–629 Provinces of Sudan

—625   Northern Province

              Class here Nubian Desert

—626   Central provinces

              Khartoum, Blue Nile

—627   Darfur Province

—628   Kordofan Province

—629   Eastern and southern provinces

              Kassala, Upper Nile, Bahr el Ghazal, Equatoria

—63   Ethiopia

—64   Northwest African coast and offshore islands

              Morocco, Spanish West Africa, Canary Islands

—65   Algeria

—66   West Africa and offshore islands

              Including Mauritania, Mali, Upper Volta, Niger, Senegal, Sierra Leone, the Gambia, Guinea republic, Portuguese Guinea, Cape Verde Islands, Liberia, Ivory Coast, Dahomey, Togo, islands of the Gulf of Guinea

              Class here Sahara Desert

—667   Ghana

—669   Nigeria

—67   Central Africa and offshore islands

> Including Cameroun, Rio Muni, Gabon, Congo (Brazzaville),
> Angola, Central African Republic, Chad, Rwanda, Burundi,
> French Somaliland, Socotra, Somalia, Mozambique
>
> Class here Negro Africa, Africa south of the Sahara
>
> Class Negroes not limited by continent [*formerly* area **67**] in
> area **174**
>
>> *For a specific country of Negro Africa, of Africa south of*
>> *the Sahara, see the subject, e.g., Nigeria area* **669**

—675   Congo (Leopoldville)

> Former Belgian Congo

—676   Uganda and Kenya

—678   Tanganyika and Zanzibar (Tanzania)

—68   South Africa

> Including Republic of South Africa, Bechuanaland
> Protectorate, Swaziland, Basutoland (Basotho)

—689   Rhodesia, Zambia, Malawi

> Formerly Southern Rhodesia, Northern Rhodesia,
> Nyasaland

—69   South Indian Ocean islands

> Including Madagascar (Malagasy Republic), Seychelles,
> Réunion, Mauritius

—7   North America

> Class Western Hemisphere [*formerly* area **7**] in area **18**

—701   Indians of North America

> Class North American Indians not limited by continent
> in area **174**

SUMMARY

—71   Canada
—72   M ddle America
—73   United States
—74   Northeastern states
—75   Southeastern (South Atlantic) states
—76   South central states
—77   North central states
—78   Western states
—79   States of Great Basin and Pacific Slope

—71   Canada

—711   British Columbia

—712   Northern territories and prairie provinces

            Including Yukon and Northwest Territories

—712 3   Alberta

—712 4   Saskatchewan

—712 7   Manitoba

—713   Ontario

—714   Quebec

            Class here Saint Lawrence River and Seaway

—715   New Brunswick

            Class here Maritime Provinces

                For Nova Scotia, see area 716; Prince Edward Island, area 717

—716   Nova Scotia

—717   Prince Edward Island

—718   Newfoundland, and Saint Pierre and Miquelon

            For Labrador territory, see area 719

—719   Labrador territory of province of Newfoundland

—72	**Middle America**
	Class here Mexico
—725	**Valley of Mexico**
	Including Mexico City
—728	**Central America**
	For Panama, see area 862
—728 1	Guatemala
—728 2	British Honduras (Belize)
—728 3	Honduras
—728 4	El Salvador
—728 5	Nicaragua
—728 6	Costa Rica
—729	**West Indies (Antilles)**

► —729 1 – 729 5 Greater Antilles

—729 1	Cuba and Isle of Pines
—729 2	Jamaica and Cayman Islands

► —729 3 – 729 4 Hispaniola and adjacent islands

—729 3	Dominican Republic
—729 4	Haiti
—729 5	Puerto Rico
—729 6	Bahama, Turks, Caicos Islands

► —729 7 – 729 8 Lesser Antilles (Caribbees)

—729 7	Leeward Islands
	Virgin Islands, Saint Christopher, Nevis, Anguilla, Sombrero, Antigua, Barbuda, Montserrat, Guadeloupe, Saint Martin, Saint Eustatius, Saba

—729 8	Windward and other southern islands

> Barbados, Martinique, Trinidad and Tobago, Dominica, Saint Lucia, Saint Vincent, Grenadines, Grenada, Carriacou, Curaçao, Aruba, Bonaire

—729 9	Bermuda
—73	United States

> *For specific states, see areas* **74–79**

▶   —74–79 Specific states of United States

> *For Hawaii, see area* **969**

—74	Northeastern states

> Class here Appalachian Mountains, Connecticut River

▶   —741–746 New England

—741	Maine
—742	New Hampshire
—743	Vermont
—744	Massachusetts
—745	Rhode Island
—746	Connecticut

▶   —747–749 Middle Atlantic states

—747	New York
—747 1	New York City
—748	Pennsylvania
—749	New Jersey
—75	Southeastern (South Atlantic) states

> Class here Southern states, Piedmont, Atlantic Coastal Plain

—751	Delaware
—752	Maryland

> Class here Potomac River

—753   District of Columbia (Washington)

—754   West Virginia

—755   Virginia

        Class here Blue Ridge, Chesapeake Bay

—756   North Carolina

—757   South Carolina

—758   Georgia

—759   Florida

—76   South central states

        Class here Old Southwest, lower Mississippi River and Valley

▶   —761–764 Gulf Coast states

        For Florida, see area 759

—761   Alabama

—762   Mississippi

—763   Louisiana

—764   Texas

        Class here Rio Grande

—766   Oklahoma

—767   Arkansas

—768   Tennessee

        Class here Tennessee River and Valley

—769   Kentucky

        Class here Ohio River

        Class Ohio Valley in area 77

—77   North central states

        Class here Middle West, Mississippi River and Valley, Ohio Valley, Great Lakes

        Class Ohio River in area 769

►   —771–776 Lake states

For New York, see area 747; Pennsylvania, area 748

—771   Ohio

—772   Indiana

—773   Illinois

—774   Michigan

—775   Wisconsin

—776   Minnesota

—777   Iowa

—778   Missouri

—78   Western states

               Class here the West, Missouri River, Rocky Mountains

                   For states of Great Basin and Pacific Slope, see area 79

—781   Kansas

—782   Nebraska

—783   South Dakota

—784   North Dakota

►   —786–789 Rocky Mountains states

For Idaho, see area 796

—786   Montana

—787   Wyoming

—788   Colorado

—789   New Mexico

—79   States of Great Basin and Pacific Slope

               Class here Pacific Coast states

—791   Arizona

               Class here New Southwest

—792	Utah
—793	Nevada
—794	California
—795	Oregon

> Class here Pacific Northwest, Cascade and Coast Ranges

—796	Idaho
—797	Washington
—798	Alaska

—8   South America

> Class here Latin America, Spanish America, the Andes
>
> *For Middle America, see area 72*

—801   Indians of South America

> Class South American Indians not limited by continent in area **174**

—81	Brazil
—82	Argentina
—83	Chile
—84	Bolivia
—85	Peru
—86	Northwestern South America and Panama
—861	Colombia
—862	Panama
—863	Panama Canal Zone
—866	Ecuador
—87	Venezuela
—88	Guiana

> British, Dutch (Surinam), French

—89	Other parts of South America
—892	Paraguay
—895	Uruguay

—9   Other parts of world

Class islands of the world [*formerly* area **9**] in area **14**

▶   **—91–96 Pacific Ocean islands (Oceania)**

For a specific island or group of islands, see the subject, e.g., Japan area **52**

▶   **—91–95 Southwest Pacific**

—91   Malay Archipelago

Including Indonesian Borneo, Celebes, Moluccas (Spice Islands)

Class here Indonesia

For Sunda Islands, see area **92**; *New Guinea, area* **95**

—911   North Borneo

Malaysian Borneo and Brunei

—914   Philippine Islands

—92   Sunda Islands

Sumatra, Java, Madura, Bali, Timor, lesser islands

Class Borneo and Celebes in area **91**

—93   New Zealand and Melanesia

Including New Caledonia territory, New Hebrides, Bismarck Archipelago; Loyalty, Solomon, Admiralty Islands

For Louisiade Archipelago, D'Entrecasteaux Islands, see area **95**; *Fiji Islands, area* **96**

—931   New Zealand

—94   Australia

—95   New Guinea (Papua)

Including Louisiade Archipelago, D'Entrecasteaux Islands

—96   **Other parts of Pacific**

Including Fiji, Easter, Pitcairn, Henderson, Ducie, Oeno, Society, Tubuai (Austral), Gambier, Rapa, Cook, Manihiki, Marquesas, Tuamotu, Line, Caroline, Marianas (Ladrone), Gilbert, Ellice, Phoenix, Marshall Islands; Tonga, Samoa, Tokelau, Nauru, Palmyra, Midway

Class here Polynesia, Micronesia

—969   **Hawaii**

—97   **Atlantic Ocean islands**

Bouvet Island, Falklands, Saint Helena, their dependencies

For a specific island or group of islands, see the subject, e.g., Azores area **469**

—98   **Arctic islands**

Svalbard (Spitsbergen), Greenland, Jan Mayen Island, Franz Josef Land, Novaya Zemlya (New Land), Severnaya Zemlya (Northern Land)

For a specific Arctic island or group of islands, see the subject, e.g., Northwest Territories of Canada area **712**

—99   **Antarctica**

Synthesis of Notation

The following numbers and sequences of numbers are used as the basis for synthesis of other sequences. Here, arranged by the secondary number or sequence, are enumerated all the "divide-like" notes that appear in the tables. The procedure for number synthesis thru division is described in the introduction, section 3.353 2.

In this list, numbers or spans of numbers preceded by asterisks are numbers whose starred subdivisions are to be divided as instructed at the place indicated.

Since every number in the tables may be built upon by the addition of the numbers of the area table, either direct (where the tables say "Add area notation . . .") or thru the use of standard subdivision 09, the "add" notes are not enumerated. Observe also that any standard subdivision may be added to *any* class number.

Like 001–999
016
Like 001–899
910.1
Like 220.1–.9
221.1–.9
225.1–.9
Like 281–289
230.1–.9
252.01–.09
264.01–.09
266.1–.9
Like 291
292
Like 351.1–.9
353.001–.009
Like 355
358.41
Like 355.1–.2
359.1–.2
Like 355.4–.8
359.4–.8
Like 420–490
572.8
Like 421–428
*430–490

Like 421–426
*430–490
Like 423
*430–490
Like 428
*430–490
Like 430–490
220.53–.59
423.3–.9
Like 439
839
Like 491
891
Like 492
892
Like 510–590
630.21–.29
Like 574
576.1
Like 574.1–.9
581.1–.9
591.1–.9
Like 574.9
560.9

Like 583–589
635.933–.939
Like 597.2–.5
799.17
Like 708.1–.9
747.21–.29
749.21–.29
Like 725–728
690.5–.8
Like 747.201–.204
749.201–.204
Like 808.1–.7
808.81–.87
809.1–.7
Like 811–817
869.1–.7
Like 970.1–.5
980.1–.5
Like area 42–48
708.2–.8
759.2–.8
Like area 73–79
708.13–.19
Like area 74–79
759.14–.19

Relative Index

Use of the Relative Index

Full instructions on use appear in the introduction, section 3.6.

A dagger (†) preceding a number means that one or more topics, not necessarily including the one named, have been relocated to this number from another number in Abridged edition 8.

An entry and number in **boldface** means that this subject and number are subdivided in the tables.

A number preceded by *"area"* may be found in the Area Table, and indicates geographical specification; a number preceded by *"s.s."* may be found in the Table of Standard Subdivisions, and indicates a form of presentation or a mode of treatment. Neither area nor standard subdivision numbers are used alone, but both may be used as required with any number from the general tables.

Abbreviations Used in the Index

ASSR	Autonomous Soviet Socialist Republic	Ia.	Iowa
admin.	administration(s)	Ida.	Idaho
Ala.	Alabama	Ill.	Illinois
anal.	analytic(al), analysis	Ind.	Indiana
arch.	architectural, architecture	ind.	industrial, industries, industry
Ariz.	Arizona	internat.	international
Ark.	Arkansas	isl(s).	island(s)
bus.	business(es)	Kan.	Kansas
bus. tech.	business technology	Ky.	Kentucky
Calif.	California	La.	Louisiana
chem. tech.	chemical technology	lit.	literary, literature(s)
co.	county	Mass.	Massachusetts
Colo.	Colorado	Md.	Maryland
comp.	comparative	Me.	Maine
Conn.	Connecticut	meas.	measures
Del.	Delaware	med.	medical, medicine
dept(s).	department(s)	med. sci.	medical sciences
econ.	economic(s)	Mich.	Michigan
econ. geol.	economic geology	mil.	military
ed.	education(al)	mil. sci.	military science
elect.	electric(al), electricity	Minn.	Minnesota
Eng.	England	Miss.	Mississippi
eng.	engineering, engineers	Mo.	Missouri
equip.	equipment	Mont.	Montana
Fla.	Florida	mt(s).	mountain(s)
Ga.	Georgia	N.C.	North Carolina
gen.	general	N.D.	North Dakota
gen. wks.	general works	N.H.	New Hampshire
geol.	geological, geology	N.J.	New Jersey
govt.	government(s), governmental	N.M.	New Mexico
		N.T.	New Testament
hist.	historical, history	N.Y.	New York
		N.Z.	New Zealand

nat.	national, natural	rel.	religion(s)
Neb.	Nebraska	res.	reservoir
Nev.	Nevada	S.C.	South Carolina
O.	Ohio	S.D.	South Dakota
O.T.	Old Testament	SSR	Soviet Socialist
Okla.	Oklahoma		Republic
Ore.	Oregon	sci.	science(s), scientific
P.E.I.	Prince Edward Island	spec.	specific
Pa.	Pennsylvania	St.	Saint
par.	parish	subj.	subject(s)
pol.	political, politics	Tenn.	Tennessee
pol. sci.	political science	Ter.	Territory
prac.	practical, practice	Tex.	Texas
prod.	producing, production,	U.S.	United States
	products	USSR	Union of Soviet
psych.	psychological,		Socialist Republics
	psychology	Va.	Virginia
pub.	public	vet.	veterinary
qual.	qualitative, quality	vet. sci.	veterinary science
quan.	quantitative, quantity	Vt.	Vermont
R.I.	Rhode Island	W.Va.	West Virginia
RSFSR	Russian Soviet Feder-	Wash.	Washington
	ated Socialist Re-	Wis.	Wisconsin
	public	Wyo.	Wyoming
reg.	regulation(s),		
	regulatory		

Relative Index

A

Aardwolves
  culture   636.9
  see also Proteles
Abandoned
  children *see* Children
Abbey
  schools *see* Monastic schools
Abbeys
  buildings *see* Monastic
      buildings
  religion *see* Religious
      congregations
Abbreviations
  linguistics
    English   421
    see also other spec.
      languages
  see also   *s.s.*–01
Abdias (O.T.) *see* Prophetic
    books
Abduction *see* Offenses
Aberdeen Scotland   *area* –412
Abnormal
  children *see* Exceptional
    children
  psychology
    animals   †156
    gen. wks.   157
    pedology   †155.45
Abnormalities *see* Teratology
Abolition
  slavery *see* Slavery
Aborigines *see* Ethnology
Abortion
  criminal *see* Offenses
  spontaneous
    animals
      vet. sci.   636.089
      zoology   591.2
      see also spec. animals
    man   618.3
    see also Miscarriage

Abortionists *see* Offenders
Absentee
  ownership
    economics
      industries   338
      land   333.4
    see also other spec. subj.
Absolute
  democracy *see* Pure
    democracy
  geometries
    gen. wks.   513
    see also   *s.s.*–01
  monarchy *see* Monarchical
    absolutism
  temperature *see* Cryogenics
Absolution
  penance *see* Sacraments
  see also other spec. rites
Absolutism
  monarchical *see* Monarchical
    absolutism
  religion *see* Predestination
Abstinence
  ethics   178
  religion *see* Religious
    experience
Abstract
  art
    gen. wks.   704.945
    see also spec. art forms
  thought
    philosophy   128
    psychology   153.2
Abstractions *see* Abstract
Abutments *see* Columns
Abyssinia *see* Ethiopia
Abyssinian
  Church
    religion   281
    see also Church buildings
  see also Ethiopic

Ammunition (continued)
  mil. sci.
    gen. wks.   355.8
    tech. forces *see* Technical
      forces
    see also spec. mil. branches
Ammunition-ships *see*
  Government vessels
Amos (O.T.) *see* Prophetic
  books
Amphibian
  planes *see* Heavier-than-air
    aircraft
Amphibians
  culture   639
  paleozoology   567
  zoology   597
  see also spec. animals
Amphibious
  landing craft *see* Warships
  warfare
    gen. wks.   †359.9
    see also hist. of spec. wars
Amphitheaters *see* Recreation
  buildings
Amulets *see* Talismans
Amusement
  park buildings *see* Park
    buildings
  parks *see* Recreational land
Amusements *see* Recreational
  activities
Amvets *see* Military societies
Ana *see* Collected writings
Anabaptists
  religion   284
  see also Church buildings
Anagrams *see* Puzzles
Analog
  instruments
    engineering   621.381 9
    managerial use   658.5
    mathematics   510.78
    office equipment 651
    see also   *s.s.*–01
Analogy
  logic   169
  psychology   †153.4
  religion
    gen. wks.   219
    see also spec. rel.

Analysis
  chemistry *see* Analytical
    chemistry
  mathematics
    calculus   **517**
    geometry   **516**
    see also   *s.s.*–01
  physics
    sound waves   534
    see also Vibrations
  see also Reasoning
Analysis situs *see* Topology
Analytic *see* Analytical
Analytical
  chemistry
    gen. wks.   543–545
    organic   547
    pharmacy
      med. sci.   615
      vet. sci.
        gen. wks.   636.089
        see also spec. animals
  geometry
    gen. wks.   **516**
    see also   *s.s.*–01
Anamnia
  paleozoology   567
  zoology   **597**
Anarchism *see* Ideal states
Anatolian
  ethnic groups   *area* –174
  language   491.9
  lingual groups   *area* –175
  see also other spec. subj.
Anatomy
  biology
    animals   591.4
    gen. wks.   574.4
    plants   581.4
    see also spec. organisms
  cells *see* Cytology
  med. sci.
    animals
      gen. wks.   636.089
      see also spec. animals
    man   611
Ancestry *see* Genealogy
Anchors *see* Nautical equipment
Ancient
  civilization *see* Ancient world

Antarctic	
waters	
geography	
gen. wks.	910.09
physical	†910.02
geology	551.4
regional subj.	
treatment	*area* –16
Antarctica	*area* –99
Anteaters *see* Edentates	
Antelopes	
conservation	639
culture	636.2
hunting	
industries	639
sports	799.27
see also Bovoidea	
Antennas	
engineering	
economics	338.4
technology	
radio	621.384 1
television	621.388 3
see also spec. applications	
Anthems *see* Choral music	
Anthologies *see* Collected	
writings	
Anthropogeography	
biology	**572.9**
psychology	†155.8
sociology	301.453
Anthropoidea *see* Primates	
Anthropology	
criminal *see* Criminal	
anthropology	
cultural *see* Culture	
physical *see* Physical	
anthropology	
social *see* Culture	
Anthropometry	
anthropology	573
crime detection	364.12
medicine	616
Anthroposophy *see* Mysticism	
Antiaircraft	
artillery	
forces *see* Artillery forces	
pieces *see* Artillery	
(pieces)	
cruisers *see* Warships	
Antichrist *see* Demonology	

Antigua West Indies	*area* –729 7
Antilles *see* West Indies	
Antimissile	
missiles *see* Guided missiles	
Antimony *see* Metals	
Antinomianism *see* Heresies	
Antiphonal	
readings *see* Responsive	
readings	
Antiques	
gen. wks.	745.1
see also spec. art forms	
Antiquities	
gen. wks. *see* Ancient world	
law	†340
Anti-Semitism	
pol. sci.	323.1
psychology	155.9
sociology	301.451
Antisocial	
compulsions *see* Personality-	
disorders	
Antitank	
artillery	
forces *see* Artillery forces	
pieces *see* Artillery	
(pieces)	
Anti-Trinitarianism *see*	
Unitarianism	
Antonyms	
English language	
lexicology	**†422–423**
usage	**†428**
see also other spec. languages	
Ants	
agricultural pests	632
culture	638
see also Hymenoptera	
Apachean *see* Na-Dene	
Apartment	
buildings *see* Residential	
buildings	
house	
districts *see* Residential	
areas	
houses *see* Public	
accommodations	
Apes	
conservation	639
culture	636.9
see also Primates	

Arachnids
  culture   639
  disease carriers *see* Disease
      carriers
  see also Arachnida
Aramaic
  ethnic groups   *area* –174
  languages   492
  lingual groups   *area* –175
  see also other spec. subj.
Araneida
  paleozoology   565
  zoology   595
Arbitrage *see* Foreign exchange
Arbitration *see* Conciliation
      practices
Arcades *see* Arches
Archangels *see* Angelology
Archbishops *see* Clergy
Archeology
  Biblical   220.93
  gen. wks.   †**913**
  modern *see geography of*
      spec. places
  prehistoric *see* Ancient world
Archery *see* Shooting
      (activities)
Arches
  architecture
    element   721
    structures   725
  construction
    economics   338.4
    technology   690.5
  engineering
    gen. wks.   624
    see also spec. branches
Architectural
  construction
    gen. wks.   721
    see also Construction
  drawing *see* Technical
      drawing
  orders *see* Columns
  subjects
    arts
      gen. wks.   704.94
      see also spec. art forms
Architecture
  art   **720**
  engineering *see* Structural
      engineering

Archive
  buildings *see* Government
      buildings
Archives (records)
  business treatment   651
  government treatment   †350
  library treatment   025.17
Arctic
  lands   *area* –98
  Ocean
    geography
      gen. wks.   910.09
      physical   †910.02
    geology   551.4
    regional subj.
      treatment   *area* –16
Arctic
  photography *see* Cold-
      weather photography
  plants
    botany   581.909
    floriculture   635.9
    see also spec. plants
Area
  planning *see* Planning
  surveying *see* Boundary
      surveying
Argentina   *area* –82
Argot *see* Dialectology
Argument *see* Persuasion
Argyll Scotland   *area* –413
Arianism *see* Heresies
Aristocracy
  class *see* Social classes
  education *see* Exceptional
      children
  gen. wks.   929.7
  heraldry *see* Heraldry
  pol. sci.   321.5
  see also spec. areas
Aristotype
  process *see* Special-process
      photography
Arithmetic
  gen. wks.   **511**
  study & teaching
    elementary ed.   372.7
    see also   *s.s.*–07
    see also   *s.s.*–01
Arizona   *area* –791
Arkansas (state)   *area* –767

Artificial (continued)
  insemination
    animals   636.08
    man   618.1
    see also Sexual ethics
  islands
    engineering
      economics   338.4
      technology   627
    see also spec. applications
  languages
    gen. wks.   †499.9
    literature   †899.9
    see also other spec. subj.
  precipitation
    physical geology   †551.6
    see also spec. applications
  satellites
    engineering
      economics   338.4
      technology
        crafts   629.46
        flights   629.43
      weather prediction   †551.6
    see also other spec.
        applications
  stones
    construction indus.
      economics   338.4
      technology   693.5
    manufacture
      economics   338.4
      technology   666
    materials
      construction   691
      engineering   620.1
    see also spec. applications
  weather control
    physical geology   †551.6
    see also spec. applications
Artigue
  process *see* Special-process
      photography
Artillery (pieces)
  art metalwork   739.7
  customs   399
  industries
    economics   338.4
    technology   623.4
  mil. sci.
    gen. wks.   355.8

Artillery (pieces)
  mil. sci. (continued)
    tech. forces *see* Technical
        forces
    see also spec. mil.
        branches
Artillery
  ammunition *see* Ammunition
  forces
    mil. sci.   358
    see also spec. kinds of
        warfare
Artiodactyla
  paleozoology   569
  zoology   599.7
Arts
  creative *see* Creative arts
  industrial *see* Industrial arts
  manual *see* Manual arts
  mil. recreation *see* Special
        services
  religion
    Christian   246–247
    gen. wks.   291.3
    see also other spec. rel.
Aruba West Indies   *area* –729 8
Aryan *see* Indo-Iranian
Asbestos
  geology
    gen. wks.   553
    mineralogy
      gen. wks.   549.6
    see also spec. minerals
  industries
    extractive *see* Mining
    manufacturing *see spec.*
        products
  properties
    construction   691
    engineering   620.1
    see also Refractory materials
Ascension
  Thursday *see* Holy days
Asceticism *see* Religious
        experience
Ash
  Wednesday *see* Holy days
Ashuanipi Ter.   *area* –719
Asia   *area* –5

354

Atlantic
  Ocean (continued)
    isls.   *area* –97
    regional subj.
      treatment   *area* –16
    region
      geography   910.09
      history   909
      subj. treatment   *area* –18
      see also spec. areas
Atlantis *see* Imaginary places
Atlases *see* Graphic
      illustrations
Atmosphere
  geology *see* Physical geology
  regional subj.
    treatment   *area* –16
Atolls *see* Islands
Atomic
  chemistry *see* Atoms
  energy *see* Nuclear energy
  power *see* Nuclear energy
  structure *see* Atoms
  theory *see* Atoms
  war
    conduct *see* Nuclear
      warfare
    planning *see* Strategy
    weapons *see* Firearms
Atomism
  philosophy   146
  science   501
Atoms
  chemistry   541
  physics   539
Atonement
  religion
    Christian   232
    gen. wks.   291.2
    see also other spec. rel.
  see also Redemption
Attacks
  mil. sci. *see* Battle tactics
Attention
  learning *see* Learning
  perception *see* Perception
Attitudes *see* Sentiments
Auction
  catalogs
    books   017–019
    see also   *s.s.*–02

Auctions *see* Distribution
    channels
Audiology
  med. sci.   617
  music   781.2
  physiology   612
  psychology
    animals   †156
    gen. wks.   †152.1
  see also Acoustics
Audio-visual
  materials
    library treatment 025.17
    teaching use
      gen. wks.   371.33
      see also spec. levels
        of ed.
    see also   *s.s.*–†022
    treatment   *s.s.*–02
Auditing
  finance *see* Financial
    administration
  public *see* Public accounting
Auditoriums *see* Recreation
    buildings
Augsburg
  Diet *see* Reformation
Augustinians *see* Religious
    congregations
Australia   *area* –94
Australian
  ethnic groups   *area* –174
  languages   499
  lingual groups   *area* –175
  see also other spec. subj.
Austria   *area* –436
Austrian
  Succession War
    gen. wks.   940.2
    see also spec. countries
Austroasian
  ethnic groups   *area* –174
  languages   495
  lingual groups   *area* –175
  see also other spec. subj.
Austronesian
  ethnic groups   *area* –174
  languages   499
  lingual groups   *area* –175
  see also other spec. subj.
Autarchy *see* Monarchical
    absolutism

Baby-sitting *see* Child care
Backgammon *see* Dice games
Bacon *see* Red meats
Bacteria *see* Schizomycetes
Bacteriological
  warfare *see* Biological
    warfare
Bacteriology *see* Schizomycetes
Badgers *see* Mustelines
Badminton *see* Racket games
Baffin Bay *see* Arctic Ocean
Bagpipes *see* Wind instruments
    (musical)
Bahai faith *see* Bahaism
Bahaism
  culture groups
    geography   910.09
    history   909
    subject treatment   *area* –176
  philosophy   181
  religion   297
Bahama Isls.   *area* –729 6
Bahr el Ghazal Sudan   *area* –629
Bahrein   *area* –53
Bakery
  products
    manufacture
      economics   338.4
      technology
        commercial   664
        home   641.8
      marketing   658.8
Baking
  ceramics *see* Ceramics
  food *see* Cooking processes
Balalaikas *see* Guitars
Bali   *area* –92
Balikesir Turkey   *area* –562
Balinese *see* Austronesian
Balkan Peninsula   *area* –496
Ball
  bearings *see* Bearings
  games
    customs   394
    ethics   175
    gen. wks.   **796.3**
Ballades *see* Choral music
Ballads
  folklore *see* Rhymes
  literature *see* Poetry
  music *see* Choral music

Ballet
  ethics   175
  music
    gen. wks.   782.9
    see also spec. mediums
  performances   **792.8**
Ballistic
  missiles *see* Guided missiles
Ballistics
  engineering   623.5
  mechanics
    solids   531
    see also spec. branches
  see also spec. applications
Ballot
  systems
    laws   †340
    pol. sci.   324
Balls (dances) *see* Dancing
Balls (sporting goods) *see*
    Recreational
    equipment
Baltic Sea *see* Atlantic Ocean
Baltic
  ethnic groups   *area* –174
  languages   491.9
  lingual groups   *area* –175
  see also other spec. subj.
Balto-Slavic *see* Slavic
Baluchi *see* Iranian
Baluchistan   *area* –†549
Bamboowork *see* Basketry
Banat   *area* –†498
Band
  music *see* Bands
  saws *see* Tools
Bandicoots *see* Marsupials
Bands
  music   785.1
  performance   785.06
  recreation
    military *see* Special
      services
    students
      gen. wks.   †371.89
      see also spec. levels
        of ed.
Banjos *see* String instruments
Bank
  buildings *see* Commercial
    buildings

Basketry
  crafts   746.4
  industry
    economics   338.4
    technology   677
  study & teaching
    elementary ed.   372.5
    see also   *s.s.–07*
Basotho *see* Basutoland
Basque
  ethnic groups   *area* –174
  language   499
  lingual groups   *area* –175
  see also other spec. subj.
Bass
  fiddles *see* String instruments
Basset
  horn *see* Wind instruments
      (musical)
  hounds *see* Hounds
Bassoons *see* Wind instruments
      (musical)
Basutoland   *area* –68
Bat
  games
    customs   394
    gen. wks.   **796.35**
Bath mitzvah *see* Rites
Bathing
  customs   391
  hygiene   613.4
  techniques
    children *see* Child care
    gen. wks.   646.7
Bathing-beaches
  civic art   711
  pub. health   614
  recreation
    gen. wks.   796.5
    see also Swimming
        activities
  see also Safety measures
Bathing-suits *see* Garments
Bathrooms *see* Lavatories
Baths *see* Bathing
Batik *see* Resist-dyeing
Bats (animals)
  agricultural aids   632
  culture   636.9
  hunting   †639
  see also Chiroptera

Bats (sporting goods) *see*
      Recreational
      equipment
Battalions *see* Organizational
      units
Batteries
  elect. eng.   621.35
  see also spec. applications
Battle
  cries *see* War customs
  songs *see* National songs
  tactics
    mil. sci.
      gen. wks.   **355.4**
      see also spec. mil.
        branches
    see also hist. of spec. wars
Battledore & shuttlecock *see*
      Racket games
Battles
  history
    gen. wks.   904
    see also spec. wars
  mil. sci.
    analysis
      gen. wks.   355.4
      see also spec. mil.
        branches
Battleships *see* Warships
Beach
  formation *see* Marine waters
  protection *see* Shore
      reclamation
Beaches
  gen. wks. *see* Coasts
  recreational *see* Bathing-
      beaches
Beadwork
  crafts   746.5
  industry
    economics   338.4
    technology   677
Beagles *see* Hounds
Bearbaiting *see* Animal
      performances
Bearings
  engineering
    economics   338.4
    technology
      gen. wks.   621.8
      see also spec. branches
  see also spec. applications

Bengal (bay) *see* Indian Ocean	
Bengali *see* Prakrits	
Berber	
ethnic groups	*area* –174
languages	493
lingual groups	*area* –175
see also other spec. subj.	
Bergen Norway	*area* –483
Bering	
Sea *see* Pacific Ocean	
Berith milah *see* Rites	
Berkshire Eng.	*area* –422
Bermuda	*area* –729 9
Bernardines *see* Religious congregations	
Berths	
docks *see* Docks	
shipyards *see* Shipyards	
Berwick Scotland	*area* –414
Beryllium *see* Metals	
Bessarabia	*area* –†477
Betatrons *see* Particle acceleration	
Betting *see* Gambling	
Beverages	
manufacture	
economics	338.4
technology	
commercial	663
domestic	641.8
marketing	
technology	658.8
see also Liquor traffic	
pub. health meas.	614
Bhagavad Gita	
literature	891.2
religion	294.5
Bhutan	*area* –†549
Bible	
literature	†809.9
religion	
gen. wks.	**220**
theology	**230**
see also Scripture readings	
Biblical	
Sabbath *see* Holy days	
Bibliographical	
centers	
management	658

Bibliographical	
centers (continued)	
planning	
civic art	711
sociology	301.3
services	†021.6
Bibliographies	
books	**010**
music scores	781.9
Bicameral	
legislatures *see* Legislative bodies	
Bicycles *see* Cycles (vehicles)	
Bicycling *see* Cycling	
Bids *see* Procurement	
Biennials	
botany	**582.1**
floriculture	635.93
landscaping	712
see also spec. plants	
Big	
businesses	
economics	338.6
management	658
game	
hunting *see* Hunting (activity)	
Bigamists *see* Offenders	
Bigamy *see* Offenses	
Bigotry *see* Evils	
Bihari *see* Prakrits	
Bill	
of Rights *see* Constitutional law	
Billeting *see* Quarters	
Billiards *see* Indoor ball games	
Billing-machines *see* Digital machines	
Bills (legislation)	
gen. wks.	328.3
spec. localities	**328.4–.9**
Bills	
of credit *see* Credit instruments	
Bindery *see* Bookbinding	
Binding	
books *see* Bookbinding	
Bio-astronautics *see* Biophysics	

Blues
music
    gen. wks.   781.5
    see also spec. mediums
Boarding
schools *see* Secondary
    schools
Boardinghouses *see* Public
    accommodations
Boars *see* Swine
Boat
racing *see* Boating
Boatbuilding *see* Boats
Boathouses *see* Recreation
    buildings
Boating
seamanship   623.88
services   **386–387**
sports   797.1
Boats
construction
    economics   338.4
    technology   623.82
mil. sci.
    gen. wks.   355.8
    see also spec. mil.
        branches
see also Transportation
    services
Bobcats *see* Cats
Bobsledding *see* Snow sports
Body
contours
    control
        hygiene   613.2
        technology   646.7
    customs   391
Bog
plants *see* Hydrophytes
Bohemian
Brethren *see* Hussites
linguistic aspects *see* Czech
Boiler-house
practices
    gen. wks.   621.1
    see also spec. applications
Boilers
engineering
    gen. wks.   621.1
    see also spec. branches
see also spec. uses

Boiling
cookery *see* Cooking
    processes
transformation *see* Physical
    transformations
Bokmaal *see* Germanic
Bolivia (country)   *area* –84
Bolshevist
states *see* Communist states
Bolts *see* Fastenings
Bolu Turkey   *area* –†563
Bolyai
geometry
    gen. wks.   513
    see also   *s.s.*–01
Bombardments
gen. wks. *see* Disasters
mil. sci.
    aerial *see* Air warfare
    gen. wks. *see* Siege
        warfare
Bombardons *see* Wind
    instruments
    (musical)
Bombers
aircraft *see* Heavier-than-air
    aircraft
Bombings *see* Bombardments
Bombproof
construction *see* Resistant
    construction
structures *see* Blastproof
    structures
Bombs *see* Ammunition
Bonaire West Indies   *area* –729 8
Bonded
debts *see* Public securities
Bonds (finance) *see* Securities
Bongos *see* Antelopes
Bonin Isls.   *area* –528
Bonsai *see* House plants
Boobies *see* Gannets
Book
rarities *see* Rare books
reviews
    gen. wks.   028.1
    see also spec. subj.
trade
    services
        domestic   381
        foreign   382
        gen. wks.   †380.1

Broadcasting			Bryophyta	
activity *see* Telecommunication			botany	588
			floriculture	635.938
stations			paleobotany	561
architecture	725		Brythonic *see* Celtic	
construction	690.5		Buccaneers *see* Pirates	
engineering			Buckingham Eng.	*area* –425
economics	338.4		Buddhism	
technology			culture groups	
radio	621.384 1		geography	910.09
television	621.388 6		history	909
see also other			subj. treatment	*area* –176
wireless systems			philosophy	181
services	**384.5**		religion	294.3
Broadsides			Budgerigars	
collections			culture	636.6
general	**†080**		disease carriers *see* Disease	
see also	*s.s.*–08		carriers	
library treatment	025.17		*see also* Psittaciformes	
Broiling			Budget (The) *see* Budgets	
cookery *see* Cooking			Budget	
processes			accounts *see* Credit	
Brokerage			Budgetary	
firms *see* Investment			control *see* Financial	
institutions			administration	
Bromoil			Budgets	
process *see* Special-process			administration *see* Financial	
photography			administration	
Broncos *see* Ponies			economics	
Bronze			private	332
Age			public	336.3
gen. wks.	†913.03		Buffaloes *see* Bison	
see also spec. subj.			Bugle	
metal *see* Metals			corps *see* Bands	
Bronzework *see*			Bugles *see* Wind instruments	
Coppersmithing			(musical)	
Brooks *see* Water bodies			Bugs	
Brotherhoods			agricultural pests	632
religion *see* Religious			culture	638
congregations			*see also* Insecta	
Brothers			Building	
children *see* Children			cooperatives *see*	
gen. wks. *see* Kinship			Cooperatives	
of the Christian Schools *see*			stones	
Religious congregations			geology	
			gen. wks.	553
Brownies (elves) *see*			mineralogy *see spec*	
Supernatural beings			*minerals*	
Brownouts *see* Camouflage			industries	
Brunch *see* Meals			construction	
Brunei	*area* –911		economics	338.4
			technology	693.1

Building
  stones
    industries (continued)
      extractive
        economics   338.2
        technology   622
      properties
        construction   691
        engineering   620.1
      see also spec. structures
Buildings
  architecture   **720**
  construction
    economics   338.4
    technology   **690**
  landscape element   717
  pub. health   614
  see also Architectural
      subjects
Bukovina   *area* –†498
Bulbs (lamps) *see*
      Illumination fixtures
Bulbs (plants)
  agricultural crops
    economics   338.1
    technology   631.5
Bulgaria   *area* –497
Bulgarian
  ethnic groups   *area* –174
  language   491.8
  lingual groups   *area* –175
  see also other spec. subj.
Bulk
  carriers *see* Merchant ships
Bull
  fiddles *see* String instruments
  Moose Party *see* Political
      parties
Bulldogs *see* Nonsporting dogs
Bulldozers *see* Tractors
Bullets *see* Small-arms
      ammunition
Bullfighting *see* Animal
      performances
Bulls *see spec. animals*
Buntings *see* Finches
Burdur Turkey   *area* –562
Bureaucracy
  government
    gen. wks.   †350
    see also spec. levels of
        govt.

Bureaucracy (continued)
    see also spec. organizations
Burglar
  alarms *see* Alarm systems
Burglars *see* Offenders
Burglary
  crime *see* Offenses
  insurance
    gen. wks.   368
    see also Financial
        institutions
  psychopathic *see* Personality-
        disorders
Burial
  places *see* Cemeteries
  rites *see* Funeral rites
Buried
  cities
    ancient *see* Ancient world
  treasure
    adventure   910.4
    fiction *see* Fiction
Burlesque (theater) *see* Drama
Burma   *area* –591
Burmese
  ethnic groups   *area* –174
  language   495
  lingual groups   *area* –175
  see also other spec. subj.
Burros *see* Asses
Bursa Turkey   *area* –563
Burundi   *area* –67
Buryat ASSR   *area* –†57
Buryat (subject) *see* Mongolic
Buses *see* Motor vehicles
Bushes *see* Shrubs
Bushman *see* Macro-Khoisan
Business
  arithmetic
    gen. wks.   511.8
    see also   *s.s.*–01
  colleges *see* Vocational
        education
  cycles
    economics
      gen. wks.   338.54
      see also spec. industries
    see also hist. of spec. areas
  districts *see* Commercial
        areas
  education *see* Vocational
        education

Business (continued)
  enterprises
    economics   **338**
    pol. status   322
    technology   **650**
    see also   s.s.–065
  ethics *see* Occupational
      ethics
  insurance
    gen. wks.   368
    see also Financial
        institutions
  law *see* Commercial law
  libraries
    gen. wks.   027.6
    see also spec. *functions*
  machines
    gen. wks.   651
    see also spec. *machines*
  see also Economic order
Buskerud Norway   *area* –482
Bute Scotland   *area* –413
Butter
  food
    gen. wks.   641.3
    see also Dairy products
  industry
    economics   338.1
    technology   637
Butterflies
  agricultural pests   632
  culture   638
  see also Lepidoptera
Buttermaking *see* Butter
      industry
Buttresses *see* Columns
Buying *see* Procurement
Buzz
  games
    entertainment   793.7
    folklore   398.8
  groups *see* Discussion
      methods
Buzzards *see* Hawks
Buzzers *see* Alarm systems
By-products
  management   658.5
  production *see* Waste
      salvage
  spec. industries *see* spec.
      industries
Byzantium *see* Istanbul

C

Cabala
  literature   809.9
  religion   296.1
  see also Occultism
Cabalistic
  traditions *see* Mystic
      traditions
Cabinets (furniture) *see*
      Furniture
Cabinets (government
      agencies)
  gen. wks.   †350
  see also spec. *levels of govt.*
Cable
  railways *see* Railways
  telegraphy *see*
      Telecommunication
Cables
  engineering
    materials   620.1
    structures   624
    see also spec. *kinds*
  manufacture
    gen. wks.   671.8
    see also spec. *metals*
  power transmission   621.319
  see also Cordage
Cabs *see* Motor vehicles
Cactales
  botany   583
  floriculture   635.933
Cactus
  plants *see* Cactales
Cadastration *see* Taxation
Cadmium *see* Metals
Caecilians *see* Amphibians
Caesarism *see* Despotic states
Cafeterias
  public *see* Public
      accommodations
  school equipment *see*
      School buildings
Caicos Isls.   *area* –729 6
Caissons (gun mounts) *see*
      Gun mounts
Caithness Scotland   *area* –411
Cakes *see* Bakery products
Calcium *see* Metals

Canada   *area* –71
Canakkale Turkey   *area* –562
Canalboats *see* Towed craft
Canals
    drainage *see* Drainage
        structures
    engineering
        economics   338.4
        technology   627
    irrigation *see* Irrigation
    transportation   386
Canapés *see* Auxiliary foods
Canaries *see* Finches
Canary Isls.   *area* –64
Candies
    marketing   658.8
    production
        economics   338.4
        technology
            commercial   664
            domestic   641.8
Candlemas *see* Holy days
Canework *see* Basketry
Canidae
    paleozoology   569
    zoology   599.7
Canine
    corps
        services   363.2
        training   636.7
Canines *see* Dogs
Cankiri Turkey   *area* –563
Canning
    food *see* Food technology
Cannons *see* Artillery (pieces)
Canoeing *see* Boating
Canoes *see* Hand-propelled
        craft
Canon
    law *see* Religious law
    music
        gen. wks.   781.4
        see also spec. mediums
Canonical
    hours *see* Divine Office
Cantatas
    sacred   783.4
    secular   782.8

Canteens
    military *see* Military
        buildings
    public *see* Public
        accommodations
Canticle of Canticles *see* Poetic
        books
Canticles *see* Songs
Canzonets *see* Choral music
Cape
    Verde Isls.   *area* –66
Capital
    goods
        gen. wks.   339
        see also Finance
    punishment
        ethics   179
        see also Punishment
Capitalism *see* Economic
        systems
Capitalization
    finance *see* Financial
        administration
Capital-surplus
    accounting *see* Financial
        accounting
Capitol
    buildings *see* Government
        buildings
Capitulations *see* Diplomacy
Cappadocia   *area* –39
Caps *see* Garments
Captains *see* Personnel
Captured
    soldiers *see* War prisoners
Capuchins *see* Religious
        congregations
Carabao *see* Water buffaloes
Caravels *see* Historic ships
Carbines *see* Small arms
Carbon
    compounds
        inorganic *see* Inorganic
            chemistry
        organic *see* Organic
            chemistry
Carbonated
    drinks *see* Soft drinks
    water *see* Mineralized
        waters

Cascades *see* Water bodies

Case
  studies
    gen. wks. †001.4
    see also s.s.–01

Cases
  internal law
    Anglo-U.S. 345–346
    other **349**

Casks
  wooden *see* Sawmill products

Casserole
  foods *see* Entrees

Cassowaries *see* Emus

Castanets *see* Percussion
      instruments

Caste
  system
    ethics 177
    sociology 301.44
    see also Discriminatory
        practices

Castes *see* Social classes

Casting
  metals
    arts
      metalwork 739
      sculpture 731.4
    technology
      gen. wks. 671.2
      see also spec. metals

Castles *see* Residential
      buildings

Castrametation
  tactics *see* Logistics
  training *see* Training
      maneuvers

Casual-migratory
  workers *see* Seasonal workers

Casualty
  insurance
    gen. wks. 368
    see also Financial
        institutions
  prevention *see* Safety
      measures

Casuariiformes *see* Palaeog-
      nathae

Casuistry *see* Conscience

Catalan
  ethnic groups *area* –174
  language 449
  lingual groups *area* –175
  see also other spec. subj.

Cataloging
  books 025.3
  museum pieces 069

Catalogs
  books **010**
  music scores 781.9
  recordings 789.9
  see also s.s.–†021

Cataracts (water) *see* Water
      bodies

Catastrophes *see* Disasters

Catboats *see* Sailing craft

Catechisms
  religion
    Christian 238
    gen. wks. 291.2
    see also other spec. rel.
  see also s.s.–076

Catering
  services
    management 658
    technology 642

Caterpillars
  agricultural pests 632
  culture 638
  see also Lepidoptera

Cathedral
  buildings
    architecture 726
    construction 690.6
    religion *see* Sacred places
  schools
    education *see* Church-
        supported schools
    rel. training *see* Religious
        training
  systems *see* Episcopal system

Catholic
  epistles
    liturgy 264
    N.T.
      gen. wks. 227
      see also Pseudepigrapha
  socialism *see* Socialistic states

Catholicism
  culture groups
    geography   910.09
    history   909
    subj. treatment   *area* −176
  religion   280
Cats
  conservation   †639
  culture   636.8
  hunting
    industries   †639
    sports   799.27
  see also Felidae
Cattle
  disease carriers *see* Disease
    carriers
  husbandry   636.2
  see also Bovoidea
Caucasian
  ethnic groups   *area* −174
  languages   499
  lingual groups   *area* −175
  see also other spec. subj.
Caucasus
  ancient   *area* −39
  modern   *area* −479
Cause *see* Occasionalism
Cavalcades *see* Pageants
Cavalry
  forces *see* Mounted forces
Cavan Ireland   *area* −416
Caverns see Caves
Caves
  geography
    gen. wks.   910.09
    physical   †910.02
  geology   551.4
  regional subj.
    treatment   *area* −14
  see also spec. areas
Cavies *see* Hystricomorphs
Cayman Isls.   *area* −729 2
Caymans *see* Crocodiles
Celebes   *area* −91
Celebrations
  customs   394
  student life
    gen. wks.   †371.89
    see also spec. levels of ed.
Celestas *see* Percussion
    instruments

Celestial
  mechanics
    astronautics   **629.4**
    astronomy   521
  navigation
    gen. wks.   527
    see also spec. applications
  physics *see* Celestial
    mechanics
Celestines *see* Religious
    congregations
Celibacy
  psychology   †155.3
  sociology   †301.41
  see also Sexual ethics
Cellophane *see* Cellulosics
Cellos *see* String instruments
Cells
  biological *see* Cytology
Celluloid *see* Cellulosics
Cellulose
  gen. wks. *see* Polysaccharides
  products *see* Cellulosics
Cellulosics
  materials
    arts   702.8
    construction   691
    engineering   620.1
  plastics *see* Plastics
  textiles *see* Textiles
Celtic
  ethnic groups   *area* −174
  languages   491.6
  lingual groups   *area* −175
  see also other spec. subj.
Cementing
  materials
    geology
      gen. wks.   553
      mineralogy *see spec.*
      minerals
    manufacture
      economics   338.4
      technology   666
    materials
      construction   691
      engineering   620.1
    see also spec. applications
Cements *see* Cementing
    materials

Chattels
  law *see* Private law
Cheating *see* Evils
Chechen *see* Caucasian
Checkers
  ethics   175
  customs   394
  gen. wks.   794.2
Checks
  financial *see* Credit
    instruments
Cheerfulness *see* Virtues
Cheese
  food   641.3
  industry
    economics   338.1
    technology   637
  see also Dairy products
Cheetahs *see* Cats
Chelonia
  paleozoology   568
  zoology   598.13
Chemical
  analysis *see* Analytical
    chemistry
  engineering *see* Chemical
    technology
  jurisprudence *see* Forensic
    chemistry
  metallurgy
    gen. wks.   669.9
    see also spec. applications
  technology
    economics   338.4
    manufactures   **660**
  warfare
    defenses
      mil. eng.   623
      welfare services   †363.35
    forces
      gen. wks.   358
    see also spec. kinds of
      warfare
Chemicals
  industrial *see* Industrial
    chemicals
Chemistry
  applied *see* Chemical
    technology
  gen. wks.   **540**
  soils *see* Soil chemistry

Chemurgy *see* Chemical
  technology
Cheremiss *see* Finno-Ugric
Cherokee (subject) *see*
  Hokan-Siouan
Cherubim *see* Angelology
Chesapeake Bay
  gen. wks.   *area* –755
  Md.   *area* –752
Cheshire Eng.   *area* –427
Chess
  customs   394
  ethics   175
  gen. wks. *see*   **794.1**
Chesterfield
  Isls. *see* New Caledonia
Cheviot Hills Eng.   *area* –428
Chevon *see* Red meats
Chevrotains
  conservation   †639
  culture   636.9
  see also Tragulida
Chewing
  tobacco
    addiction *see* Addictions
    customs
      private   392
      public   394
Chewing-tobacco *see* Tobacco
  products
Chicken
  eggs *see* Eggs
Chickens
  culture   636.5
  disease carriers *see* Disease
    carriers
  food *see* Poultry
  see also Galliformes
Chief
  executives
    government
      gen. wks.   †350
    see also spec. levels of
      govt.
Chiggers
  agricultural pests   632
  culture   †639
  disease carriers *see* Disease
    carriers
  see also Acari
Chihuahuas *see* Miniature dogs

Choral
  music
    gen. wks. — 784.1–.2
    religious — 783.4
  speaking
    rhetoric — 808.55
  texts
    collections — 808.855
    criticism — 809.55
  see also spec. *lit.*
Chordata *see* Vertebrates
Choruses *see* Choral music
Choses
  law *see* Private law
Chow chows *see* Nonsporting
    dogs
Christ
  Jesus *see* Christology
Christening
  religion *see* Sacraments
  soc. customs — 392
Christian
  art *see* Religious art
  Brothers *see* Religious
    congregations
  Church *see* Disciples of
    Christ
  religion
    culture groups
      geography — 910.09
      history — 909
      subject treatment — *area* –176
    gen. wks. — **201–209**
    spec. elements — **220–280**
  Science churches *see*
    Church of Christ,
    Scientist
  socialism *see* Socialistic states
  Sunday *see* Holy days
  symbolism *see* Symbolism
  year *see* Liturgical year
Christianity *see* Christian
    religion
Christians — *area* –176
Christmas
  carols *see* Christmas music
  Day *see* Holy days
  music
    gen. wks.
      liturgical — 783.2
      nonliturgical — 783.6
    see also spec. *mediums*

Christmas (continued)
  religion *see* Liturgical year
Christology
  gen. wks. — 232
  Trinity — 231
  see also New Testament
Chromocollographic
  printing *see*
    Photomechanical
    printing
Chromolithographs *see* Prints
Chromolithography *see*
    Planographic
    processes
Chromophotography *see* Color-
    photography
Chromotype
  process *see* Special-process
    photography
Chromoxylography *see* Relief
    (surface) printing
Chronicles (O.T.) *see*
    Historical books
    (O.T.)
Chronology
  astronomy — 529
  history — 902
Chronometers *see* Timepieces
Chuckwallas *see* Lizards
Chukchi *see* Paleosiberian
Church (organization)
  pol. status — 322
  see also Church history
Church
  administration
    central *see* Ecclesiology
    local *see* Parishes
  buildings
    architecture — 726
    construction — 690.6
    religion *see* Sacred places
  calendars *see* Calendars
  fathers *see* Apostolic Church
  furniture *see* Sacred
    furniture
  government *see* Church
    administration
  history
    gen. wks. — 270
    see also Christian religion
  law *see* Religious law

Civic
  art *see* Planning
    communities
  centers
    planning
      civic art   711
      sociology   301.3
Civics *see* Citizenship
Civil
  defense
    administration
      government
        gen. wks.   †350
        see also spec. levels
          of govt.
      private   658
      services   †363.35
    engineering
      gen. wks.   624
      see also spec. branches
    government
      church relations
        pol. sci.   322
        religion
          Christian   261.7
          gen. wks.   291
          see also other spec.
            rel.
      see also Government
        (state)
    rights
      law   342
      pol. sci.   323.4
    service
      gen. wks.   †350
      see also spec. levels of
        govt.
    war
      international law   341.3
      mil. sci.   355
      societies *see* Hereditary
        societies
    wars
      crime *see* Offenses
      ethics   172
      history
        U.S.   973.7
      see also other spec.
        countries

Civilization
  gen. wks.   901.9
  see also spec. places
Clackmannan Scotland   *area* –413
Clairaudience *see* Extrasensory
    perception
Clairvoyance *see* Extrasensory
    perception
Clams
  fisheries
    economics   338.3
    technology   †639
  food *see* Seafood
  see also Mollusca
Clans
  biology *see* Ecology
  sociology *see* Kinship
Clare Co.
  Ireland   *area* –419
Clarinet *see* Wind instruments
      (musical)
Classical
  high schools *see* Secondary
      schools
  languages
    gen. wks.   †480
    see also spec. languages
  religions
    culture groups
      geography   910.09
      history   909
      subject treatment   *area* –176
    gen. wks.   292
Classical-language
  literature
    gen. wks.   880
    see also spec. literatures
Classification
  systems
    knowledge   112
    library services   025.4
    see also   *s.s.* –01
Classified
  catalogs
    books   017
    see also   *s.s.* –†021
Clavichords *see* Keyboard
      string instruments
Clay
  industries *see* Ceramics

Coats of arms *see* Heraldic
design
Cockateels *see* Parrots
Cockatoos *see* Parrots
Cockfighting *see* Animal
performances
Cocktail
parties *see* Hospitality
Cocktails *see* Spirits
(alcoholic)
Coconscious *see* Depth
psychology
Cocos Isls. Indian
Ocean   *area* –69
Codes
cryptography *see*
Cryptography
internal law *see* Statutes
religion
Christian   241.5
gen. wks.   291.5
see also other spec. rel.
Cogwheels *see* Gears
Coiffures *see* Hairdressing
Coinage
finance   332.4
see also Coins
Coins
manufacture
economics   338.4
technology
gen. wks.   671.8
see also spec. metals
numismatics   **737.4**
Coke *see* Coals
Colchis
ancient   *area* –39
modern   *area* –479
Cold
creams *see* Cosmetics
storage
food *see* Food technology
war
activities *see* Psychological
warfare
Cold-weather
photography
gen. wks.   778.7
see also spec. applications
warfare *see* Battle tactics

Cold-working
operations
metals
gen. wks.   671.3
see also spec. metals
see also other products
Coleoptera
paleozoology   565
zoology   595.76
Collected
writings
gen. wks.   **†080**
literature
gen. wks.   **808.8**
see also spec. lit.
see also   *s.s.*–08
Collecting
museum sci.   069
recreation   790.023
research methodology   †001.4
see also   *s.s.*–075
Collective
bargaining *see* Employer-
employee
relationships
groups *see* Behavior-groups
security *see* International
relations
Collectivism
economics
production   **338**
systems   **335**
pol. sci. *see spec. types of*
state
College
buildings
architecture   727
construction   690.7
libraries
gen. wks.   027.7
see also spec. functions
preparatory schools *see*
Secondary schools
songs *see* Student songs
Colleges
gen. wks.   378.1
govt. control
education   379
pub. admin.
gen. wks.   †350
see also spec. levels of
govt.

Commerce
  departments *see* Executive
    departments
Commercial
  areas
    geography *see spec. areas*
    planning
      civic art   711
      sociology   301.3
  arithmetic *see* Business
    arithmetic
  art
    advertising   659.13
    drawings   **741.6**
  buildings
    architecture   725
    construction
      economics   338.4
      technology   690.5
  credit *see* Credit
  education *see* Vocational
    education
  land
    economics
      gen. wks.   333.7
      see also Real-estate
    see also Commercial
      areas
  law
    internal   †347.7
    international   †341.5
  paper *see* Credit
    instruments
  policy *see* Trade (activity)
Commissary
  services *see* Special services
Commission
  houses *see* Investment
    institutions
  merchants *see* Wholesale
    marketing
Commissions
  government
    gen. wks.   †350
    see also spec. levels of
      govt.
  see also spec. professions
Committees *see* Organizations
Commodities (goods) *see*
  Consumer goods

Commodity
  exchanges *see* Investment
    institutions
  taxes *see* Taxation
Common
  land
    economics   333.2
    landscaping   712–719
    see also   *area* –14
  law
    criminal   343
    gen. wks.   **347**
Commoners *see* Social classes
Commons (land) *see*
  Recreational land
Commonwealths *see* Central
  governments
Communication
  engineering *see*
    Communication
    systems
  gen. wks.   †001.5
  govt. control
    gen. wks.   †350
    see also spec. levels of
      govt.
  services   380.3
  sociology   †301.16
  systems
    architecture   729
    engineering
      gen. wks.
        economics   338.4
        technology   **621.382–.389**
      military   623.7
      ships   623.85
    executive management   658.4
    mil. sci.
      gen. wks.   358
      see also spec. kinds of
        warfare
    office services   651.7
    see also spec. systems &
      applications
  see also Language
Communion
  music *see* Mass (religion)
  religion *see* Sacraments
Communism *see* Communist
  states

Concerti
  grossi *see* Orchestras
Concertinas *see* Accordions
Concertos *see* Orchestras
Concerts
  gen. wks.   780.73
  see also spec. mediums
Conchology *see* Mollusca
Conciliation
  practices
    ind. relations   331.15
    international relations
      law   341.6
      pol. sci.   **327**
    management *see*
      Employer-employee
      relationships
Concourses *see* Trafficways
Concrete
  blocks *see* Artificial stones
  masonry *see* Masonry
    (construction)
  music *see* Musique concrète
Condemned
  books *see* Prohibited books
Conditioned
  reflexes *see* Reflex actions
Conduct
  of life *see* Ethics
  of war *see* Warfare
Conduits
  drainage *see* Drainage
    structures
  irrigation *see* Irrigation
Confectionery *see* Candies
Conferences
  organizations *see*
    Organizations
  teaching *see* Discussion
    methods
Confession
  penance *see* Sacraments
Confessions
  of faith *see* Creeds
Configuration
  psychology *see* Gestalt
    psychology
Confinement
  childbirth *see* Parturition
Confirmation *see* Sacraments

Conformity
  psychology   †153.8
  sociology   301.15
Confucianism
  culture groups
    geography   910.09
    history   909
    subject treatment   *area* −176
  philosophy   181
  religion   299
Congo (Brazzaville)   *area* −67
Congo (Leopoldville)   *area* −675
Congregational
  Christian Churches *see*
    Congregationalism
  Methodist Church *see*
    Methodist churches
  singing *see* Hymnology
  system   262
Congregationalism
  religion   285
  see also Church buildings
Congregations
  denominational *see* Parishes
  religious *see* Religious
    congregations
Congresses
  legislative *see* Legislative
    bodies
  organizations *see*
    Organizations
Congressional
  immunity *see* Political
    immunity
Conies *see* Hyracoideans
Conjuring *see* Magic arts
Connacht Ireland   *area* −417
Connaught Ireland *see*
    Connacht
Connecticut (state)   *area* −746
Consanguinity
  gen. wks. *see* Kinship
  law *see* Family (institution)
Conscience
  ethics   171
  religion
    Christian   241
    gen. wks.   291.5
    see also other spec. rel.

Continents
  geography
    gen. wks.   910.09
    physical   †910.02
  geology   551.4
  regional subj.
    treatment   *area* –14
  see also spec. continents
Continuation
  schools
    gen. wks.   374.8
    govt. control
      gen. wks.   †350
      *see also spec. levels of
        govt.*
Contour
  band saws *see* Tools
Contouring
  cultivation methods   631.5
  erosion control   631.4
Contrabasses *see* String
      instruments
Contrabassoons *see* Wind
      instruments
      (musical)
Contract
  law *see* Private law
  systems
    labor
      economics   331.5
      penology   365
Contracting
  practices
    economics   338.4
    technology   692
Contracts
  business   658.7
  government
    gen. wks.   †350
    *see also spec. levels of
      govt.*
Control
  devices
    engineering *see spec.
      branches*
    engineering *see* Automatic
      control
  towers
    engineering
      airport   629.136
      space   629.47

Control
  towers (continued)
    services *see*
        Transportation
        services
Controllers
  engineering *see spec.
      branches*
Conundrums *see* Puzzles
Convalescent
  homes
    management   658
    services   362.1
Convent
  education
    gen. wks.   376
    see also Church-
        supported schools
Conventions
  customs *see* Customs
      (conventions)
  organizations *see*
      Organizations
Convents
  religion *see* Religious
      congregations
Conventuals *see* Religious
      congregations
Conversion
  religion *see* Religious
      experience
Converted
  household
    garbage *see* Fertilizers
  paper products
    manufacture
      economics   338.4
      technology   676
    marketing   658.8
Conveying
  systems *see* Materials-
        handling equipment
Convict
  labor
    economics   331.5
    penology   365
Convicts *see* Inmates
Cook
  Isls.   *area* –96
Cookbooks *see* Cookery

Cookery
 commercial
  economics   338.4
  technology   664
 home   641.5–.8
Cookies *see* Bakery products
Cooking
 oils *see* Fixed oils
 processes
  commercial   664
  home   641.7
Cookouts *see* Outdoor meals
Cooperage *see* Sawmill
   products
Cooperation
 library functions   †021.6
 psychology   †158
 sociology   301.2
 see also Cooperatives
Cooperative
 cataloging *see* Cataloging
 management *see* Employer-
   employee
   relationships
 welfare
  agencies *see* Community
   welfare
Cooperatives
 economics   334
 managerial control   658.1
Coordinate
 geometry *see* Analytical
   geometry
Coos (subject) *see* Macro-
   Penutian
Coots *see* Rails (birds)
Copper
 Age
  gen. wks.   †913.03
  see also spec. subj.
 alloys *see* Metals
 coinage *see* Coinage
 engravings *see* Prints
 geology
  gen. wks.   553
  mineralogy
   element   549.2
   minerals *see spec.*
    minerals

Copper (continued)
 industries
  manufacturing *see*
   Coppersmithing
  mining *see* Mining
 products *see spec. subj.*
 properties
  chemistry   546
  engineering   620.1
  metallography   669.9
  see also Physical chemistry
Copperplate
 printing *see* Metal engraving
Coppersmithing
 arts   739
 manufacturing
  economics   338.4
  technology   673
Copperwork *see*
   Coppersmithing
Coptic
 Church
  religion   281
  see also Church buildings
 ethnic groups   area –174
 language   493
 lingual groups   area –175
 see also other spec. subj.
Copyright
 deposits   021.8
 law   †340
Copywriting
 advertising   659.13
 journalism   070.4
Coraciiformes
 paleozoology   568
 zoology   598.89
Cordage
 manufacture
  economics   338.4
  technology   677
 materials
  engineering   620.1
  nautical   623.88
 see also spec. applications
Corgis *see* Working dogs
Corinthians (N.T.) *see* Pauline
   epistles
Cork Ireland   area –419

Crafts (continued)
  mil. recreation *see* Special
    services
  see also spec. crafts
Craftsmen
  economics
    labor   331.7
    production   338.1–.4
  see also spec. subj.
Cranes (birds)
  culture   636.6
  see also Gruiformes
Cranes (mechanical)
  engineering
    economics   338.4
    technology
      gen. wks.   621.8
      see also spec. branches
  see also spec. applications
Craniology
  anthropometry   573
  phrenology   139
Crates
  wooden *see* Sawmill products
Crayfish
  fisheries
    economics   338.3
    technology   †639
  food *see* Seafood
  see also Macrura
Creation
  of man *see* Cosmology
Creative
  activities
    children *see* Child play
  arts
    gen. wks.   **700–800**
    study & teaching
      elementary schools   372.5
    see also   *s.s.*–07
Creativity *see* Imagination
Credit
  administration
    gen. wks.   †350
    see also spec. levels of
      govt.
  bonds *see* Public securities
  economics
    gen. wks.   332.7
    public   336.3

Credit (continued)
  institutions *see* Financial
    institutions
  instruments
    economics   332.7
    see also spec. applications
  management   658.88
  unions *see* Financial
    institutions
Credos *see* Creeds
Cree *see* Algonkian-Mosan
Creeds
  religion
    dogmatics
      Christian   238
      gen. wks.   291.2
      see also other spec. rel.
    liturgy
      Christian   264
      gen. wks.   291.3
      see also other spec. rel.
Creek (subject) *see* Hokan-
  Siouan
Creeks *see* Water bodies
Cremation
  rites *see* Funeral rites
Crests
  heraldic *see* Heraldic design
Crete
  ancient   *area* –39
  modern   *area* –499
Cricket *see* Bat games
Crickets *see* Grasshoppers
Crimea   *area* –477
Crimes *see* Offenses
Criminal
  abortion *see* Offenses
  anthropology
    gen. wks.   364.2
    see also Abnormal
      psychology
  anthropometry *see*
    Anthropometry
  law
    internal   343
    international   341.4
  libel *see* Offenses
Criminals *see* Offenders
Criminology
  gen. wks.   **364**
  see also Personality disorders

Cuitlatec *see* Miskito-
    Matagalpan
Culinary
  arts *see* Cookery
Cultivation
  techniques
    gen. wks. — 631.5
    see also spec. crops
Cultural
  anthropology *see* Culture
  areas
    geography *see spec. areas*
    landscaping — 712
    planning
      civic art — 711
      sociology — 301.3
Culture
  anthropology — †390
  govt. control
    gen. wks. — †350
    see also spec. levels of
      govt.
  sociology — 301.2
  see also Civilization
Culverts *see* Drainage
    structures
Cumberland Eng. — *area* –428
Curates *see* Clergy
Curb
  exchanges *see* Investment
    institutions
Curbs (pavements) *see*
    Auxiliary pavements
Curlews
  culture — 636.6
  see also Charadriiformes
Curling (sport) *see* Ice sports
Curling
  hair *see* Hairdressing
Currents
  oceanic *see* Marine waters
Curriculums
  gen. wks. — 375
  see also spec. levels of ed.
Curses
  folklore *see* Superstitions
Cursing *see* Profanity
Curtains
  interior decoration
    art — 747
    home economics — 645

Curtains (continued)
  manufacture
    economics — 338.4
    technology — 684.3
Cushitic
  ethnic groups — *area* –174
  languages — 493
  lingual groups — *area* –175
  see also other spec. subj.
Customhouses *see*
    Government
    buildings
Customs (conventions)
  military
    gen. wks. — 355.1
    see also spec. services
  social *see* Social customs
Customs (taxes)
  economics — 336.2
  gen. wks. — †382
  govt. control
    gen. wks. — †350
    see also spec. levels of
      govt.
Cut
  flowers
    arrangement — †745.92
    culture
      gen. wks. — 635.96
      see also spec. plants
  stock *see* Sawmill products
Cutlery
  manufacture
    economics — 338.4
    technology — 683
  table decor *see* Table decor
Cutters
  revenue *see* Government
    vessels
  sailing ships *see* Sailing craft
Cutting
  hair
    men *see* Barbering
    women *see* Hairdressing
  metals
    arts — 739
    technology
      gen. wks. — 671.5
      see also spec. metals
Cutting-machinery *see* Tools

Dikes (structures) *see* Flood
    control
Dining
  places *see* Public
    accommodations
  service *see* Meals
Dinners *see* Meals
Diocesan
  schools *see* Church-
    supported schools
Dioceses *see* Episcopal system
Diplomacy
  administration   †350
  law   341.7
  pol. sci.   327
Diplomatic
  conduct *see* Diplomacy
  immunity *see* Political
    immunity
Diplomatics *see* Paleography
Diptera
  paleozoology   565
  zoology   595.77
Direct-current
  machinery
    economics   338.4
    engineering   621.313
    manufacture   681
    see also spec. applications
  motors
    generators *see* Direct-
      current machinery
    prime movers   621.4
  transmission
    engineering
      economics   338.4
      technology   621.319
Direction
  finders
    engineering
      economics   338.4
      technology
        radar   621.384 8
        radio   621.384 19
    navigation
      aircraft   629.132
      ships   623.89
    see also Magnetic
      compasses
  finding *see* Navigation

Direct-mail
  advertising
    economics   338.4
    technology   659.13
  marketing *see* Retail
    marketing
Dirigibles *see* Lighter-than-air
    aircraft
Dirks *see* Side arms
Disability
  insurance
    govt. sponsored   368.4
    voluntary   368.3
    see also Financial
      institutions
  pensions *see* Pension systems
Disabled
  children *see* Exceptional
    children
  people
    labor economics 331.5
    service institutions 362.4
  veterans
    benefits *see* Postmilitary
      benefits
    gen. wks. *see* Disabled
      people
Disarmament *see* Armament
    limitation
Disasters
  history   †904
  psych. effects   †155.9
  relief
    administration
    government
      gen. wks.   †350
      see also spec. levels
        of govt.
      private   658
    police planning   363.3
    services   361.5
    technology   **614.8**
Disciples
  of Christ
    churches
      religion   286
      see also Church
        buildings
Discography *see* Catalogs

Diving
  aerodynamics *see*
      Aerodynamics
  hydraulic eng. *see*
      Underwater
      operations
  sports
      hygiene   †613.7
      performance   797.2
Divinities *see* Deities
Divinity *see* God
Divorce
  ethics
      philosophy   173
      religion
          Christian   241
          see also other spec. rel.
  laws   347.6
  psychology   †155.6
  sociology   301.42
  statistics *see* Demography
Diyarbakir Turkey   *area* −566
Doberman
  pinschers *see* Working dogs
Docks
  eng. & construction
      economics   338.4
      technology
          gen. wks.   627
          military   623.6
  see also Transportation
      services
Doctrinal
  theology *see* Dogmatism
Documentation
  equipment *see* Computers
  library sci.   †029.7
  see also Records
      management
Documents
  collections
      general   †080
      see also   *s.s.*−08
  library treatment   025.17
Dodecanese Greece
  ancient   *area* −39
  modern   *area* −499
Dogmas *see* Dogmatism

Dogmatism
  philosophy   148
  religion
      Christian   230
      comp. rel.   291.2
      see also other spec. rel.
Dogs
  culture   636.7
  disease carriers *see* Disease
      carriers
  see also Canidae
Dolls *see* Toys
Dolphins (mammals) *see*
      Odontocetes
Dolphins (mooring structures)
      see Port installations
Domestic
  animals *see* Livestock
  art *see* Folk art
  arts
      customs   392
      technology   640
  cats *see* Cats
  commerce *see* Trade
      (activity)
  fowls *see* Poultry
  science *see* Domestic arts
  see also Family
Dominica West Indies   *area* −729 8
Dominican Republic   *area* −729 3
Dominicans *see* Religious
      congregations
Dominion
  Day *see* Holidays
Dominoes *see* Counter games
Donegal Ireland   *area* −416
Donkeys *see* Asses
Dorset Eng.   *area* −423
Double
  basses *see* String instruments
Double-reed
  instruments *see* Wind
      instruments
      (musical)
Doubt *see* Skepticism
Doves *see* Pigeons
Down Ireland   *area* −416
Dowry *see* Marriage

Drinking
  customs
    private   392
    public   394
  hygiene   613.3
  songs *see* Folk songs
  see also Addictions
Drinks *see* Beverages
Drives (psychology) *see*
        Motivation
Drives (roads) *see* Trafficways
Driveways *see* Auxiliary
        pavements
Dromedaries *see* Camels
Drug
  addictions *see* Addictions
  traffic
    govt. control
      gen. wks.   †350
      police services   363.4
      see also spec. levels of
        govt.
    offense *see* Offenses
Drugs *see* Pharmacology
Drum
  majoring *see* Bands
Drum & bugle
  corps *see* Bands
Drums *see* Percussion
        instruments
Drunkenness
  crime *see* Offenses
  psychopathic *see* Addictions
Dry
  cleaning
    commercial   667
    domestic   646.6
Drypoint
  engraving
    arts   767
    industry   655.3
  engravings *see* Prints
Dualism
  philosophy   147
  religion
    heresy   273
    gen. wks.   291
    see also spec. rel.
Dual-purpose
  animals *see* Multiple-
        purpose animals

Dublin Ireland   *area* –418
Ducie Isl.   *area* –96
Duckbills *see* Platypuses
Ducks
  culture   636.59
  food *see* Poultry
  hunting
    sports   799.24
  see also Anseriformes
Dude
  ranching *see* Outdoor life
Dueling
  crime *see* Offenses
  ethics   179
  soc. customs   394
Dugongs *see* Sea cows
Dumfries Scotland   *area* –414
Dunbarton Scotland   *area* –413
Dunkers *see* Baptist churches
Duplicating-machines
  marketing   658.8
  office equipment   651
  see also spec. applications
Duplication
  functions
    libraries   025.1
    museums   069
  see also Printing processes
Durham Eng.   *area* –428
Dust
  gen. wks. *see* Particulates
  storms *see* Storms
Dusting-on
  processes *see* Special-
        process photography
Dutch *see* Germanic
Duties (obligations)
  philosophy   **170**
  religion
    Christian   241
    gen. wks.   291.5
    see also other spec. rel.
Duties (taxes) *see* Customs
        (taxes)
Dyeing
  hair *see* Hairdressing
  textiles
    commercial   667
    domestic   640

Edentates		Eggs		
conservation	†639	food		
culture	636.9	cookery	641.6	
see also Edentata		gen. wks.	641.3	
Edible		marketing	658.8	
plants		production		
agriculture *see* Agriculture		economics	338.1	
(activity)		technology	637	
botany *see* Economic		zoology *see spec. animals*		
biology		Egoism		
Editing		philosophy		
gen. wks.	†808.02	ethics	171	
journalism	070.4	metaphysics	126	
Edom	*area* –39	*see also* Subconscious		
Education		Egrets		
govt.		conservation	†639	
control		culture	636.6	
gen. wks.	†350	*see also* Ciconiiformes		
see also spec. levels of		Egypt		
govt.		ancient	*area* –32	
supervision	379	modern	*area* –62	
of veterans *see* Postmilitary		Egyptian		
benefits		modern *see* Arabic		
religious *see* Religious		old *see* Old Egyptian		
training		Elamitic		
science	370	ethnic groups	*area* –174	
see also	*s.s.*–07	language	499	
Educational		lingual groups	*area* –175	
functions		*see also other spec. subj.*		
libraries	021.2	Elands *see* Antelopes		
museums	069	Elasig Turkey	*area* –566	
guidance *see* Counseling		Elasticity		
programs		engineering		
personnel management		materials	620.1	
business	658.3	structures	624	
government		mechanics		
gen. wks.	†350	gases	533	
see also spec. levels		liquids	532	
of govt.		solids	531	
see also spec. institutions		Elastomers		
psychology *see* Learning		manufacture		
sociology		economics	338.4	
gen. wks.	370.19	technology	678	
see also spec. levels of ed.		materials		
tests *see* Mental tests		arts	702.8	
Education-departments *see*		engineering	620.1	
Executive		*see also spec. products*		
departments		Elderly		
Edward Nyanza		people *see* Aged people		
gen. wks.	*area* –675	Elders *see* Clergy		
see also other areas				

Embryology
  biology
    animals   591.3
    gen. wks.   574.3
    plants   581.3
    see also spec. organisms
  med. sci.
    animals
      gen. wks.   636.089
      see also spec. animals
    man
      anatomy   611
      physiology   612.64
    see also Pregnancy
Emeralds *see* Precious stones
Emergency
  labor *see* Drafted labor
  money *see* Noncommodity
    money
Emicons *see* Electronic
    musical instruments
Emigration *see* Population
    movement
Eminent
  domain *see* Expropriation
Emotionally
  disturbed
    children *see* Exceptional
      children
    people
      psychology *see*
        Abnormal
        psychology
      treatment *see*
        Psychoneuroses
      welfare service   362.2
Emotions
  psychology
    animals   †156
    gen. wks.   †152.4
  religion   200.1
Empire
  Day *see* Holidays
Empires
  geography   910.09
  history   909
  pol. sci.   321
  subj. treatment   *area* –171
  see also spec. areas
Empiricism *see* Positivism

Employees
  labor economics   331.1
  management *see* Personnel
    management
Employer-employee
  relationships
    business   658.31
    government
      gen. wks.   †350
      see also spec. levels of
        govt.
    labor   **331.1**
Employment
  labor economics   331.1
  management
    gen. wks.   658.31
    see also Civil service
  see also Postmilitary
    benefits
Emus
  conservation   †639
  culture   636.6
  see also Palaeognathae
Enamels
  arts
    ceramics   738.4
    metals   739
  manufacture
    economics   338.4
    technology
      ceramics   666
      metals *see* Surface
        finishing
Encyclicals *see* Religious law
Encyclopedias
  gen. wks.   **030**
  see also   *s.s.*–03
Endowment
  education
    schools   379
    students   **378.3**
  research   †001.4
Energism
  philosophy   146
  psychology *see*
    Reductionism
Engineer
  forces
    mil. sci.
      gen. wks.   358
      see also spec. kinds of
        warfare

Eyeglasses (continued)
  manufacture
    economics   338.4
    technology   681
  marketing   658.8
  optometry *see* Optometry
Ezechiel (O.T.) *see* Prophetic
    books
Ezekiel (O.T.) *see* Prophetic
    books
Ezra (O.T.) *see* Historical
    books (O.T.)

F

Fables *see* Mythology
Fabrication *see* Manufactures
Fabrics *see* Textiles
Facsimile
  production *see*
        Photoduplication
  telegraphy *see*
        Telecommunication
Factory
  buildings *see* Industrial
    buildings
  management *see* Production
    management
  operations
    economics   338.4
    technology
      gen. wks.   621.7
      see also spec. branches
  ships *see* Merchant ships
  systems *see* Big businesses
Faculty (schools) *see* School
    organization
Faculty psychology
  gen. wks.   150.19
  see also spec. aspects
Fads *see* Group behavior
Faeroes   *area* –491
Fair
  buildings *see* Public
    buildings
Fairies *see* Supernatural beings
Fairs
  business *see* Distribution
    channels
  description   **914–919**
  soc. customs   394
  see also   *s.s.*–074

Fairy
  tales *see* Mythology
Faith
  metaphysics   121
  religion
    Christian   234
    gen. wks.   291.2
    see also other spec. rel.
Falangist
  state *see* Fascist states
Falconiformes
  paleozoology   568
  zoology   598.9
Falcons *see* Hawks
Falkland Isls.   *area* –97
Falling
  bodies *see* Gravity
Family (institution)
  customs   392
  ethics   173
  law   347.6
  sociology
    gen. wks.   301.42
    welfare services †362.8
Family
  counseling *see* Counseling
  histories *see* Genealogy
  libraries
    gen. wks.   027
    see also spec. functions
  prayer
    Christian religion 249
    gen. wks.   291.4
    see also other spec. rel.
Famines *see* Disasters
Fancywork *see* Embroidery
Fan-jet
  engines *see* Internal-
      combustion engines
Fans
  mechanical *see* Blowers
  ornamental
    arts   736
    customs   391
Far East   *area* –5
Farce *see* Drama
Farm
  animals *see* Livestock
  buildings
    architecture   728

Feeble-minded
  children *see* Exceptional
    children
Feeblemindedness *see* Mental
  deficiency
Feedback
  electronics *see* Circuitry
  systems *see* Automatic control
Feeding
  boilers *see* Boiler-house
    practices
  children
    gen. wks.   649.3
    see also Cookery
  invalids
    cookery *see* Cookery
    gen. wks. *see* Nursing
  livestock
    gen. wks.   636.08
    see also spec. animals
Feelings
  psychology
    animals   †156
    gen. wks.   †152.4
  religion   200.1
Fees
  compensation *see* Wages
  revenue *see* Taxation
Felidae
  paleozoology   569
  zoology   599.7
Fellowships
  education   378.33
  gen. wks.   †001.4
  see also   *s.s.*–079
Felonies *see* Offenses
Femininity *see* Sex differences
Feminism *see* Women
Fencing
  ethics   175
  mil. sci. *see* Training
    maneuvers
  sports   796.8
Fens Eng.   *area* –425
Fermanagh Ireland   *area* –416
Ferroconcrete
  blocks *see* Artificial stones
Ferroprussiate
  process *see* Special-process
    photography

Ferrotype
  process *see* Special-process
    photography
Ferryboats *see* Small craft
Fertilizers
  agriculture
    gen. wks.   631.8
    see also spec. crops
  manufacture
    economics   338.4
    technology   668
  marketing   658.8
Festivals
  gen. wks. *see* Pageants
  religion *see* Holy days
Fêtes *see* Pageants
Feudal
  states
    pol. sci.   321.3
    see also spec. areas
  tenure *see* Private land
Fezzan   *area* –61
Fiction
  collections   **808.83**
  criticism   **809.3**
  rhetoric   **808.3**
  see also spec. lits.
Field
  athletics *see* Track athletics
  crops
    agriculture
      economics   338.1
      technology   633
    processing *see spec.*
      products
  hockey *see* Mallet games
  service
    mil. sci.
      gen. wks.   355.4
      see also spec. services
      see also hist. of spec. wars
  work *see* Laboratory
    methods
Fife Scotland   *area* –413
Fifes *see* Wind instruments
  (musical)
Fighters (aircraft) *see*
    Heavier-than-air
    aircraft
Fighting
  sports *see* Boxing

Floors (continued)
  construction
    carpentry   694.2
    economics   338.4
    painting   698.1
    see also spec. structures
Floral
  arts
    arrangements   †745.92
    landscape design   715–716
Floriculture
  economics   338.1
  technology   **635.9**
Florida (state)   *area* –759
Flower
  arrangement
    gen. wks. *see* Floral arts
    table decor *see* Table
      decor
  gardening *see* Floriculture
Flowering
  plants
    floriculture   **635.93**
    landscaping   715–716
    see also Angiospermae
Flow-of-funds
  accounts *see* National
      accounting
Flues
  heating eng.   697.8
  see also spec. applications
Fluid-power
  engineering
    gen. wks.   621.1–.2
    see also spec. branches
Fluids
  physics
    mechanics   **532**
    see also spec. branches
    see also spec. applications
Fluorescent
  lighting *see* Electric lighting
Fluoridation
  water supply
    engineering
      economics   338.4
      technology   628
    pub. health   614.5
Fluorination *see* Fluoridation
Fluoroscopy *see* Radiography
Flutes *see* Wind instruments
  (musical)

Flying
  aircraft
    gen. wks. *see* Flight
      engineering
    sports *see* Air sports
Foliage-plants
  botany   **581**
  culture   635.97
  landscaping   712–716
  see also spec. plants
Folk
  art
    gen. wks.   **745.5–.9**
    see also spec. art forms
  music *see* Ethnic music
  songs
    customs   **394**
    folklore   398.8
    music   784.4
    singing   784.9
  tales *see* Mythology
Folklore *see* Mythology
Food
  analysis
    pub. health *see* Food-&-
      drug control
  animals
    culture   636.08
    zoology   591.6
    see also spec. animals
  cookery *see* Cookery
  customs *see* Eating-customs
  folklore
    hist. & criticism   398.3
    legends   398.2
  microbiology
    gen. wks.   576.16
    see also   *s.s.*–01
  preservation *see* Food
    technology
  salts
    nutrition   641.1
    see also spec. uses
  supply
    economics   †338.1
    mil. sci.
      administration   355.6
      gen. wks.   355.8
      see also spec. mil.
        branches
    see also Agriculture
      (activity)

Fuel
  cells
    engineering
      economics   338.4
      technology   621.35
    see also spec. applications
  oils *see* Petroleum products
  ships
    commercial *see* Merchant
      ships
    govt. *see* Government
      vessels
  systems
    engineering
      gen. wks.   621.43
      see also spec. applications
    heating *see* Heating-
      systems
Fuels
  gaseous *see* Industrial gases
  processing
    economics   338.4
    technology   662
  see also spec. applications
Fugues (music)
  gen. wks.   781.4
  see also spec. mediums
Fulah *see* Chari-Nile
Fulmars *see* Pelagic birds
Functionalism
  philosophy   144
  psychologies
    gen. wks.   150.19
    see also spec. aspects
Fund
  raising *see* Financial
    administration
Fundamental
  education
    gen. wks.   370.19
    see also spec. subj.
Funded
  debts *see* Public securities
Funeral
  rites
    etiquette   395
    gen. wks.   393
    mil. sci. *see* Official
      ceremonies

Funeral
  rites (continued)
    religion
      Christian   265
      gen. wks.   291.3
      see also other spec. rel.
Funicular
  railways *see* Railroads
Fur
  animals
    culture
      economics   †338.1
      technology
        gen. wks.   †636.08
        see also spec. animals
      see also Mammals
  coats *see* Fur garments
  farming *see* Fur animals
  garments
    manufacture
      economics   338.4
      technology   685
    marketing   658.8
    see also spec. applications
  processing
    economics   338.4
    technology   675
  seals *see* Eared seals
Fur-bearing
  animals *see* Fur animals
Furcrafts
  art   745.53
  industry
    economics   338.4
    technology   685
Furnishings
  households *see* Household
    furnishings
Furniture
  arts   **749**
  home economics   645
  manufacture
    economics   338.4
    technology   684.1
  ships *see* Nautical equipment
  specific kinds
    churches *see* Sacred
      furniture
    libraries   022
    museums   069

Furs *see* Fur garments
Future
  life
    metaphysics   129
    religion
      Christian   †236
      comparative   291.2
      gen. wks.   218
      see also other spec. rel.

G

Gabon   *area* –67
Gaelic *see* Celtic
Gaetulia   *area* –39
Gaining
  weight *see* Body contours
Galápagos Isls.   *area* –86
Galatia   *area* –39
Galatians (N.T.) *see* Pauline
        epistles
Galicia (eastern Europe)
  gen. wks.   *area* –†438
  Ukraine   *area* –†477
Galla *see* Cushitic
Galleries *see* Museums
Gallflies
  agricultural pests   632
  culture   638
  see also Hymenoptera
Galli *see* Galliformes
Gallia (ancient country)
  Cisalpina   *area* –37
  Transalpina *see* Gaul
Galliformes
  paleozoology   568
  zoology   598.6
Gallium *see* Metals
Galloway Scotland   *area* –414
Galls
  agriculture   632
  botany   581.2
Galvanizing
  metals *see* Surface finishing
Galway Ireland   *area* –417
Gambia   *area* –66
Gambier Isls.   *area* –96
Gamblers *see* Offenders
Gambling
  crime *see* Offenses

Gambling (continued)
  customs   394
  ethics   175
  govt. control
    gen. wks.   †350
    police services   363.4
    see also spec. levels of govt.
  mathematics   519
  recreation
    gen. wks.   795
    see also spec. activities
Game
  food
    cookery   641.6
    gen. wks.   641.3
    preservation
      commercial   664
      home   641.4
  hunting *see* Hunting
      (activity)
  reserves *see* Wildlife reserves
Games *see* Recreational
      activities
Gamma
  rays
    engineering   621.381
    physics
      electronics   537.5
      nuclear   539.7
    see also Ionizing radiation
Gangs *see* Behavior groups
Gangsterism *see* Offenses
Gannets
  conservation   †639
  culture   636.6
  see also Pelecaniformes
Garbage
  disposal
    units
      manufacture *see*
        Household appliances
    plumbing   696
  treatment
    engineering
      economics   338.4
      technology
        gen. wks.   628
        military   623.7
Garbage-fertilizers *see* Fertilizers

Garden
  crops
    agriculture
      economics   338.1
      technology   **635**
    sculpture
      arts   731.7
    landscaping
      fountains   714
      gen. wks.   717
Gardens
  horticulture   **635**
  landscaping   712
  see also Garden crops
Gargoyles
  architecture   729
  sculpture   731.5
Garmentmaking *see* Garments
Garments
  customs   391
  fur *see* Fur garments
  home sewing   646.2–.6
  hygiene   613.4
  leather *see* Leather goods
  manufacture
    economics   338.4
    technology   687
  marketing   658.8
Garnishes
  food *see* Auxiliary foods
Gas (utility)
  economics
    manufactured   338.4
    natural   338.2
  govt. control
    gen. wks.   †350
    services   363.6
  see also spec. levels of govt.
Gas
  lighting
    engineering
      economics   338.4
      technology   621.32
    home econ.   644
  mains *see* Utility lines
  warfare *see* Chemical warfare
  see also Natural gas
Gaseous
  fuels *see* Industrial gases
  illuminants *see* Industrial
    gases

Gases
  industrial *see* Industrial gases
  physics
    gen. wks.   530.4
    mechanics   **533**
    sound transmission   534
Gasolines *see* Petroleum
    products
Gastropoda *see* Mollusks
Gas-turbine
  engines *see* Internal-
    combustion engines
Gaul   *area* –36
Gauntlets *see* Handwear
Gaviiformes
  paleozoology   568
  zoology   598.4
Gavleborg Sweden   *area* –487
Gazelles *see* Antelopes
Gazetteers
  geography   910.3
  see also   *s.s.*–03
Gaziantep Turkey   *area* –564
Gears
  engineering
    economics   338.4
    technology
      gen. wks.   621.8
      see also spec. branches
  see also spec. applications
Geckos *see* Lizards
Geese
  culture   636.59
  food *see* Poultry
  hunting
    sports   799.24
  see also Anseriformes
Geez *see* Ethiopic
Gelatin
  desserts *see* Puddings
Gelatins
  manufacture
    economics   338.4
    technology
      crude   668
      edible   664
  see also spec. applications
Gemara *see* Talmud
Gems
  natural *see* Precious stones
  synthetic *see* Synthetic
    minerals

Gestalt
  psychology
    gen. wks.   †150.19
    see also spec. aspects
Geysers
  geography
    gen. wks.   †910.02
    see also spec. places
  geology   551.2
Ghana   *area* −667
Ghosts
  folklore
    hist. & criticism   398.4
    legends   398.2
  occultism   133.1
Giants
  natural
    phys. anthropology   573
  supernatural *see* Supernatural
    beings
Gibbons *see* Apes
Gibraltar   *area* −46
Gifted
  children *see* Exceptional
    children
Gifts
  books
    library functions   025.2
    state aid   021.8
  see also Procurement
Gila
  monsters *see* Lizards
Gilbert Isls.   *area* −96
Gilyak *see* Paleosiberian
Gipsy
  ethnic groups   *area* −174
  languages   491.4
  lingual groups   *area* −175
  see also other spec. subj.
Giraffes
  conservation   †639
  culture   636.2
  see also Cervoidea
Giresun Turkey   *area* −565
Girl
  Guides *see* Young people
    organizations
  Scouts *see* Young people
    organizations
Girls (children) *see* Children

Girls'
  clothing *see* Garments
  clubs *see* Young people
    organizations
Glaciology
  geography
    gen. wks.   †910.02
    see also spec. places
  geology   551.3
Glass
  arts
    arch. decoration   729
    gen. wks.   **748**
  manufacture
    economics   338.4
    technology   666
  properties
    construction   691
    engineering   620.1
Glassware
  production *see* Glass
  table decor *see* Table decor
Glees *see* Choral music
Gliders *see* Heavier-than-air
    aircraft
Gliding
  eng. *see* Aerodynamics
  sports *see* Air sports
Glires
  paleozoology   569
  zoology   599.3
Glockenspiel *see* Percussion
    instruments
Gloucester Eng.   *area* −424
Gloves *see* Handwear
Glues
  manufacture
    economics   338.4
    technology   668
  materials
    engineering   620.1
    see also spec. applications
Gluttony
  ethics   178
  religion
    Christian   241.3
    see also other spec. rel.
Glyptics
  arts   736
  industry   688

Grade-school
  children *see* Children
  libraries *see* School libraries
Graduate
  schools *see* Universities
Graft *see* Offenses
Grail
  legends *see* Mythology
Grammar
  gen. wks.   415
  study & teaching
    elementary ed.   372.6
    see also   s.s.–07
  see also spec. languages
Grammar-school
  children *see* Children
  libraries *see* School libraries
Grammar-schools *see*
        Elementary schools
Grampian Mts. Scotland   *area* –412
Grand
  Army of the Republic *see*
      Patriotic societies
  juries *see* Judicial system
  Old Party *see* Political parties
Granite
  geology
    deposits   553
    petrology   552
    see also spec. minerals
  industries
    construction
      economics   338.4
      technology   693.1
    extractive
      economics   338.2
      technology   622
  properties
    construction   691
    engineering   620.1
Graphic
  arts
    creative   **760**
    industrial
      economics   338.4
      technology   655.1–.3
  expressions
    psychology
      animals   †156
      gen. wks.   †152.3
  see also spec. forms

Graphic (continued)
  illustrations
    geography   **912**
    see also   s.s.–†022
  statics *see* Statics
Graphology
  crime detection   364.12
  diagnostic   †155.28
  divinatory   137
Grasshoppers *see* Insects
Grasslands
  economics
    gen. wks.   333.7
    see also Real-estate
  geography
    gen. wks.   910.09
    physical   †910.02
  history   909
  subj. treatment   *area* –15
  see also spec. areas
Graves *see* Cemeteries
Graveyards *see* Cemeteries
Gravies *see* Auxiliary foods
Gravitation
  astronomy   521
  physics   531
Gravity
  determinations
    geodesy   526
    physics   531
  railways *see* Railroads
Gravure
  printing *see* Metal engraving
Gray
  Friars *see* Religious
      congregations
Grazing
  land *see* Grasslands
Greasing *see* Lubrication
Great
  Basin U.S.   *area* –79
  Britain   *area* –42
  Lakes
    Canada   *area* –713
    gen. wks.   *area* –77
    see also spec. lakes
Great
  Danes *see* Working dogs
  Pyrenees
    dogs *see* Working dogs

Guarani *see* Amerindians
Guard
    animals *see* Working animals
    duty *see* Logistics
Guardhouses *see* Quarters
Guatemala   *area* –728 1
Guerrilla
    warfare
        international law   341.3
        mil. sci.   355.4
        see also hist. of spec. wars
Guessing
    games
        entertainment   793.5–.7
        folklore   398.8
Guiana   *area* –88
Guidance
    counsel *see* Counseling
    systems *see* Command systems
Guided
    aircraft *see* Heavier-than-air
        aircraft
    missiles
        manufacture
            economics   338.4
            technology   623.4
        mil. sci.
            gen. wks.   355.8
            see also spec. mil. forces
Guinea
    coast
        lower   *area* –67
        upper   *area* –66
    gulf *see* Atlantic Ocean
    isls.   *area* –66
Guinea
    fowl
        culture   636.59
        food *see* Poultry
        see also Galliformes
    pigs *see* Hystricomorphs
Guitars *see* String instruments
Gujarati-Rajasthani *see* Prakrits
Gulf Coast states U.S.   *area* –76
Gulfs *see* Marine waters
Gulls
    culture   636.6
    see also Charadriiformes
Gum-bichromate
    process *see* Special-process
        photography

Gumusane Turkey   *area* –565
Gun
    carriages *see* Gun mounts
    dogs
        culture   636.75
        use
            hunting   799.2
            see also other purposes
        see also Canidae
    mounts
        art metalwork   739.7
        industries
            economics   338.4
            technology   623.4
        mil. sci.
            gen. wks.   355.8
            see also spec. mil.
              branches
Gunboats *see* Warships
Gunnery
    engineering   623.5
    training
        gen. wks.   355.5
        see also spec. mil. branches
Guns *see* Artillery (pieces)
Gunsmithing *see* Small arms
Gymnasiums
    gen. wks. *see* Recreation
        buildings
    school equipment *see* School
        buildings
Gymnastics
    customs   394
    gen. wks.   796.4
    hygiene   †613.7
    see also Circuses
Gymnospermae
    botany   585
    floriculture   635.935
    paleobotany   561
Gymnosperms
    forestry   634.9
    see also Gymnospermae
Gynecology
    medicine   618.1
    vet. sci.
        gen. wks.   636.089
        see also spec. animals
    see also Obstetrics
Gypsy *see* Gipsy

Heroes
  biographies *see* Biographies
  history *see history of spec.*
        areas
  legends *see* Mythology
Heroism *see* Courage
Herons
  conservation   †639
  culture   636.6
  see also Ciconiiformes
Herpetology *see* Reptilia
Hertford Eng.   *area* –425
Hertzian
  waves
    biophysics
      gen. wks.   574.1
      see also spec. organisms
    engineering *see* Radio
          engineering
    physics   537.5
    see also spec. applications
Hesped *see* Funeral rites
Hibernia (ancient region)   *area* –36
Hiding
  games *see* Child play
Hierarchy
  management   †658.4
  mil. sci.
    gen. wks.   355.3
    see also spec. branches
Hieroglyphics
  gen. wks.   †411
  see also spec. languages
Hi-fi
  systems *see* Electroacoustical
        devices
High
  schools *see* Secondary
        schools
Higher
  education
    gen. wks.   **378**
    govt. control
      gen. wks.   †350
      see also spec. levels of
        govt.
    see also   *s.s.*–071
High-fidelity
  sound *see* Electroacoustical
        devices

High-school
  libraries *see* School libraries
  songs *see* Student songs
High-speed
  photography
    gen. wks.   778.3
    see also spec. applications
High-temperature
  effects *see* Temperature
        effects
Highway
  maintenance
    operations   625.7
    see also Trafficways
  patrols *see* Police
  safety *see* Safety measures
  traffic control *see* Traffic
        management
Highways *see* Trafficways
Hiking *see* Outdoor life
Himalayan *see* Tibeto-Burman
Himalayas
  gen. wks.   ***area* –54**
  see also other areas
Himyaritic *see* South Arabic
Hinayana *see* Buddhism
Hindi *see* Prakrits
Hinduism
  culture groups
    geography   910.09
    history   909
    subject treatment   *area* –176
  philosophy   181
  religion   294.5
Hindustani *see* Prakrits
Hippopotamuses
  conservation   †639
  culture   636.9
  hunting   799.27
  see also Suiformes
Hispania   *area* –36
Hispaniola   *area* –729 3
Histochemistry *see* Biochemistry
Histology
  biology
    animals   591.8
    gen. wks.   574.8
    plants   581.8
    see also spec. organisms

Housing-renewal *see* Slums
    redevelopment
Howland Isl.   *area* –96
Hudson
    Bay *see* Arctic Ocean
    Strait *see* Arctic Ocean
Huguenots *see* Reformed
    churches
Hull
    construction
        ships
            economics   338.4
            technology   623.84
Human
    ecology *see* Adaptability
    figure
        arts
            gen. wks.   704.94
            see also spec. art forms
        see also Anatomy
    races *see* Ethnology
    relations
        psychology   †158
        sociology   **301.1**
Humanism
    philosophy   144
    religion
        gen. wks.   211
        see also spec. rel.
Humanitarian
    philosophy *see* Humanism
    socialism *see* Ideal states
Humanities
    gen. wks.   001.3
    see also spec. branches
Hummingbirds *see* Apodiformes
Humor
    literature
        collections   808.87
        criticism   809.7
        rhetoric   808.7
        see also spec. lit.
    see also Collected writings
Humpback
    whales *see* Mysticetes
Hungarian *see* Finno-Ugric
Hungary   *area* –439
Hunting (activity)
    industries
        technology   639
        see also Primary industries
    sports   **799.2**

Hunting-animals *see* Working
    animals
Hunting-dogs *see* Sporting dogs
Huntingdon Eng.   *area* –425
Hunting-guns *see* Small arms
Hunting-songs *see* Folk songs
Huon Isls. *see* New Caledonia
Hurdy-gurdies *see* Mechanical
    musical instruments
Huron (lake)
    gen. wks.   *area* –774
    Ont.   *area* –713
Huron (subject) *see* Hokan-
    Siouan
Hurricanes
    disasters *see* Disasters
    meteorology *see* Storms
Hurricane-warning
    systems *see* Alarm systems
Hussites
    religion   284
    see also Church buildings
Hutterian
    Brethren *see* Mennonites
Hyaenidae
    paleozoology   569
    zoology   599.7
Hydraulic
    engineering
        economics   338.4
        technology   627
        see also Fluids
Hydraulic-power
    engineering
        gen. wks.   621.2
        see also spec. operations
Hydraulics *see* Fluids
Hydrodynamics
    engineering
        gen. wks.   627
        see also spec. branches
    mechanics   532
    see also spec. applications
Hydrogenated
    oils *see* Fats
Hydrographic
    biology
        animals   **591.92**
        gen. wks.   **574.92**
        plants   **581.92**
    see also spec. organisms

Imagination
art   701.15
literature   801
psychology   †153.3
Imams *see* Clergy
Imbibition
process *see* Special-process
       photography
Imbros
ancient   *area* –39
modern   *area* –499
Immaculate
Conception *see* Mariology
Immigrants
labor economics   331.6
see also Population movement
Immigration *see* Population
       movement
Immortality
metaphysics   129
religion
    Christian   †236
    comparative   291.2
    gen. wks.   218
    see also other spec. rel.
Immunity
political *see* Political
       immunity
Impasto
painting *see* Painting arts
paintings *see* Paintings
Impeachment
executive branch
    gen. wks.   †350
    see also spec. levels of govt.
legislative   328.3
Import
taxes *see* Customs (taxes)
trade *see* Trade (activity)
Imprisonment
corrective *see* Reformatories
punitive *see* Prisons
Imroz Turkey *see* Imbros
Inactive
files *see* Archives (records)
Inaugurations *see* Official
       ceremonies
Incarnation
metaphysics   129
religion
    Christian   232

Incarnation
religion (continued)
    gen. wks.   291.2
    see also other spec. rel.
Incest
crime *see* Offenses
sex *see* Sex relations
Inclined
planes *see* Simple machines
railways *see* Railroads
Income (money)
economics
    gen. wks.   **339**
    see also spec. elements
    see also spec. applications
Income
taxes *see* Taxation
Incunabula
gen. wks.   094
library treatment   025.17
Indebtedness
private *see* Credit
public *see* Public debts
Indentured
labor *see* Contract systems
Independence
personal *see* Personality
political *see* National
       independence
Indeterminism
metaphysics   123
religion
    Christian   234
    comparative   291.2
    see also other spec. rel.
Indexing
library sci.   029.5
museum sci.   069
India
ancient   *area* –34
modern   *area* –54
Indian
Ocean
    geography
       gen. wks.   910.09
       physical   †910.02
    geology   551.4
    isls.
       south   *area* –69
       see also spec. isls.
    regional subj.
       treatment   *area* –16

Inns *see* Public
accommodations
Inorganic
chemistry
applied | 661
pure | 546
Input-output
accounts *see* National
accounting
Insecta
paleozoology | 565
zoology | **595.7**
Insecticides *see* Pesticides
Insectivora
paleozoology | 569
zoology | 599.3
Insectivores
agricultural pests | 632
culture | 636.9
hunting | †639
see also Insectivora
Insectivorous
plants *see* Carnivorous
plants
Insects
agricultural pests | 632
culture | 638
disease carriers *see* Disease
carriers
see also Insecta
Insignias
religious
Christian | 247
gen. wks. | 291.3
see also other spec. rel.
secular
gen. wks. | **929**
military
gen. wks. | 355.1
see also spec. branches
Inspiration
art | 701.15
Bible | 220.1
psychology | †153.2
see also | s.s.–01
Installment
plans *see* Credit
Institutes (education) *see*
Extension

Institutional
cookery *see* Cookery
household *see* Public
accommodations
Instrumentalism
philosophy | 144
see also | s.s.–01
Instruments
manufacture
economics | 338.4
technology | 681
see also spec. applications
Insulated
construction *see* Resistant
construction
Insulating
materials
construction | 691
engineering
gen. wks. | 620.1
see also spec. branches
see also spec. applications
Insulation
electric conductors | 621.319
see also Thermology
Insurance
gen. wks. | **†368**
see also Financial institutions
Intaglio
processes
arts | 765–767
industry | 655.3
see also Carving-
techniques
Intaglios
gems *see* Carvings
prints *see* Prints
Integration
racial *see* Racial integration
Intellectual
guidance *see* Counseling
occupations *see* Professional
occupations
processes
animals | †156
children | †155.41
gen. wks. | **†153**
see also Intellectualism
Intellectualism
gen. wks. | 001.2
philosophy | 149

Italy	
ancient	area –37
modern	**area –45**
Ivory Coast	area –66
Ivory	
carvings	736
products	
manufacture	
economics	338.4
technology	679
see also spec. applications	
Izmir Turkey	area –562

J

Jacamars *see* Piciformes	
Jacanas *see* Charadriiformes	
Jackasses *see* Asses	
Jacobite	
Church *see* Monophysite churches	
Jade	
mineralogy	549.6
see also Semiprecious stones	
Jaguars *see* Cats	
Jai alai *see* Racket games	
Jail	
buildings *see* Prison buildings	
Jails *see* Prisons	
Jainism	
culture groups	
geography	910.09
history	909
subject treatment	area –176
philosophy	181
religion	294.4
Jamaica (West Indian island)	area –729 2
James (N.T.) *see* Catholic epistles	
Jams	
cookery	641.6
production	
commercial	†664
home	641.8
Jamtland Sweden	area –488
Jan Mayen Isl.	area –98
Jansenist	
Church *see* Schismatic churches	
religion *see* Heresies	

Japan (country)	**area –52**
Japan (sea) *see* Pacific Ocean	
Japanese	
ethnic groups	area –174
language	495.6
lingual groups	area –175
wrestling *see* Unarmed combat	
see also other spec. subj.	
Japanning *see* Lackering	
Japans	
manufacture	
economics	338.4
technology	667
see also spec. applications	
Java	area –92
Javanese *see* Austronesian	
Javelin	
throwing *see* Track athletics	
Jays	
agricultural pests	632
see also Passeriformes	
Jazz	
gen. wks.	781.5
see also spec. mediums	
Jehovah *see* God	
Jehovah's Witnesses *see* Recent Christian sects	
Jellies	
cookery	641.6
production	
commercial	664
home	641.8
Jeremiah (O.T.) *see* Prophetic books	
Jeremias (O.T.) *see* Prophetic books	
Jeremy (Apocrypha) *see* Epistle of Jeremy	
Jesuits *see* Religious congregations	
Jesus	
Christianity *see* Christology	
Islam *see* Koran	
Jet	
aircraft *see* Heavier-than-air aircraft	
engines *see* Internal-combustion engines	
streams *see* Winds	

Judith
Apocrypha 229
liturgy
Christianity 264
Judaism 296.4
Judo *see* Unarmed combat
Jugatae *see* Lepidoptera
Juggling *see* Magic arts
Jujitsus *see* Unarmed combat
Jumping *see* Track athletics
June
beetles
agricultural pests 632
culture 638
see also Coleoptera
Jungle
warfare *see* Battle tactics
Junior
college
libraries *see* College
libraries
colleges *see* Colleges
high school
libraries *see* School
libraries
high schools *see* Secondary
schools
misses' clothing *see*
Garments
republics
management 658
services 362.7
Juries *see* Judicial system
Jurisprudence *see* Law
Jury
trials
civil cases 347.9
criminal cases 343
Justice
departments *see* Executive
departments
govt. control
gen. wks. †350
*see also spec. levels of
govt.*
law *see* Law
Juvenile
delinquents
criminology *see* Offenders
gen. wks. *see* Exceptional
children
Juveniles *see* Young people

K

Kabyle *see* Berber
Kallitype
process *see* Special-process
photography
Kalmar Sweden area −486
Kalmyk (subject) *see*
Mongolic
Kanarese *see* Dravidian
Kandh *see* Dravidian
Kangaroos *see* Marsupials
Kannada *see* Dravidian
Kansas area −781
Kantianism
gen. wks. †142
see also spec. philosophers
Kanuri *see* Chad
Karate *see* Unarmed combat
Karelian *see* Finnic
Karpathos Greece
ancient area −39
modern area −499
Kars Turkey area −566
Karting *see* Motoring
Kartvelian *see* Caucasian
Kashubian *see* Polish
Kastamonu Turkey area −563
Katharevusa *see* Greek
Katydids *see* Insects
Kayseri Turkey area −564
Kazakhstan USSR area −584
Kechua *see* Amerindians
Keeshonden *see* Nonsporting
dogs
Keewatin area −712
Kennels *see* Shelters
Keno *see* Counter games
Kent Eng. area −422
Kentucky area −769
Kenya area −676
Kerguelen Isls. Indian
Ocean area −69
Kerosenes *see* Petroleum
products
Ket *see* Paleosiberian
Kettledrums *see* Percussion
instruments
Key
bugles *see* Horns (musical
instruments)

Knightly	
customs	
folklore	
hist. & criticism	398.3
legends	398.22
gen. wks.	394
orders *see* Knighthood	
Knights (heraldry) *see*	
Knighthood	
Knitwear *see* Garments	
Knowledge	
gen. wks.	**001**
philosophy	
classification	112
gen. wks.	121
psychology	
animals	†156
gen. wks.	153.4
religion *see* Intellectualism	
see also Education	
Koalas *see* Marsupials	
Kocaeli Turkey	*area* –563
Kodagu *see* Dravidian	
Kolarian *see* Austroasian	
Konya Turkey	*area* –564
Kopparberg Sweden	*area* –487
Koran	
literature	809.9
religion	297
Korea	*area* –519
Korean	
ethnic groups	*area* –174
language	495.7
lingual groups	*area* –175
see also other spec. subj.	
Koryak *see* Paleosiberian	
Kota *see* Dravidian	
Krasnodar RSFSR	*area* –479
Krimmer	
Brueder Gemeinde *see*	
Mennonites	
Kristianstad Sweden	*area* –486
Kronoberg Sweden	*area* –486
Kudus *see* Antelopes	
Kurdish *see* Iranian	
Kurdistan	*area* –566
Kurile Isls.	*area* –†57
Kurukh *see* Dravidian	
Kutahya Turkey	*area* –562
Kuwait	*area* –53

L

Labor (childbirth) *see*	
Parturition	
Labor	
control	
governmental	
gen. wks.	†350
see also spec. levels of	
govt.	
political	322
Day *see* Holidays	
departments *see* Executive	
departments	
economics	**331**
movements	
pol. sci.	322
sociology	301.15
relations *see* Employer-	
employee	
relationships	
songs *see* Topical songs	
unions *see* Unions	
Laboratories	
school equipment *see* School	
buildings	
spec. subj.	*s.s.* –028
Laboratory	
animals *see* Experimental	
animals	
methods	
teaching	
gen. wks.	371.38
see also spec.	
levels of ed.	
see also	*s.s.* –01
Laboring	
classes	
economics	**331**
sociology	301.44
welfare services	†362.8
Labor-management	
disputes *see* Union-	
management disputes	
relationships *see* Employer-	
employee	
relationships	
Labrador	*area* –719
Laccadive Isls. India	*area* –54
Lacertilia *see* Lepidosauria	

458

Larceny
  criminal *see* Offenses
  psychopathic *see* Personality
      disorders
Lard *see* Fats
Larks *see* Passeriformes
Lasers
  engineering
    economics 338.4
    technology 621.32
  physics 535.5
  see also spec. applications
Lasethi Greece .... *area* –499
Last
  judgment *see* Judgment
  Supper
    of Jesus Christ 232.95
    see also Sacraments
  things *see* Eschatology
Latexes *see* Elastomers
Lathwork
  economics 338.4
  technology 693.6
Latin America .... *area* –8
Latin
  ethnic groups .... *area* –174
  language **471–478**
  lingual groups .... *area* –175
  see also other spec. subj.
Latin grammar schools *see*
      Secondary schools
Latter-Day Saints
  Church
    religion 289.3
    see also Church buildings
Latvia .... *area* –47
Latvian
  ethnic groups .... *area* –174
  language 491.9
  lingual groups .... *area* –175
  see also other spec. subj.
Launches *see* Small craft
Laundering
  commercial 667
  domestic 648
Lavatories
  equipment
    homes 643
    schools *see* School
        buildings
    see also other spec.
        structures

Lavatories (continued)
  public *see* Sanitation
Law
  Biblical 220.8
  gen. wks. .... **†340**
  military
    gen. wks. 355.1
    see also spec. services
Law enforcement *see* Police
      services
Law of nations *see*
      International
      relations
Lawlessness *see* Offenses
Lawmaking *see* Legislation
Lawn
  billiards *see* Mallet games
  bowling *see* Simple ball
      games
  tennis *see* Racket games
Laws *see* Statutes
Laz *see* Caucasian
Lazarists *see* Religious
      congregations
Lead *see* Metals
Leadership
  psychology .... †158
  sociology 301.15
Leaf
  beetles
    agricultural pests 632
    culture 638
    see also Coleoptera
  hoppers
    agricultural pests 632
    culture 638
    see also Insecta
League
  of Nations
    gen. wks. 341.12
    see also spec. services
Learned
  societies
    gen. wks. **060**
    library services
      gen. wks. .... †027.6
      see also spec. functions
Learning
  education
    gen. wks. 370.15
    techniques **371.3**

Line-&-staff
  organization *see* Hierarchy
Liners (ships) *see* Merchant
    ships
Lingual
  regions
    geography   910.09
    history   909
    subj. treatment   *area* –175
    see also spec. regions
Linguistics
  gen. wks.   410
  see also spec. languages
Linoleum-block
  printing *see* Printing
    processes
  prints *see* Prints
Linoleums
  interior decoration
    art   747
    home economics   645
  manufacture *see* Textiles
Linseed
  oil *see* Fixed oils
Lions *see* Cats
Liquidation
  accounting *see* Financial
    accounting
Liquidations *see* Financial
    administration
Liquids
  engineering
    gen. wks.   621.2
    see also spec. branches
  physics
    gen. wks.   530.4
    mechanics   532
    see also other spec.
      branches
Liquor
  traffic
    govt. control
      gen. wks.   †350
      see also spec. levels of
        govt.
    police services   363.4
  see also Addictions
Liquors
  alcoholic *see* Spirits
    (alcoholic)

Litanies
  music
    gen. wks.   783.2
    see also spec. mediums
  religion *see* Prayers
Literary
  composition *see* Rhetoric
  criticism
    gen. wks.   809
    see also spec. lit.
  games *see* Puzzles
Literature
  gen. wks.   800
  study & teaching
    elementary ed.   †372.8
    see also   *s.s.*–07
Lithographs *see* Prints
Lithography *see* Planographic
    processes
Lithology *see* Petrology
Lithozincographs *see* Prints
Lithozincography *see*
    Planographic
    processes
Lithuania   *area* –47
Lithuanian
  ethnic groups   *area* –174
  language   †491.9
  lingual groups   *area* –175
  see also other spec. subj.
Little
  Church of France *see*
    Schismatic churches
Liturgical
  music
    gen. wks.   783.2
    see also spec. mediums
  year
    religion
      Christian
        gen. wks.   263
        liturgy   264
        prayers   242.3
        sermons   252
        gen. wks.   291.3
      see also other spec. rel.
    see also Holy days
Liturgies *see* Public worship
Livestock
  husbandry
    economics   338.1
    technology   636

Lotteries
  advertising *see* Contest
      advertising
  games *see* Gambling
  investments *see* Interest
      lotteries
  revenue *see* Nontax
      revenues
Lotto *see* Counter games
Louisiade Archipelago   *area* –95
Louisiana   *area* –763
Louth Ireland   *area* –418
Love
  psychology *see* Emotions
  sexual *see* Courtship
Low Archipelago *see* Tuamotu
    Isls.
Low
  German *see* Germanic
Loyalty Isls.   *area* –93
Loyalty
  employee *see* Employer-
      employee
      relationships
  ethics   179
  military
    gen. wks.   355.1
    see also spec. branches
  social   301.15
Lubricants
  gen. *see* Fixed oils
  petroleum *see* Petroleum
      products
Lubrication
  engineering
    economics   338.4
    technology
      gen. wks.   621.8
      see also spec. branches
    see also spec. applications
Luchu *see* Ryukyu Isls.
Lucrative
  capital *see* Finance
Ludo *see* Dice games
Luggage
  manufacture
    economics   338.4
    technology   685
  see also spec. applications

Luke (N.T.) *see* Gospels
Lullabies *see* Folk songs
Lumber
  industries
    logging *see* Logging
      (trees)
    processing
      economics   338.4
      technology   674
  see also Woods (substance)
Lunar
  astronomy *see* Moon
  flights *see* Space
    (extraterrestrial)
    flights
Lunchroom
  meals
    cookery *see* Cookery
    service   642
Lunchrooms
  public *see* Public
      accommodations
  school equipment *see*
      School buildings
Luorawetlin *see* Paleosiberian
Lusitania   *area* –36
Lutes *see* String instruments
Lutheran
  churches
    religion   **284**
    see also Church buildings
Lutheranism *see* Lutheran
    churches
Luxembourg (grand
      duchy)   *area* –493
Lycia   *area* –39
Lydia   *area* –39
Lying
  ethics   177
  psychopathology *see*
      Personality-disorders
  religion
    Christian   241.3
    see also other spec. rel.
Lynching
  ethics   179
  see also Offenses
Lynx *see* Cats
Lyres *see* String instruments

M

Magicians
religion
  gen. wks.   291.6
  see also spec. rel.
  see also Magic arts
Magna Carta *see*
  Constitutional law
Magnetic
compasses
  physics   538
  see also Direction finders
Magnetism
chemistry *see* Physical
  chemistry
physics   **538**
Magnetochemistry *see* Physical
  chemistry
Magyar *see* Finno-Ugric
Mahabharata
literature   891.2
religion   294.5
Mahayana *see* Buddhism
Mah-jongg *see* Counter games
Mahomet *see* Prophets
Mahri   *area* –53
Mahri-Sokotri *see* South Arabic
Mail
services *see* Postal
  communication
Mail-order
catalogs *see* Direct-mail
  advertising
houses *see* Retail marketing
Maine (state)   *area* –741
Malachi (O.T.) *see* Prophetic
  books
Malachias (O.T.) *see* Prophetic
  books
Maladjusted
children *see* Exceptional
  children
Maladjustments
prod. economics
  gen. wks.   338.54
  see also spec. industries
psychology *see* Abnormal
  psychology
Malagasy Republic *see*
  Madagascar
Malatya Turkey   *area* –565
Malawi *see* Nyasaland

Malay Archipelago   *area* –91
Malaya   *area* –595
Malayalam *see* Dravidian
Malayan *see* Austronesian
Malay-Javanese *see*
  Austronesian
Malayo-Polynesian *see*
  Austronesian
Malaysia (archipelago) *see*
  Malay Archipelago
Malaysia (country)   *area* –595
Maldive Isls.   *area* –†549
Malfeasance *see* Offenses
Malformations *see* Teratology
Mali   *area* –66
Mallet
games
  customs   394
  gen. wks.   796.35
Malmohus Sweden   *area* –486
Malpractice *see* Quackery
Malta
ancient   *area* –37
modern   *area* –458
Malted
beverages
  alcoholic *see* Beers
  nonalcoholic *see* Soft
    drinks
Maltese
dogs *see* Miniature dogs
Mammalia
paleozoology   569
zoology   **599**
Mammals
conservation practices   †639
hunting
  industries   †639
  sports   799.27
husbandry   **636**
see also Mammalia
Mammoths *see* Proboscidea
Man (isle) Eng.   *area* –428
Man
biology *see* Hominidae
metaphysics   128
religious doctrines
  Christian   233
  gen. wks.   291.2
  see also other spec. rel.
see also Men

Materials (continued)
  engineering
    gen. wks.   620.1
    see also spec. branches
    see also spec. subj.
Materials-control
  equipment *see* Materials-
       handling equipment
  management   658.7
  see also Supply
     administration
Materials-handling
  equipment
    engineering
      economics   338.4
      technology
        gen. wks.   621.8
        mines   622
        see also other spec.
          branches
      see also spec. applications
Materiel
  mil. sci.
    gen. wks.   355.8
    tech. forces *see* Technical
      forces
    see also spec. mil.
      branches
    see also spec. kinds of
      institutions
Maternity
  homes
    management   658
    services   †362.8
  hospitals
    management   658
    services   362.1
Mathematical
  games *see* Puzzles
  geography
    gen. wks.   **526**
    see also spec. applications
  logic *see* Reasoning
Mathematics
  gen. wks.   **510**
  study & teaching
    elementary ed.   372.7
    see also   *s.s.*–07
  see also   *s.s.*–01
Matrimony *see* Sacraments

Matter
  metaphysics   117
  science   **500**
Matthew (N.T.) *see* Gospels
Matzevah *see* Funeral rites
Maundy
  Thursday *see* Holy days
Mauretania   *area* –39
Mauritania   *area* –66
Mauritius   *area* –69
Mausoleums *see* Tombs
Maxims *see* Proverbs (general)
May
  Day *see* Holidays
Maya *see* Macro-Penutian
Mayas *see* Amerindians
Mayflower
  Descendants *see* Hereditary
     societies
Mayo Ireland   *area* –417
Mayors *see* Chief executives
Mazdaism *see* Zoroastrianism
Meals
  cookery   641.5
  customs *see* Eating-customs
  service
    management   658
    technology   642
Measurement
  standards *see* Metrology
Measurements
  engineering
    chemical   660
    electrical   621.37
    see also other spec.
      branches
  physics *see spec. branches*
  see also other spec. subj.
Measures *see* Metrology
Meath Ireland   *area* –418
Meats
  cookery   641.6
  gen. wks.   641.3
  preservation
    commercial   **664**
    home   **641.4**
Mechanical
  drawing *see* Technical
    drawing

Meditation (continued)
  religion
    Christian   †248.3
    gen. wks.   291.4
    see also other spec. rel.
Meditations
  religion
    Christian   †242
    gen. wks.   291.4
    see also other spec. rel.
    see also other spec. subj.
Mediterranean
  region
    geography   910.09
    history   909
    subj. treatment   *area* –†18
    see also spec. areas
  Sea *see* Atlantic Ocean
Melanesia   *area* –93
Melanesian *see* Austronesian
Meliorism
  philosophy   149
  see also spec. philosophers
Melodeons *see* Wind
    instruments (musical)
Melodrama *see* Drama
Melody *see* Composition
Membranophones *see*
    Percussion
    instruments
Memel   *area* –47
Memoirs *see* Biographies
Memorial
  Day *see* Holidays
Memory
  aids *see* Mnemonics
  games   793.7
  processes
    education   370.15
    psychology   †153.1
Men
  psychology   †155.6
  sociology   †301.4
  see also other spec. aspects
Mende *see* Niger-Congo
Mending
  books   025.7
  clothes   646.2
Mennonites
  religion
    gen. wks.   289.7

Mennonites
  religion (continued)
    see also Church buildings
    see also Social classes
Menstruation
  disorders   618.1
  physiology   612.66
Mensuration
  arithmetic *see* Business
    arithmetic
  weights & measures *see*
    Metrology
Mental
  deficiency
    welfare services   362.3
    see also Abnormal
      psychology
  diseases
    medicine *see* Psychiatry
    psychology *see* Abnormal
      psychology
  health *see* Mental hygiene
  hospitals
    management   658
    services   362.2
  hygiene
    gen. wks.   †614.58
    hospital services   362.2
  illness
    medicine *see* Psychiatry
    psychology *see* Abnormal
      psychology
    physiology *see* Physiological
      psychology
  retardation *see* Mental
    deficiency
  tests
    education   371.26
    psychology   †153.9
Mentally
  deficient
    children *see* Exceptional
      children
    people
      med. treatment *see*
        spec. diseases
      welfare services   362.3
  ill
    children *see* Exceptional
      children

Meters
  engineering (continued)
    see also other spec.
      branches
    see also spec. applications
Methodist
  churches
    religion   287
    see also Church buildings
Methodology
  gen. wks.   †001.4
  philosophy   112
  see also   *s.s.–01*
Metrology
  gen. wks.   389
  govt. control
    gen. wks.   †350
    see also spec. levels of
      govt.
  science   502
  see also spec. applications
Metropolitan
  areas *see* Communities
  governments *see* Local
    governments
Mexican
  hairless
    dogs *see* Miniature dogs
Mexico (country)   *area –72*
Mexico (gulf) *see* Atlantic
  Ocean
Mezzotinting
  arts   766
  industry   655.3
Mezzotints *see* Prints
Micah (O.T.) *see* Prophetic
  books
Mice *see* Myomorphs
Micheas (O.T.) *see* Prophetic
  books
Michigan (lake)
  gen. wks.   *area –774*
  see also other areas
Michigan (state)   *area –774*
Microbiology
  gen. wks.   **576**
  see also   *s.s.–01*
Microcards *see* Micro-
    reproductions
Microfilms *see*
    Microreproductions

Microminiaturization *see*
  Miniaturization
Micronesia   *area –96*
Micronesian *see* Austronesian
Microorganisms
  gen. wks. *see* Microbiology
  pathogenic *see* Pathogenic
    microorganisms
Microphotography
  gen. wks.   778.3
  see also Duplication
Microprints *see*
  Microreproductions
Microreproductions
  business records   651
  communication   †001.5
  library treatment   025.17
  production *see*
    Microphotography
Microscopes
  biology   578
  physics   535
  see also spec. applications
Microscopic
  books *see* Miniature editions
Microwaves
  engineering
    economics   338.4
    technology
      gen. wks.   621.381
      see also Radar
  physics   537.5
Middle
  America   *area –72*
  Atlantic states U.S. *area –74*
  Congo *see* Congo
    (Brazzaville)
  East
    ancient   *area –39*
    modern   *area –56*
  West U.S.   *area –77*
Middle
  Ages
    church hist.   270.2–.5
    gen. hist.   940.1
  Low
    German *see* Germanic
  management
    business   658.43
    military
      gen. wks.   355
      see also spec. branches

Models
  manufacture
    economics   338.4
    technology   688
  see also Operations research
Moesia   *area* –39
Mohammed *see* Prophets
Mohammedanism *see* Islam
Molding
  metals
    arts
      metalwork   739
      sculpture   731.4
    technology
      gen. wks.   671.2
      see also spec. metals
    see also other spec. materials
Moldlofts *see* Shipyards
Molecular
  compounds *see* Salts
  structure *see* Molecules
Molecules
  chemistry   541
  physics   539
Moles (animals) *see*
    Insectivores
Molinism *see* Heresies
Mollusca
  culture   639
  paleozoology   564
  zoology   594
Mollusks
  fisheries
    economics   338.3
    technology   †639
  see also Mollusca
Moluccas   *area* –91
Mon *see* Austroasian
Monaco   *area* –449
Monaghan Ireland   *area* –416
Monarchical
  absolutism
    pol. sci.   321.6
    see also spec. areas
Monarchies
  absolute *see* Monarchical
    absolutism
  limited *see* Constitutional
    monarchies

Monasteries
  buildings *see* Monastic
    buildings
  religion *see* Religious
    congregations
Monastic
  buildings
    architecture   726
    construction
      economics   338.4
      technology   690.6
  life
    Christian religion   †248.8
    gen. wks.   291.4
    see also other spec. rel.
  orders *see* Religious
    congregations
  schools
    education   377
    see also Church-
      supported schools
Money
  economics   332.4–.5
  govt. control
    gen. wks.   †350
    see also spec. levels of
      govt.
  numismatics *see*
    Numismatics
  see also Financial
    administration
Mongolia   *area* –51
Mongolic
  ethnic groups   *area* –174
  languages   494
  lingual groups   *area* –175
  see also other spec. subj.
Mongooses *see* Viverrines
Monism
  philosophy   147
  science   501
Monkeys
  conservation   †639
  culture   636.9
  experimental med.
    animals   636.089
    man   619
  see also Primates
Mon-Khmer *see* Austroasian
Monmouth Eng.   *area* –424

Mosaic (continued)
  laws *see* Ethics
  ornaments *see* Mosaics
Mosaics
  arts
    architectural design   729
    jewelry   738.5
    painting
      collections   **759**
      process   751.4
Mosan *see* Algonkian-Mosan
Moscow RSFSR   *area* –473
Moslems
  ethnic group   *area* –174
  religion *see* Islam
Mosques
  architecture   726
  construction   690.6
  religion *see* Sacred places
Mosquitoes
  agricultural pests   632
  culture   638
  disease carriers *see* Disease
      carriers
  see also Orthorrhapha
Motacillidae *see* Passeriformes
Motels *see* Public
      accommodations
Moth
  flies
    agricultural pests   632
    culture   638
    see also Orthorrhapha
Mother
  Goose *see* Rhymes
Motherhood *see* Parenthood
Moths
  agricultural pests   632
  culture   638
  see also Lepidoptera
Motion (activity)
  astronomy   521
  metaphysics   116
  physics   531–533
Motion-picture
  education *see* Extension
  films
    communication
      gen. wks.   †001.5
      services   †384.8
    library treatment   025.17

Motion-picture (continued)
  music
    gen. wks.   782.8
    see also spec. mediums
  photography
    gen. wks.   778.5
    see also spec. applications
  plays *see* Drama
  programs
    ethics   175
    production
      gen. wks.   791.43
      management   658
Motion-pictures *see* Audio-
      visual materials
Motivation
  psychology
    animals   †156
    gen. wks.   †152.5
    learning factors
      animals   †156
      gen. wks.   †153.1
  research
    marketing *see* Market
      research & analysis
    spec. subj.   *s.s.*–01
Motives *see* Motivation
Motmots *see* Coraciiformes
Motor
  bicycles *see* Cycles (vehicles)
  buses *see* Motor vehicles
  cars *see* Motor vehicles
  courts *see* Public
      accommodations
  fuels *see* Petroleum products
  functions
    biology *see* Physiology
    psychology
      animals   †156.2
      gen. wks.   †152.3
  generators *see* Motors
  launches *see* Small craft
  learning *see* Habit formation
  trucks *see* Motor vehicles
  vehicles
    agricultural use
      gen wks.   631.3
      see also spec. crops
    architecture   725

Motor
  vehicles (continued)
    construction
      economics   338.4
      technology
        gen. wks.   **629.2**
        military   623.7
    marketing   658.8
    see also Transportation
      services
Motorboating *see* Boating
Motorboats *see* Small craft
Motorcycle
  cavalry *see* Mechanized
    cavalry
  racing *see* Motoring
Motorcycles *see* Cycles
  (vehicles)
Motorcycling *see* Motoring
Motoring
  instruction   **629.28**
  recreation   796.7
  see also Transportation
Motors
  generators   621.313
  prime movers   621.4
  see also spec. applications
Mountain
  climbing *see* Outdoor life
  railways *see* Railroads
  ranges *see* Mountains
Mountaineering *see* Outdoor
  life
Mountains
  geography
    gen. wks.   910.09
    physical   †910.02
  geology   551.4
  regional subj.
    treatment   *area* –14
  see also spec. areas
Mounted
  forces
    mil. sci.
      gen. wks.   357
    see also spec. kinds of
      warfare
    see also hist. of spec. wars
Mourning
  customs *see* Funeral rites
Mouth organs *see* Wind
  instruments (musical)

Movement *see* Motion
  (activity)
Movements
  horological *see* Timepieces
  mechanical *see* Motion
    (activity)
  physiological *see* Motor
    functions
Movies *see* Motion-picture
Moving vans *see* Motor
  vehicles
Mucilages *see* Glues
Muffs *see* Handwear
Mugla Turkey   *area* –562
Muhammad *see* Prophets
Mulches
  agriculture *see* Mulching
  manufacture
    economics   338.4
    technology   668
    marketing   658.8
Mulching
  erosion control   631.4
  soil improvement   631.8
  water conservation   631.7
  see also spec. plants
Mules (animals)
  husbandry   636.1
  see also Equidae
Mules (footwear) *see*
  Footwear
Multiple-loop
  systems *see* Automatic
    control
Multiple-purpose
  animals
    culture
      gen. wks.   636.08
      see also spec. animals
Munda *see* Austroasian
Mundari *see* Austroasian
Municipal
  buildings *see* Government
    buildings
  engineering
    economics   338.4
    technology   628
  governments *see* Local
    governments
  law *see* Internal law
  planning *see* Planning
    communities

Neutral
nations
 geography   910.09
 history   909
 subj. treatment   *area –171*
 see also spec. nations
Neutrality
 administration   †350
 law   341.3
 pol. sci.   327
 see also hist. of spec.
    countries
Nevada (state)   *area –793*
Nevis West Indies   *area –729 7*
Nevsehir Turkey   *area –564*
New
 Brunswick (province)   *area –715*
 Caledonia   *area –93*
 England   ***area –74***
 Guinea   *area –95*
 Hampshire   *area –742*
 Hebrides   *area –93*
 Jersey   *area –749*
 Land *see* Novaya Zemlya
 Mexico   *area –789*
 York   ***area –747***
 Zealand   *area –931*
New
 Economics (The) *see*
   Economic systems
 Jerusalem churches *see*
   Church of the New
   Jerusalem
 Testament
  apocrypha &
   pseudepigrapha   229
  gen. wks.   **225**
  theology   **230**
  see also Scripture readings
 Thought *see* Recent Christian
   sects
 Year's
  Day *see* Holidays
Newborn
 infants *see* Children
Newfoundland   *area –718*
Newfoundlands *see* Working
   dogs
News
 journalism   070.4
 publishing *see* Publishing

Newscasts
 broadcasts *see*
   Telecommunication
 journalism *see* Journalism
Newspapers
 general   071–079
 publishing *see* Publishing
 see also Serials
Newts *see* Salamanders
Niagara
 Falls
  gen. wks.   *area –713*
  N.Y.   *area –747*
Nicaragua   *area –728 5*
Nickel *see* Metals
Nicknames *see* Personal names
Niger (country)   *area –66*
Niger-Congo
 ethnic groups   *area –174*
 languages   496
 lingual groups   *area –175*
 see also other spec. subj.
Nigeria   *area –669*
Night
 baseball *see* Bat games
 clothes *see* Garments
 schools *see* Adult education
Nightclub
 shows *see* Drama
Nightclubs *see* Public
   accommodations
Nightingales *see* Passeriformes
Nihilism
 philosophy   149
 see also spec. philosophers
Nile River
 gen. wks.   ***area –62***
 see also other areas
Ninepins *see* Indoor ball games
Nirvana *see* Eschatology
Noise
 control
  govt. control
   gen. wks.   †350
   see also spec. levels of
     govt.
  pub. health   614
  see also Acoustics
Nominalism
 philosophy   149

Nuclear
  accidents *see* Disasters
  energy
    engineering   621.48
    physics   **539.7**
    see also spec. applications
  engineering
    economics   338.4
    technology
      gen. wks.   621.48
      see also spec.
        applications
  engines *see* Nuclear reactors
  fission *see* Nuclear energy
  fusion *see* Thermonuclear
      fusion
  heating
    gen. wks.   697.7
    see also spec. applications
  physics
    gen. wks.   **539.7**
    see also spec. applications
  reactors *see* Nuclear
      engineering
  war *see* Strategy
  warfare
    defenses
      mil. eng.   623
      welfare services   †363.35
    forces
      gen. wks.   358
      see also spec. kinds of
        warfare
Nudes *see* Human figure
Number
  metaphysics   119
  see also spec. philosophers
Numbers (O.T.) *see* Historical
      books (O.T.)
Numbers (symbols)
  algebra *see* Algebra
  occultism *see* Divination
Numbers-game *see* Gambling
Numeration
  systems *see* Arithmetic
Numerology *see* Divination
Numidia   *area* −39
Numismatics
  gen. wks.   †737
  see also Paper money

Nunneries *see* Religious
      congregations
Nurseries (children) *see*
      Rooms
Nurseries (plants)
  agriculture
    gen. wks.   635.9
    see also spec. plants
  management
    economics   338.4
    technology   658
  see also Nursery stock
Nursery
  rhymes *see* Rhymes
  schools *see* Elementary
      schools
  stock
    gen. wks.   631.5
    see also spec. crops
Nurses *see* Nursing
Nursing
  home economics   649.8
  med. sci.   610.73
  mil. sci. *see* Special services
Nursing-homes *see*
      Convalescent homes
Nuthatches *see* Passeriformes
Nutrition
  biology
    animals   591.1
    gen. wks.   574.1
    plants   581.1
    see also spec. organisms
  practices
    animals
      gen. wks.   636.089
      see also spec. animals
    man
      home econ.   **641**
      hygiene   613.2
Nuts (mechanics) *see*
      Fastenings
Nyasaland   *area* −689
Nygde Turkey   *area* −564

O

Oases
  geography
    gen. wks.   910.09
    physical   †910.02

Oases (continued)
geology	551.4
history	909
subj. treatment	*area* –15

see also spec. areas
Obadiah (O.T.) *see* Prophetic
    books
Obedience
| ethics | 179 |

theology
| Christian | 234 |
| gen. wks. | 291.2 |

see also other spec. rel.
see also spec. applications
Obesity *see* Overweight people
Oblates *see* Religious
    congregations
Oboes *see* Wind instruments
    (musical)
Obscenity
  crime *see* Offenses
| ethics | 179 |

religion
| Christian | 241.3 |

see also other spec. rel.
see also Sexual ethics
Observants *see* Religious
    congregations
Observatories
| astronomy | 522 |

school equipment *see*
    School buildings
Obstetrics
| medicine | 618.2 |

vet. sci.
| gen. wks. | 636.089 |

see also spec. animals
Ocarinas *see* Wind instruments
    (musical)
Occasionalism
| gen. wks. | 147 |
| metaphysics | 122 |

see also spec. philosophers
Occident *see* Atlantic region
Occult
  sciences *see* Occultism
Occultism
| **folklore** | **398** |
| **gen. wks.** | **133** |

Occupational
  education *see* Vocational
    education
ethics
| philosophy | †174 |

religion
| **Christian** | **241** |

see also other spec. rel.
rehabilitation *see* Educational
    programs
Occupations
economics
| **labor** | **331.7** |
| production | 338.1–.4 |

technology *see* spec. subj.
see also Social classes
Ocean
  currents *see* Marine waters
floor
| geography | †910.02 |
| geology | 551.4 |

see also spec. oceans
liners *see* Merchant ships
transportation *see*
    Transportation
    services
| **Oceania** | *area* –9 |

Oceanography *see* Marine
    waters
Oceans *see* Marine waters
Ocelots *see* Cats
Ocular
disorders
animals
| vet. sci. | 636.089 |
| zoology | 591.2 |

see also spec. animals
| man | 617 |

Odes
  of Solomon *see* Poetic books
Odobenidae
| paleozoology | 569 |
| zoology | 599.7 |

Odonata *see* Insects
Odontocetes
| culture | 636.9 |

see also Odontoceti
Odontoceti
paleozoology	569
zoology	599.5
Oeno Isl.	*area* –96

Offaly Ireland   *area* –418
Offenders
  criminology   †364.3
  law *see* Criminal law
  see also Personality-disorders
Offenses
  criminology   †364.3
  govt. control
    gen. wks.   †350
    see also spec. levels of govt.
  law *see* Criminal law
  military   355.1
  protective services   363.2–.4
Office
  buildings *see* Commercial
              buildings
  equipment
    gen. wks.   651
    manufacture *see spec.*
      items
  personnel
    gen. wks.   651
    labor economics   331.7
    management   †658.3
  services
    economics   338.4
    technology   651
Official
  ceremonies
    customs   394
    history *see history of spec.*
      areas
  mil. sci.
    gen. wks.   355.1
    see also spec. branches
Offset
  lithography *see* Planographic
              processes
  printing
    economics   338.4
    technology   655.3
Ogres *see* Supernatural beings
Ohio (state)   *area* –771
Ohio
  River
    gen. wks.   *area* –769
    see also other areas
  Valley
    gen. wks.   *area* –77
    see also other areas

Oil
  gas *see* Industrial gases
  painting *see* Painting arts
  paintings *see* Paintings
  varnishes *see* Japans
Oils
  cooking *see* Fixed oils
  edible *see* Fixed oils
  essential *see* Essential oils
  fixed *see* Fixed oils
  industrial *see* Fixed oils
  mineral *see* Mineral oils
  nonvolatile *see* Fixed oils
  petroleum *see* Petroleum oils
  saponifying *see* Fixed oils
  vegetable *see* Fixed oils
  volatile *see* Essential oils
Oil-transfer
  photography *see* Special-
              process photography
Ojibway *see* Algonkian-Mosan
Okapis
  conservation   †639
  culture   636.2
  hunting
    sports   799.27
  see also Cervoidea
Okhotsk Sea *see* Pacific Ocean
Oklahoma (state)   *area* –766
Old
  age *see* Old-age
  Catholic Church *see*
              Schismatic churches
  Egyptian
    ethnic groups   *area* –174
    language   493
    lingual groups   *area* –175
    see also other spec. subj.
  English *see* Anglo-Saxon
  Frisian *see* Germanic
  Icelandic *see* Germanic
  Low
    Franconian *see* Germanic
    German *see* Germanic
  Norse *see* Germanic
  Prussian
    ethnic groups   *area* –174
    language   491.9
    lingual groups   *area* –175
    see also other spec. subj.
  Saxon *see* Germanic

Orange
  Free State South
      Africa   *area* –68
Orangutans *see* Apes
Orâon *see* Dravidian
Orations *see* Speeches
Oratories *see* Chapels
Oratorios
  sacred   783.3
  secular   782.8
Oratory *see* Speeches
Orbits
  astronautics   629.4
  astronomy
    descriptive   **523**
    theoretical   521
Orchards
  agriculture
    economics   338.1
    technology   634
Orchestras
  music   785.1–.8
  performance   785.06
Orchestrions *see* Mechanical
    musical instruments
Order
  work
    library functions   025.2
    museum functions   069
    see also other spec.
      organizations
Ordnance (firearms) *see*
    Firearms
Ordu Turkey   *area* –565
Orebro Sweden   *area* –487
Oregon (state)   *area* –795
Ores
  geology
    gen. wks.   553
    see also spec. minerals
  industries
    extractive
      economics   338.2
      technology
        metallurgy   **669**
        mining   622
Organic
  chemistry
    applied   †661
    pure   547
    see also spec. products

Organic (continued)
  evolution
    animals   591.3
    gen. wks.   **575**
    man   573.2
    plants   581.3
    see also other spec.
      organisms
  fertilizers *see* Fertilizers
Organization
  of American States
    gen. wks.   341.18
    see also spec. services
Organizational
  units
    mil. sci.
      gen. wks.   355.3
      see also spec. mil.
       branches
    see also Combat units
Organizations
  employee *see* Employer-
    employee
    relationships
  gen. wks.   **060**
  international peace **341.1**
  religion *see* Religious
    organizations
  social & welfare   **366–369**
  sociology *see* Behavior-
    groups
  students
    gen. wks.   **371**
    see also spec. levels of ed.
  see also   *s.s.*–06
Organs (instruments)
  manufacture
    economics   338.4
    technology   681
  music   786.6
Orient   *area* –5
Oriental
  churches
    religion   281
    see also Church buildings
Origami *see* Paper sculpture
Orinoco River
  gen. wks.   *area* –87
  see also other areas
Oriya *see* Prakrits
Orkney Isls.   *area* –411

494

Ownership
  marks
    husbandry   636.08
    spec. items   s.s.–027
Oxen *see* Cattle
Oxford Eng.   *area* –425
Oysters
  fisheries
    economics   338.3
    technology   †639
  food *see* Seafood
  marketing   658.8
  processing *see spec.*
        products
  see also Mollusca
Ozalid
  process *see* Special-process
        photography
Ozobrome
  process *see* Special-process
        photography
Ozotype
  process *see* Special-process
        photography

P

PAX *see* Private exchanges
PBX *see* Private exchanges
Pacific
  Coast states U.S.   *area* –79
  Ocean
    geography
      gen. wks.   910.09
      physical   †910.02
      geology   551.4
      history   909
    isls. *see* Oceania
    regional subj.
        treatment   *area* –16
    region
      geography   910.09
      history   909
      subject treatment   *area* –18
    see also spec. areas
Pacifism
  ethics   172
  see also Peace movements
Pack
  animals *see* Draft animals
Packaging *see* Shipment

Packing (operation) *see*
        Shipment
Pacts *see* Treaties
Paddling *see* Boating
Paenungulata
  paleozoology   569
  zoology   599.6
Pageantry *see* Pageants
Pageants
  customs   394
  music   782.9
  performance   791.6
  see also Water pageants
Pahari *see* Prakrits
Pahlavi *see* Iranian
Painless
  childbirth *see* Parturition
Paint
  shop practice *see* Surface
        finishing
Painted
  glass
    arts   748.5
    technology *see* Surface
        finishing
Painting
  arts
    fine   **751**
    minor
      ceramics   738.1
      glassware   748.5
    see also other art
        forms
    study & teaching
      elementary ed.   372.5
    see also   s.s.–07
  crafts
    gen. wks.   745.7
    interior decoration   747
    textiles   746.6
  industries *see* Surface
        finishing
  trades
    buildings
      economics   338.4
      technology   698.1
    see also other spec.
        structures
    woodwork *see* Trims
  see also Graphic expressions

Pathology (continued)
man
  gen. wks. 616.07
  psych. effects †155.9
plants
  agriculture 632
  botany 581.2
Patience (virtue) *see* Virtues
Patio
  furniture *see* Furniture
  lighting *see* Illumination
Patriotic
  holidays *see* Holidays
  societies
    gen. wks. 369
    see also spec. activities
  songs *see* National songs
Patternmaking
  foundries
    gen. wks. 671.2
    see also spec. metals
  garment industries
    commercial 687
    domestic 646.4
Pauline
  epistles
    liturgy 264
    N.T.
      gen. wks. 227
      see also Pseudepigrapha
Paupers *see* Poor people
Pavements
  engineering
    economics 338.4
    technology 625.8
  see also Trafficways
Pawnshops *see* Financial
      institutions
Pay
  plans *see* Wages
Paymaster's
  department *see* Payroll
      administration
Payroll
  administration
    business †658.32
    government
      gen. wks. †350
      see also spec. levels of
        govt.

Peace
  corps
    soc. planning *see* Planning
    spec. operations *see spec.*
        subj.
  movements
    international law **341.1**
    religion
      Christian †261.8
      see also other spec. rel.
Peacocks *see* Peafowl
Peafowl
  conservation †639
  culture 636.59
  food *see* Poultry
  see also Galliformes
Peahens *see* Peafowl
Peasant
  art *see* Folk art
Peasants *see* Social classes
Peccaries
  conservation †639
  culture 636.9
  see also Suiformes
Pederasty
  crime *see* Offenses
  sex *see* Sexual disorders
Pediatrics
  hygiene 613.97
  medicine
    gen. wks. 618.92
    surgery 617
Pedigrees
  stockbreeding
    gen. wks. 636.08
    see also spec. animals
  see also Genealogy
Pedology (child study) *see*
      Children
Pedology (soils) *see* Soils
Peebles Scotland *area* –414
Pekingese
  dogs *see* Miniature dogs
Pelagianism *see* Heresies
Pelagic
  birds
    conservation †639
    culture 636.6
    see also Procellariiformes

Political (continued)
  science
    ethics · 172
    gen. wks. · **320**
    law · **†340**
    pub. administration · **†350**
  songs *see* National songs
  unions
    geography · 910.09
    history · 909
    pol. sci. · 321
    subj. treatment · *area* –†171
Politics *see* Political science
Polity
  church *see* Ecclesiology
  gen. wks. *see* Political science
Poll
  taxes *see* Taxation
Pollution
  air *see* Air pollution
  soil *see* Soil pollution
  water *see* Water supply
Polo *see* Mallet games
Poltergeists *see* Ghosts
Polyandry *see* Marriage
Polygamy *see* Marriage
Polyglot
  dictionaries
    gen. wks. · 413
    see also · *s.s.*–03
Polygraphy *see* Collected
    writings
Polymerization
  plastics *see* Plastics
  process
    chem. tech. · 660
    chemistry · 547
    see also spec. products
  textiles *see* Textiles
Polynesia · *area* –96
Polynesian *see* Austronesian
Polyphaga *see* Coleoptera
Polyphonic
  music *see* Choral music
Polysaccharides
  chemistry · 547
  manufacture
    economics · 338.4
    technology · 664

Polysaccharides (continued)
  nutrition
    home econ. · 641.1
    physiology
      gen. wks. · 574.1
    see also spec. organisms
Polytheism
  philosophy · 110
  religion
    comparative · 291
    gen. wks. · 212
    see also spec. rel.
Pomeranian
  dogs *see* Miniature dogs
Ponds *see* Water bodies
Pongidae *see* Primates
Ponies
  husbandry · 636.1
  see also Equidae
Pontus · *area* –39
Poodles *see* Nonsporting dogs
Pool (game) *see* Indoor ball
    games
Pools (combinations)
  gambling *see* Gambling
  industrial *see* Combinations
  transportation *see*
    Transportation
    services
Pools (water)
  natural *see* Water bodies
  swimming *see* Swimming
    pools
Poor
  Clares *see* Religious
    congregations
  people
    psychology · †155.9
    sociology · 301.44
    welfare services · 362.5
Poploca *see* Macro-
    Otomanguean
Population
  density *see* Demography
  movement
    pol. sci. · **325**
    sociology · 301.3
  statistics *see* Demography
Porcelain
  arts · 738.2
  industries · 666

Privy
  councils *see* Cabinets
    (government
    agencies)
Prize
  fighting *see* Boxing
Prizes *see* Awards
Probabilities
  mathematics   519
  see also   *s.s.*–01
Probate
  law *see* Succession law
Probation *see* Reformative
    measures
Problem
  children *see* Exceptional
    children
Proboscidea *see* Paenungulata
Procellariiformes
  paleozoology   568
  zoology   598.4
Processions *see* Pageants
Procurement
  business   658.7
  government
    gen. wks.   †350
    see also spec. levels of
      govt.
  see also Acquisitions
Procyonidae
  paleozoology   569
  zoology   599.7
Procyonines
  conservation   †639
  culture   636.9
  see also Procyonidae
Prodigies *see* Superior
    intelligence
Producers'
  cooperatives *see* Production
Product
  research
    marketing *see* Market
      research & analysis
    technology
      gen. wks.   607
      see also spec. products
Production
  economics
    cooperatives   334
    gen. wks.   338

Production (continued)
  govt. control
    gen. wks.   †350
    see also spec. levels of
      govt.
  management
    economics   338.4
    technology   658.5
  technology *see spec.*
    industries
Profanity
  ethics   179
  religion
    Christian   241.3
    see also other spec. rel.
Professional
  education
    gen. wks.   378
    govt. control
      gen. wks.   †350
      see also spec. levels of
        govt.
    see also   *s.s.*–071
  ethics *see* Occupational ethics
  occupations
    economics
      labor   331.7
      production   338.4
    technology *see spec. subj.*
    see also Social classes
  writing *see* Rhetoric
Program
  music
    gen. wks.   781.5
    see also spec. mediums
  notes
    music
      gen. wks.   780.15
      see also spec. mediums
    see also other spec.
      performing arts
Programed
  learning *see* Individualized
    instruction
Programing *see* Operations
    research
Prohibited
  books
    book rarities   098
    library treatment 025.17

Protective
  adaptations *see* Ecology
  coatings
    application *see* Surface
      finishing
    manufacture *see spec.*
      kinds
  tariff
    economics 338
    govt. control 351.8
    pol. sci. 327
    taxation *see* Customs
      (taxes)
Protectorates *see* Dependent
    states
Proteles
  paleozoology 569
  zoology 599.7
Protestant
  Episcopal Church *see*
    Anglican churches
  sects *see* Protestantism
Protestantism
  religion †280
  see also *area* –176
Protestants *area* –176
Protocol
  diplomatic *see* Diplomacy
  social *see* Etiquette
Protozoa
  culture †639
  paleozoology 563
  zoology 593
Provençal
  ethnic groups *area* –174
  language 449
  lingual groups *area* –175
  see also other spec. subj.
Proverbs (general)
  folklore 398.9
  gen. wks. *see* Collected
    writings
  literature 808.88
Proverbs (O.T.) *see* Poetic
    books
Providence
  Isl. Indian Ocean *area* –69
Provincial
  governments *see* Central
    governments
  libraries *see* Government
    libraries

Proving
  grounds *see* Testing grounds
Prussia *area* –43
Psalmody *see* Hymnology
Psalms
  liturgy
    Christian 264
    see also other spec. rel.
  O.T. *see* Poetic books
  see also Hymnology
Pseudepigrapha
  Bible 229
  liturgy 264
Pseudo
  gospels *see* Gospels
Pseudopsychology
  gen. wks. 131
  personality 137–139
Psittaciformes
  paleozoology 568
  zoology 598.7
Psychiatric
  hospitals *see* Mental
    hospitals
  jurisprudence *see* Forensic
    medicine
  social work
    gen. wks. 362.2
    see also spec. services
Psychiatry
  gen. wks. †616.89
  pediatrics 618.92
  surgery 617
  see also Mental hygiene
Psychical
  research *see* Parapsychology
Psychoanalysis
  gen. wks. †150.19
  medicine †616.89
Psychological
  warfare
    administration 355.3
    pol. sci. 327
Psychology
  gen. wks. 150
  see also *s.s.* –01
Psychoneuroses
  med. sci.
    gen. wks. 616.85–.86
    pediatrics 618.92

Public
  education
    government (continued)
      support   379
    see also Public schools
  entertainment
    gen. wks.   **791**
    see also spec. activities
  expenditure
    administration *see*
      Financial
      administration
    economics   336.3
  finance *see* Finance
  health
    engineering *see* Sanitation
      engineering
    govt. control
      gen. wks.   †350
      see also spec. levels of
        govt.
    med. sci.
      animals
        gen. wks.   636.089
        see also spec. animals
      man   **614**
  information
    services
      gen. wks. *see*
        Communication
        services
      mil. sci. *see* Special
        services
  land
    economics   333.1
    landscaping   712–719
    see also   *area* –14
  libraries
    gen. wks.   **027.4**
    see also spec. functions
  morals
    govt. control
      gen. wks.   †350
      see also spec. levels of
        govt.
    police services   363.4
  opinion
    practical pol.   329
    sociology   301.15

Public (continued)
  order
    govt. control
      gen. wks.   †350
      see also spec. levels of
        govt.
    police services   363.3
  parks *see* Recreational land
  relations
    advertising *see*
      Advertising
    business
      economics   338.4
      technology   659.2
    effects
      psychology   †155.9
      sociology   301.15
    religion
      Christian   254.4
      gen. wks.   291.6
      see also other spec. rel.
  schools
    gen. wks.   371
    see also spec. levels of ed.
  securities
    administration
      gen. wks.   †350
      see also spec. levels of
        govt.
    economics
      investments   332.63
      transactions   336.3
  servants
    economics
      labor   331.7
      production   338.1–.4
    management *see*
      Personnel
    see also Civil service
  spending *see* Public
    expenditure
  utilities
    departments *see* Executive
      departments
    govt. control
      gen. wks.   †350
      see also spec. levels of
        govt.
    services   †363.6

Quantum
  mechanics
    gen. wks.   530.12
    see also spec. applications
  statistics
    gen. wks.   530.13
    see also spec. branches
Quarantine
  disease control
    animals
      gen. wks.   636.089
      see also spec. animals
    man   614
    plants
      gen. wks.   632
      see also spec. plants
    see also spec. diseases
  govt. control
    gen. wks.   †350
    see also spec. levels of
      govt.
Quarter
  horses *see* Ponies
Quartermasters *see* Special
      services
Quarters
  gen. wks. *see* Housing
    (dwellings)
  mil. sci.
    administration   355.6
    gen. wks.   355.7
    see also spec. mil.
      branches
Quartz
  mineralogy   549.6
  see also spec. forms
Quasi
  contract law *see* Private law
Quays *see* Docks
Quebec (province)   *area* –714
Queen's Birthday *see* Holidays
Quiche *see* Macro-Penutian
Quilting
  crafts   746.4
  industry
    economics   338.4
    technology   677
Quiz
  programs
    advertising *see* Broadcast
      advertising

Quiz (continued)
    entertainment *see spec.*
      mediums
Quizzes
  games *see* Puzzles
  tests *see spec. kinds*
Quoits *see* Pitching games
Quotations
  literature
    gen. wks.   808.88
    see also spec. lit.
  see also Collected writings
Quran *see* Koran

R

Rabbi *see* Clergy
Rabbinical
  writings
    literature *see spec.*
      literatures
  religion   296.1
Rabbits *see* Lagomorphs
Raccoons *see* Procyonines
Race
  animals *see* Sporting
    animals
  horses *see* Horses
Races
  domestic animals *see*
    Genetics
  human *see* Ethnology
Racial
  differences *see* Ethnology
  discrimination *see*
    Discriminatory
    practices
  groups *see* Ethnic groups
  integration
    education
      gen. wks.   †370.19
      see also spec. levels
      of ed.
    ethics   177
    pol. sci. *see* Civil rights
    sociology   **301.45**
  music *see* Ethnic music
  segregation
    education
      gen. wks.   †370.19
      see also spec. levels
      of ed.

Racial
  segregation (continued)
    ethics   177
    pol. sci. *see* Civil rights
    sociology   **301.45**
    see also Discriminatory
      practices
Racing
  aircraft *see* Air sports
  animals
    customs   394
    ethics   175
    gen. wks.   798
  boats *see* Boating
  horses *see* Equestrian sports
  motor vehicles *see* Motoring
  people *see* Track athletics
Racing-games *see* Child play
Racing-yachts *see* Sailing
    craft
Racket
  games
    customs   394
    gen. wks.   796.34
Racketeering *see* Offenses
Racketeers *see* Offenders
Racon
  engineering *see* Radar
  navigation
    aircraft   629.132
    ships   623.89
Radar
  astronomy
    gen. wks.   523.01
    see also spec. celestial
      bodies
  engineering
    economics   338.4
    technology
      gen. wks.   621.384 8
      military   623.7
    see also spec. branches
  platforms *see* Artificial
    islands
  see also Telecommunication
Radiant
  panel heating
    gen. wks.   697.7
    see also spec. applications

Radiation
  ionizing *see* Ionizing
    radiation
  paraphotic *see* Paraphotic
    phenomena
  radio waves *see* Hertzian
    waves
  solar *see* Solar radiation
  terrestrial
    gen. wks.   525
    meteorology   551.5
    see also Paraphotic
      phenomena
  thermal *see* Heat transfer
  visible light *see* Light
    (radiation)
Radiative
  heating
    engineering
      central   697.4–.5
      local   697.1
      see also Radiant panel
        heating
    see also spec. applications
Radiesthesia *see* Divination
Radio
  advertising *see* Broadcast
    advertising
  astronomy
    gen. wks.   523.01
    see also spec. celestial
      bodies
  beacons *see* Position finders
  classes *see* Extension
  compasses *see* Direction
    finders
  engineering
    economics   338.4
    technology
      gen. wks.   621.384
      military   623.7
  music *see* Theater music
  physics   537.5
  plays *see* Drama
  programs
    ethics   175
    production
      gen. wks.   791.44
      management   658
  teaching *see* Audio-visual
    materials
  see also Telecommunication

Rasp
  carving *see* Wood carvings
Ratchets *see* Gears
Rationalism
  philosophy   149
  psychology
    gen. wks.   †150.19
    see also spec. aspects
  religion
    gen. wks.   211
    see also spec. rel.
Rationing *see* Restricted
      consumption
Rats *see* Myomorphs
Rattanwork *see* Braiding
Rayon *see* Cellulosics
Reaction-time
  studies *see* Quantitative
      psychology
Reactors
  engineering
    electrical   621.313
    nuclear   621.48
  physics
    electrical   537.6
    nuclear   **539.75–.76**
  see also spec. kinds
Reader
  advisory services
    libraries   †025.5
    see also other spec.
      institutions
Readers
  elementary ed.   372.4
  linguistics
    English   428.6
    see also other spec.
      languages
Reading
  gen. wks.   **028**
  linguistics
    English   428.4
    see also other spec.
      languages
  psychology   †153.7
  study & teaching
    elementary schools 372.4
    see also   *s.s.–07*
Real
  property
    gen. wks. *see* Real-estate
  law *see* Private law

Real-estate
  business
    economics   338.4
    management   658
  economics   333.3
  law *see* Private law
  taxes *see* Taxation
Realism
  arts   709.03
  literature   808.8
  philosophy   149
  religion
    gen. wks.   291
    see also spec. rel.
Realization
  accounting *see* Financial
      accounting
Realty
  law *see* Private law
Reasoning
  philosophy   **160**
  psychology
    animals   †156
    gen. wks.   †153.4
Rebellion *see* Civil war
Recent
  Christian sects
    religion   289.9
    see also Church buildings
Receptions *see* Hospitality
Recipes
  food *see* Cookery
  formulas   *s.s.–021*
Recitals
  gen. wks.   780.73
  see also spec. mediums
Reclamation
  land *see* Land reclamation
  soil *see* Soil conservation
  water *see* Water
      reclamation
Recollects *see* Religious
      congregations
Recording
  accounting *see* Bookkeeping
  printed matter *see*
      Cataloging
Recordings
  gen. wks. *see*
      Electroacoustical
      devices

Recordings (continued)	
library treatment	025.17
see also	*s.s.–02*
Records	
management	
services	651
supplies *see* Supply	
administration	
Recreation (activity) *see*	
Recreational	
activities	
Recreation	
buildings	
architecture	725
construction	
economics	338.4
technology	690.5
pub. health	614
Recreational	
activities	
customs	**394**
ethics	175
folklore	398.8
mil. sci. *see* Special	
services	
performance	**790**
student life	
gen. wks.	†371.89
see also spec. levels	
of ed.	
see also Child play	
equipment	
manufacture	
economics	338.4
technology	688.7
marketing	658.8
see also spec. applications	
land	
geography *see spec. areas*	
land economics	333.7
landscaping	712
planning	
civic art	
cities	711
gen. wks.	719
sociology	301.3
see also spec. activities	
parks *see* Recreational land	
Recruitment	
employees	
business	658.31

Recruitment	
employees (continued)	
government	
gen. wks.	†350
see also spec. levels of	
govt.	
soldiers	
gen. wks.	355.2
see also spec. mil.	
branches	
Rectors *see* Clergy	
Red	
Sea *see* Indian Ocean	
Red	
meats	
cookery	641.6
gen. wks.	641.3
preservation	
commercial	664
home	641.4
Redemption	
religion	
Christian	234
gen. wks.	291.2
see also other spec. rel.	
see also Atonement	
Redemption of first-born male	
see Rites	
Redemptorists *see* Religious	
congregations	
Redistricting *see*	
Representation	
Reducing	
of overweight *see* Body	
contours	
salons *see* Slenderizing-	
salons	
Reductionism	
philosophy	146
psychologies	
gen. wks.	150.19
see also spec. aspects	
Reed	
instruments *see* Wind	
instruments (musical)	
organs	
manufacture	
economics	338.4
technology	681
music	786.9

Reemployment
  labor economics †331.1
  management 658.31
Reference
  libraries *see* Research
    libraries
  services
    libraries †025.5
    museums 069
    see also other spec.
      institutions
Reflection
  light *see* Light (radiation)
  radio waves *see* Hertzian
    waves
  sound waves 534
  thermal *see* Heat transfer
Reflex
  actions
    biology
      animals 591.1
      gen. wks. 574.1
      plants 581.1
      see also spec. organisms
    psychology
      animals †156
      gen. wks. †152.3
Reflexology *see* Reductionism
Reforestation *see* Forestation
Reform
  movements
    pol. status 322
    see also Group behavior
  schools *see* Reformatories
Reformation
  church history 270.6
  gen. history 940.2
Reformative
  measures
    criminology 364.6
    penology 365
Reformatories
  administration
    gen. wks. †350
    see also spec. levels of
      govt.
  criminology 364.7
Reformatory
  buildings *see* Prison
    buildings
  labor *see* Prison labor

Reformed
  churches
    religion
      American 285
      European 284
    see also Church buildings
Refractory
  materials
    manufacture
      economics 338.4
      technology 666
      metallurgical use 669.8
    see also other spec.
      applications
Refrigerators
  engineering
    economics 338.4
    technology
      gen. wks. 621.5
      see also spec. branches
  home economics 643
  see also spec. applications
Refuge
  programs *see* Wildlife
    reserves
Refugees *see* Displaced
    persons
Refuse
  disposal
    operations *see* Waste
      disposal
    structures *see* Sanitary
      engineering
    treatment *see* Garbage
      treatment
Regattas *see* Boating
Regencies *see* Executive
    departments
Regenerated
  cellulose *see* Cellulosics
Regeneration
  religion *see* Salvation
Regimentation *see* Group
    behavior
Regiments *see* Organizational
    units
Regional
  libraries *see* Public libraries
  planning *see* Planning

Sacrificial

  offerings

    customs 392–394

    religion

      gen. wks. 291.3

      see also spec. rel.

Saddlery

  economics 338.4

  technology 685

Saddles

  livestock equipment

    gen. wks. 636.08

    see also spec. animals

  manufacture *see* Saddlery

Sadism *see* Sexual disorders

Safe

  driving *see* Motoring

Safes

  manufacture *see*

    Locksmithing

  office equipment 651

  see also other spec.

    applications

Safety

  belts

    manufacture

      economics 338.4

      technology 688

    see also Safety measures

  equipment

    ind. management 658.2

    manufacture *see spec.*

      items

  measures

    govt. control

      gen. wks. †350

      see also spec. levels of

        govt.

    personnel management *see*

      Health programs

    schools *see* Hygiene

    technology

      gen. wks. **614.8**

      mining 622

    see also Industrial

      hygiene

Sagas *see* Mythology

Saguia el Hamra *area –64*

Sahara

  Algeria *area –65*

  gen. wks. *area –66*

Sailboating *see* Boating

Sailboats *see* Sailing craft

Sailing (activity) *see* Boating

Sailing

  craft

    engineering 623.82

    see also Transportation

      services

Sailors'

  songs *see* Folk songs

  yarns

    adventure *see* Seafaring

      life

    fiction *see* Fiction

Saint

  Christopher West

    Indies *area –729 7*

  Eustatius West

    Indies *area –729 7*

  Helena (isl.) *area –97*

  Lucia West Indies *area –729 8*

  Martin West Indies *area –729 7*

  Paul Isl. Indian

    Ocean *area –69*

  Pierre & Miquelon

    (isls.) *area –718*

  Vincent West Indies *area –729 8*

Saint

  Bernards *see* Working dogs

Saints

  folklore

    hist. & crit. 398.3–.4

    legends 398.2

  religion

    Christian 235

    gen. wks. 291.2

    see also other spec. rel.

Saints' days *see* Holy days

Sakarya Turkey *area –563*

Sakhalin *area –†57*

Salads

  cookery 641.8

  food tech. 664

Salamanders *see* Amphibians

Salaries *see* Wages

Sales

  catalogs

    books 017–019

    see also *s.s.–02*

  contracts

    bus. management *see*

      Salesmanship

    law *see* Private law

Sculpture (continued)
  religion
    Christian — 246
    gen. wks. — 291.3
    see also other spec. rel.
  study & teaching
    elementary ed — 372.5
    see also — *s.s.–07*
Scythia — *area* –39
Sea
  bears *see* Eared seals
  biology *see* Hydrographic
    biology
  cows
    culture — 636.9
    hunting
      industries — †639
      sports — 799.27
    see also Sirenia
  fishing *see* Salt-water fishing
  forces *see* Naval forces
  laws *see* Commercial law
  lions *see* Eared seals
  serpents *see* Imaginary
    animals
  warfare
    international law — 341.3
    mil. sci. — **359**
    see also hist. of spec. wars
  waters *see* Marine waters
Seadromes *see* Airports
Seafaring
  life
    gen. wks. — 910.4
    see also spec. aspects
Seafood
  cookery — 641.6
  gen. wks. — 641.3
  marketing — 658.8
  preservation
    commercial — 664
    home — 641.4
Seals (animals)
  eared *see* Eared seals
  earless *see* Earless seals
Seals (heraldry) *see* Heraldic
  design
Seals (stamps)
  manufacture
    gen. wks. — 671.8
    see also spec. metals

Seals (stamps) (continued)
  numismatics — †737
  see also spec. applications
Sealyhams *see* Terriers
Seamanship
  engineering — 623.88
  services — 387
Seaplanes *see* Heavier-than-air
  aircraft
Seaports *see* Harbors
Seas *see* Marine waters
Seasonal
  workers
    labor economics — 331.6
    see also Social classes
Seasons
  astronomy — 525
  meteorology — 551.5–.6
Sea-water
  conversion
    economics — 338.4
    technology
      gen. wks. — 628
      naval — 623.85
    see also spec. applications
Second
  coming of Jesus Christ *see*
    Advent
Secondary
  education
    gen. wks. — 373
    govt. control
      gen. wks. — †350
      see also spec. levels of
      govt.
  industries
    economics — 338.4
    govt. control
      gen. wks. — †350
      see also spec. levels of
      govt.
    management — 658
    technology *see spec.*
      industries
  school
    libraries *see* School
      libraries
  schools
    gen. wks. — 373.1–.2

Semiprecious
stones (continued)
industries
extractive
economics   338.2
technology   622
glyptics   736
Semiquantitative
analysis *see* Qualitative
analysis
Semiskilled
occupations *see* Occupations
Semisovereign
states *see* Dependent states
Semitic
ethnic groups   *area* –174
languages   **492**
lingual groups   *area* –175
see also other spec. subj.
Senates *see* Legislative bodies
Senegal   *area* –66
Senility *see* Gerontology
Senior
citizens *see* Aged people
colleges *see* Colleges
high schools *see* Secondary
schools
Sensation
physiology *see* Physiology
psychology *see* Perception
Sensationalism
philosophy   145
see also Perception
Sentiments
psychology   †152.4
see also Personality
Septic
tanks *see* Unsewered
structures
Serbia Yugoslavia   *area* –†497
Serbian *see* Serbo-Croatian
Serbo-Croatian
ethnic groups   *area* –174
language   491.8
lingual groups   *area* –175
see also other spec. subj.
Serenades
customs   392
music *see spec. mediums*
Serfs *see* Social classes

Serial
advertising
economics   338.4
technology   659.13
publications
printing   655.1–.3
publishing   655.5
see also Serials
Serials
general   **050**
library treatment   025.17
see also   *s.s.* –05
Series
writings *see* Collected
writings
Serigraphy *see* Silk-screen
printing
Sermons
Christian religion
gen. wks.   †252
pub. worship   264
gen. wks.   291.3
see also other spec. rel.
Serpentes
paleozoology   568
zoology   598.12
Serpents *see* Snakes
Service
club
songs *see* Fraternal songs
occupations see Occupations
stations (motor vehicles)
management   658
services
gen. wks.   388.3
repairs   629.28
Servomechanisms *see* Automatic
control
Session
laws *see* Statutes
Setters *see* Gun dogs
Setting-up
exercises *see* Gymnastics
Seven
Years' War
gen. wks.   940.2
see also spec. countries
Seventh-day
observance *see* Holy days
schools *see* Religious training

Sheep (continued)
  husbandry   636.3
  see also Bovoidea
Sheepdogs *see* Working dogs
Sheet-metal
  work
    gen. wks.
      economics   338.4
    technology
      gen. wks.   671.8
      see also spec. metals
    shipbuilding *see* Hull
      construction
    see also other spec.
      products
Shell
  carvings   736
  parakeets *see* Budgerigars
Shellac *see* Varnishes
Shellcrafts
  arts   745.55
  industry
    economics   338.4
    technology   679
Shellfish
  crustaceans *see* Crustaceans
  food *see* Seafood
  mollusks *see* Mollusks
Shells (artillery) *see*
    Ammunition
Shells (mollusks) *see* Mollusca
Shelters
  air raid *see* Blastproof
    structures
  livestock
    gen. wks.   636.08
    see also Farm buildings
  see also Welfare
Shepherd
  dogs *see* Working dogs
Sherbets *see* Frozen desserts
Sheriffs *see* Police
Shetland Isls.   *area* –411
Shibah *see* Funeral rites
Shields
  heraldic *see* Heraldry
  military *see* Armor
Shintoism
  culture groups
    geography   910.09
    history   909
    subject treatment   *area* –176

Shintoism (continued)
  philosophy   181
  religion   299
Ship
  canneries *see* Merchant
    ships
  engineering *see* Naval
    engineering
  handling *see* Seamanship
  railways *see* Railroads
Shipbuilding *see* Ships
Shipfitting *see* Hull
    construction
Shipment
  management   658.7
  services *see* Transportation
    services
Ships
  construction
    economics   338.4
    technology   623.82
  mil. sci.
    gen. wks.   355.8
    see also spec. mil. branches
  see also Transportation
    services
Ship-to-shore
  stations *see* Broadcasting
    stations
Shipworms *see* Mollusks
Shipwrecks
  rescue *see* Rescue operations
  travel   910.4
  see also Commercial law
Shipyards
  construction
    economics   338.4
    technology   627
    naval eng.   623.8
Shoats *see* Swine
Shock-resistant
  construction *see* Resistant
    construction
Shoes *see* Footwear
Shooting (activities)
  mil. sci.
    tactics *see* Tactics
    training *see* Training
      maneuvers
  sports   799.3
  see also Hunting (activity)
Shoplifters *see* Offenders

Small
  arms
    art metalwork   739.7
    manufacture
      economics   338.4
      technology
        gen. wks.   683
        military   623.4
    mil. sci.
      gen. wks.   355.8
      practice *see* Training
        maneuvers
      see also spec. mil.
        branches
  businesses
    economics   338.6
    management   †658
  craft
    engineering   623.82
    see also Transportation
      services
  forge work
    economics   338.4
    technology   682
Small-arms
  ammunition
    manufacture
      economics   338.4
      technology   623.4
    mil. sci.
      gen. wks.   355.8
      see also spec. mil.
        branches
    see also spec. applications
Small-boat
  installations *see* Docks
Smog *see* Air pollution
Smokers'
  supplies
    manufacture
      economics   338.4
      technology   688
    see also spec. applications
Smoking
  tobacco
    customs
      private   392
      public   394
    habit *see* Addictions
Smuggling *see* Offenses
Smyrna Turkey *see* Izmir

Snack
  bars *see* Public
    accommodations
Snakes
  agricultural pests   632
  culture   †639
  see also Serpentes
Snow
  formations
    climatology   †551.6
    meteorology   †551.5
  precipitation
    climatology   †551.6
    meteorology   †551.5
  removal
    highways *see* Highway
      maintenance
    runways *see* Runways
    streets
      economics   338.4
      technology   628
  sculpture   736
  sports
    customs   394
    gen. wks.   796.9
Snowfall *see* Snow precipitation
Snowshoeing *see* Snow sports
Snowshoes *see* Footwear
Snuff *see* Tobacco products
Soap
  sculpture
    arts   736
    study & teaching
      elementary ed.   372.5
      see also   s.s.–07
Soaps
  manufacture
    economics   338.4
    technology   668
  marketing   658.8
  see also spec. applications
Soaring
  engineering *see*
    Aerodynamics
  sports *see* Air sports
Soccer *see* Football
Social
  accounting *see* National
    accounting
  anthropology *see* Culture

Socioeconomic
  problems
    religion
      Christian   261.8
      gen. wks.   291
      see also other spec. rel.
    sociology   301.4–.5
  regions & groups   *area* –17
Sociology
  gen. wks.   301
  see also spec. applications
Socotra   *area* –67
Sodermanland Sweden   *area* –487
Sodomy
  crime *see* Offenses
  sex *see* Sexual disorders
Soft
  drinks
    drinking *see* Drinking
    manufacture
      economics   338.4
      technology
        commercial   663
        domestic   641.8
    marketing   658.8
Softball *see* Bat games
Sogdiana   *area* –39
Sogn og Fjordane
    Norway   *area* –483
Soil
  chemistry
    agriculture   631.4
    mineralogy   549.6–.7
  conditioners
    agriculture
      gen. wks.   631.8
      see also spec. crops
    manufacture
      economics   338.4
      technology   668
  conservation
    economics
      policies   333.7
      production   338.2
    practices   631.4
  erosion
    control meas.
      agriculture   631.4
      botany   581.5
    geology   551.3

Soil (continued)
  microbiology
    agriculture   631.4
    biology   576.16
  pollution
    countermeasures
      economics   338.4
      technology   628
      pub. health   614
  surveys
    agriculture   631.4
    engineering
      foundations   624
    see also spec. applications
  see also   *area* –†14
Soilless
  culture
    gen. wks.   631.5
    see also spec. crops
Soils
  agriculture
    gen. wks.   631.4
    see also spec. crops
  engineering
    gen. wks.   620.1
    see also Soil surveys
  geology
    gen. wks.   553
    mineralogy   549.6–.7
Sokotri *see* South Arabic
Solar
  astronomy
    descriptive   **523.7**
    tables   525
    theoretical   521
  batteries *see* Solar-energy
    engineering
  engines *see* Solar-energy
    engineering
  furnaces *see* Solar-energy
    engineering
  heating
    gen. wks.   697.7
    see also spec. applications
  houses *see* Residential
    buildings
  radiation
    astronomy   525
    chemistry *see*
      Photochemistry
    meteorology   551.5

Sporades Greece
  northern
    ancient   *area* –39
    modern   *area* –499
  southern *see* Dodecanese
Sport
  cars *see* Motor vehicles
Sporting
  animals
    culture
      gen. wks.   †636.08
      see also spec. animals
    dogs
      culture   636.75
      use
        hunting   799.2
        see also other spec.
          purposes
      see also Canidae
  goods *see* Recreational
    equipment
Sports (biological) *see*
    Genetics
Sports (recreation)
  customs   394
  equipment *see* Recreational
    equipment
  ethics   175
  gen. wks.   †796
  military *see* Special services
  student life
    gen. wks.   †371.89
    see also spec. levels of ed.
Sportmanship *see* Recreational
    activities
Sportswear *see* Garments
Springs (mechanical)
  engineering
    economics   338.4
    technology
      gen. wks.   621.8
      see also spec. branches
    see also Structural forms
    see also spec. applications
Springs (water) *see* Ground
    waters
Sprinkling
  streets *see* Street cleaning
Sprinting *see* Track athletics
Sprites *see* Supernatural
    beings

Squabs *see* Pigeons
Squadrons *see* Organizational
    units
Squash (sport) *see* Racket
    games
Squirrels *see* Sciuromorphs
Stabiles
  interior decoration   747
  sculpture   731.5
Stadiums *see* Recreation
    buildings
Staff
  organization *see* Hierarchy
Stafford Eng.   *area* –424
Stage
  animals *see* Stunt animals
  presentations *see* Theater
  scenery
    paintings   751.7
    stage presentations   792
Stained
  glass
    arts
      arch. decoration   729
      gen. wks.   748.5
    manufacture
      economics   338.4
      technology   666
    religion
      Christian   247
      gen. wks.   291.3
      see also other spec. rel.
Stairs
  architecture   721
  construction
    economics   338.4
    technology
      carpentry   694.6
      gen. wks.   690
    see also spec. structures
Stallions *see* Horses
Stammering *see* Speech
    disorders
Stamp
  taxes *see* Taxation
Stamps
  metallic *see* Seals (stamps)
  postage *see* Postage stamps
Standard
  of living *see* Cost of living

Storehouses
  gen. wks. *see* Storage
      buildings
  military *see* Military
      buildings
Stores *see* Commercial
      buildings
Storks
  conservation   †639
  culture   636.6
  see also Ciconiiformes
Storms
  climatology   †551.6
  history
    gen.wks.   †904
    see also spec. places
  meteorology   551.5
  see also Disasters
Storytelling
  library services   027.62
  rhetoric   808.54
  schools   †372.6
Strains (biological) *see*
      Genetics
Strains (mechanical)
  engineering
    materials   620.1
    structures   624
    see also spec. kinds
  mechanics
    solids   531
    see also spec. branches
Strategy
  mil. sci.
    gen. wks.   355.4
    see also spec. mil. branches
  see also hist. of spec. wars
Stratigraphy
  geology   551.7
  paleontology   560.17
Streams *see* Water bodies
Street
  cleaning
    engineering
      economics   338.4
      technology   628
      pub. health   614
  fighting *see* Battle tactics
  lighting *see* Illumination
  organs *see* Mechanical
        musical instruments
  songs *see* Folk songs

Streetcar
  advertising *see*
        Transportation
        advertising
Streets *see* Trafficways
Strength
  tests
    engineering
      materials   620.1
      structures   624
      see also spec. kinds
    physics   531
Stresses (mechanical) *see*
      Strains (mechanical)
Strikes (work stoppage)
  labor *see* Union-
        management
        disputes
  sociology *see* Group
        behavior
String
  bands *see* Orchestras
  basses *see* String instruments
  instruments
    manufacture
      economics   338.4
      technology   681
    music   787
Strings *see* Cordage
Structural
  analysis
    engineering
      gen. wks.   624
      see also spec. branches
    ships *see* Naval
        architecture
  clay products
    materials
      construction   691
      engineering   620.1
      see also spec. applications
  design *see* Structural analysis
  elements
    architecture   721
    area planning   711
    engineering *see* Structural
        analysis
  engineering
    gen. wks.   624
    see also spec. structures

Submarines *see* Warships
Submerged
  lands
    economics   333.9
    law   †340
Subnormal
  children *see* Exceptional
    children
Subscription
  libraries *see* Proprietary
    libraries
Subsonics
  engineering
    gen. wks.   †620.2–.3
    see also spec. branches
  physics   534.5
Substandard
  wage earners
    economics   331.5
    see also Social classes
Subsurface
  minerals *see* Mineral
    resources
  structures *see* Utility lines
  waters *see* Ground waters
Suburban
  communities
    geography   *area* –173
    planning *see* Planning
      communities
    see also spec. areas
  governments *see* Local
    governments
  land
    economics   333.7
    see also Real-estate
  living
    psychology   †155.9
    sociology   301.3
  parishes
    govt. & admin.   254.2
    see also spec. aspects
Subversive
  activities *see* Offenses
  groups
    pol. status   323.2
    sociology *see* Behavior-
      groups
Subways *see* Rapid transit
  railways

Successful
  living
    pseudopsychology   131.3
    psychology   †158
Succession
  law
    internal   347.6
    international   †341.5
Sudan   *area* –624
Sudanese *see* Chari-Nile
Sudanic *see* Chari-Nile
Suffolk Eng.   *area* –426
Suffrage
  laws   †340
  pol. sci.   324
Sufism *see* Personal religion
Sugars
  chemistry   547
  food
    cookery   641.6
    gen. wks.   641.3
  manufacture
    economics   338.4
    technology   664
  see also spec. products
Suicidal
  compulsions *see* Personality-
    disorders
Suicide
  crime *see* Offenses
  ethics   179
  soc. customs   394
Suiformes
  paleozoology   569
  zoology   599.7
Suites (music)
  gen. wks.   781.5
  see also spec. mediums
Sukkoth *see* Holy days
Sulpicians *see* Religious
  congregations
Sulu Archipelago   *area* –914
Sumatra   *area* –92
Sumerian
  ethnic groups   *area* –174
  language   499
  lingual groups   *area* –175
  see also other spec. subj.

Surface (continued)
  phenomena
    chemistry *see* Chemistry
    mechanics
      gases   533
      liquids   532
    piloting *see* Navigation
    tension *see* Surface
            phenomena
    treatment *see* Surface
            finishing
Surfboard
  riding *see* Boating
Surgery
  gen. medicine   617
  vet. sci.
    gen. wks.   636.089
    see also spec. animals
Surinam   *area* –88
Surnames *see* Personal names
Surrey Eng.   *area* –422
Sürt Turkey   *area* –566
Survey
  methods *see* Statistical
          method
Surveying
  engineering
    military   623.7
    public works   625
    see also other spec.
            branches
  gen. wks.   526.9
Surveys
  geography   910.4
  science   508.3
  soc. conditions   **309.1**
  soils *see* Soil surveys
  see also   *s.s.*–01
Survival
  training
    gen. wks.   †613.6
    mil. sci. *see* Training
            maneuvers
Survivors
  insurance   368.4
  welfare services   362.6
Survivorship
  law *see* Succession law
Susanna
  Apocrypha   229
  liturgy   264

Sussex Eng.   *area* –422
Sutherland Scotland   *area* –411
Suttees *see* Funeral rites
Svalbard   *area* –98
Svanetian *see* Caucasian
Svealand Sweden   *area* –487
Svetambara *see* Jainism
Swahili
  ethnic groups   *area* –174
  language   496
  lingual groups   *area* –175
  see also other spec. subj.
Swallows *see* Passeriformes
Swans
  culture   636.6
  see also Anseriformes
Swaziland   *area* –68
Sweden   *area* –485
Swedenborgianism *see* Church
            of the New Jerusalem
Swedish *see* Germanic
Sweets *see* Candies
Swifts *see* Passeriformes
Swimming
  activities
    hygiene   613.7
    sports   **797.2**
  pools
    architecture   725
    construction
      economics   338.4
      technology   690.5
    school equipment *see*
            School buildings
Swindlers *see* Offenders
Swindles *see* Defrauding
Swine
  disease carriers *see* Disease
            carriers
  husbandry   636.4
  see also Suiformes
Swing
  music *see* Jazz
Switzerland (country)   *area* –494
Swords *see* Side arms
Syllogism *see* Reasoning
Sylviidae *see* Passeriformes
Symbioses *see* Ecology
Symbolism
  art
    gen. wks.   704.94
    see also spec. art forms

Technical (continued)
services
    libraries   025
    museums   069
writing *see* Rhetoric
Techniques   *s.s.*–028
Technology
  gen. wks. *see* Industrial arts
  sociological effects   301.2
Tectonic
  geology *see* Structural
    geology
Tectonophysics *see* Structural
    geology
Teen
  agers *see* Young people
Tekirdag Turkey   *area* –496
Telautography *see*
    Telecommunication
Telecommunication
  gen. wks.   †001.5
  govt. control
    gen. wks.   †350
    see also spec. levels of
      govt.
  services   384.1–.7
  sociology   †301.16
  systems
    engineering
      economics   338.4
      technology
        gen. wks.   621.382–.389
        military   623.7
      see also spec. applications
    mil. sci.
      gen. wks.   358
      see also spec. kinds of
        warfare
    see also Language
Telegraphy *see*
    Telecommunication
Telemark Norway   *area* –482
Teleology
  metaphysics   124
  religion
    gen. wks.   210
    see also spec. rel.
Teleostei
  paleozoology   567
  zoology   597.5

Telepathy *see* Extrasensory
    perception
Telephonographs *see*
    Telecommunication
Telephony *see*
    Telecommunication
Telephotography
  gen. wks.   778.3
  see also spec. applications
Teleprinting *see*
    Telecommunication
Telescopes
  astronomy   522
  manufacture
    economics   338.4
    technology   681
  physics   535
  see also spec. applications
Telescopic
  sights *see* Range finders
Teletype
  telegraphy *see*
    Telecommunication
Teletypesetter
  composition *see* Machine
    typesetting
Teletypewriting *see*
    Telecommunication
Television
  advertising *see* Broadcast
    advertising
  cameras
    engineering
      economics   338.4
      technology   621.388 3
    photography *see*
      Television programs
  classes *see* Extension
  music *see* Theater music
  plays *see* Drama
  programs
    ethics   175
    production
      gen. wks.   791.45
      management   658
  teaching aids *see* Audio-
    visual materials
  see also Telecommunication
Telugu *see* Dravidian
Tempera
  painting *see* Painting arts
  paintings *see* Paintings

Thrushes *see* Passeriformes
Thysanoptera *see* Insects
Thysanura *see* Insects
Tibet   *area* –515
Tibetan *see* Tibeto-Burman
Tibeto-Burman
  ethnic groups   *area* –174
  languages   495
  lingual groups   *area* –175
  see also other spec. subj.
Ticks
  agricultural pests   632
  culture   †639
  disease carriers *see* Disease
      carriers
  see also Acari
Tidal
  waves
    gen. wks. *see* Marine
      waters
    history
      gen. wks.   †904
      see also spec. places
      see also Disasters
Tide
  tables
    astronomy   525
    navigation   623.89
Tidelands *see* Submerged
     lands
Tides
  astronomy   525
  oceans *see* Marine waters
Tie-dye
  techniques *see* Resist-dyeing
Tierra del Fuego
  Chile   *area* –83
  gen. wks.   *area* –82
Tigers *see* Cats
Tigris Valley *see* Mesopotamia
    (Middle East)
Tiles
  arts   738.6
  manufacture
    economics   338.4
    technology   666
  see also spec. applications
Tillage *see* Crop production
Time (duration)
  metaphysics   115
  see also Chronology

Time (rhythm) *see*
    Composition
Time
  studies
    production *see*
      Operational
      management
    psychology *see*
      Quantitative
      psychology
Timepieces
  art   739.3
  chronology   529
  manufacture
    economics   338.4
    technology   681
  see also spec. applications
Timor   *area* –92
Timothy (N.T.) *see* Pauline
    epistles
Timpani *see* Percussion
    instruments
Tinamiformes *see*
    Palaeognathae
Tinamous
  culture   636.6
  see also Palaeognathae
Tinsmithing
  arts   739
  manufacturing
    economics   338.4
    technology   673
  see also spec. products
Tinted
  etching *see* Aquatinting
  etchings *see* Prints
Tintype
  process *see* Special-process
    photography
Tinwork *see* Tinsmithing
Tipperary Ireland   *area* –419
Tires
  manufacture *see* Elastomers
  motor vehicles *see* Motor
    vehicles
Tishah b'Ab *see* Holy days
Titanium *see* Metals
Tithing *see* Financial
    administration

Topology (continued)
  geometry
    gen. wks. — 513
    see also — *s.s.*–01
Torah *see* Historical
      books (O.T.)
Tornadoes
  effects *see* Disasters
  meteorology *see* Storms
Tortoises *see* Turtles
Torts
  internal law — 347.5
  international law — †341.5
Tosefta *see* Talmud
Totalitarian
  states
    economics
      Marxian — **335.4**
      nationalist — 335.6
    pol. sci. — †321.9
    see also spec. areas
Totemism
  religion
    gen. wks. — 291.2
    see also spec. rel.
  soc. customs — 392
Totems *see* Totemism
Toucans
  culture — 636.6
  see also Piciformes
Touracos *see* Plantain eaters
Touring
  travel — 910.4
  see also Motoring
Tourist
  guides *see* Travels
  inns *see* Public
      accommodations
Tournaments
  soc. customs *see* Knightly
      customs
  sports *see spec. sports*
Tours *see* Travels
Towboats *see* Small craft
Towed
  craft
    construction
      economics — 338.4
      technology — 623.82
    see also Transportation
      services

Town
  governments *see* Local
      governments
  halls *see* Government
      buildings
  libraries *see* Public libraries
  meeting
    government *see* Pure
      democracy
Towns *see* Communities
Townships *see* Communities
Toy
  dogs *see* Miniature dogs
  theater *see* Miniature theater
Toys
  child play *see* Child play
  crafts — 745.59
  manufacture
    economics — 338.4
    technology — 688.7
  marketing — 658.8
Trabzon Turkey *see* Trebizond
Track
  athletics
    customs — 394
    gen. wks. — 796.4
  racing
    horses *see* Equestrian
      sports
Tracking
  game *see* Hunting (activity)
Traction
  systems *see* Electric traction
Tractors
  agriculture — 631.3
  engineering
    economics — 338.4
    technology
      gasoline — 629.22
      steam — 621.1
    see also spec. applications
Trade (activity)
  govt. control
    gen. wks. — †350
    *see also spec. levels of
      govt.*
  management — **†658.8**
  services
    gen. wks. — †380.1
    see also spec. kinds

Trade
  catalogs
    books *see* Publishers'
      catalogs
    spec. subj.   *s.s.*–02
  lanes *see* Transportation
    services
  schools *see* Vocational
    education
Trading
  procedures
    commerce *see* Commerce
      (activity)
    finance
      economics   332.6
      govt. control
        gen. wks.   †350
      see also spec. levels
        of govt.
Traditionalism *see* Dogmatism
Traditions *see* Customs
  (conventions)
Traffic
  flow *see* Traffic management
  management
    ind. plants   658.7
    trafficways   388.3
  safety *see* Safety measures
  violations *see* Offenses
Trafficways
  eng. & construction
    gen. wks.   625.7
    military   623.6
  farm structures   631.2
  govt. control
    gen. wks.   †350
    see also spec. levels of
      govt.
  landscaping   713
  planning   711
  see also Transportation
    services
Tragedy *see* Drama
Tragulida
  paleozoology   569
  zoology   599.7
Trailer
  camps *see* Public
    accommodations
  travel *see* Motoring

Trailers
  architecture   728
  construction
    economics   338.4
    technology   629.22
  see also spec. applications
Trailing
  game *see* Hunting (activity)
Training
  maneuvers
    gen. wks.   355.5
    see also spec. mil.
      branches
Trains
  eng. & construction
    economics   338.4
    technology
      gen. wks.   625.2
      military   623.6
  see also Transportation
    services
Traitors *see* Offenders
Trajectories
  ballistics   623.5
  mechanics
    gen. wks.   531
    see also Orbits
Trampolining *see* Gymnastics
Transcendentalism
  philosophy
    gen. wks.   141
    metaphysics   **111.8**
  psychology *see* Occultism
Transcription (music) *see*
    Arrangement
    (music)
Transfiguration
  of Jesus Christ
    feast *see* Holy days
    gen. wks.   232.95
    meditations   242.3
Transformers
  elect. eng.
    economics   338.4
    technology   621.31
  see also spec. applications
Transit
  taxes *see* Customs (taxes)
Transits
  astronomy
    descriptive   523.9

Troop (continued)
  carriers *see* Heavier-than-air
    aircraft
  movements *see* Logistics
  ships *see* Government vessels
Troops *see* Organizational units
Tropic
  birds *see* Gannets
  photography *see* Hot-
    weather photography
Tropical
  plants
    botany   581.909
    floriculture   635.9
    see also spec. plants
Tropics
  climatology   †551.6
  geography   910.09
  history   909
  subj. treatment   *area* –13
  see also spec. areas
Troy (ancient city)   *area* –39
Trucial Oman   *area* –53
Trucks *see* Motor
  vehicles
Trumpets *see* Wind instruments
  (musical)
Trunks *see* Luggage
Trust Territory of the Pacific
  Isls.   *area* –96
Trust
  companies
    banks *see* Financial
      institutions
    industrial *see*
      Combinations
  services
    banks   †332.1
    courts   347.9
  territories *see* Dependent
    states
Truth
  metaphysics   111.8
  religion
    gen. wks.   210
    see also spec. rel.
Truthfulness
  ethics   177
  religion
    Christian   241.4
    see also other spec. rel.

Tsimshian *see* Macro-Penutian
Tuamotu Isls.   *area* –96
Tuareg *see* Berber
Tuataras *see* Lepidosauria
Tubas *see* Wind instruments
  (musical)
Tubes
  manufacture
    economics   338.4
    technology   671.8
  materials
    engineering
      gen. wks.   620.1
      see also spec.
        applications
    see also Materials-handling
Tubuai Isls.   *area* –96
Tugboats *see* Small craft
Tulu *see* Dravidian
Tumbling *see* Gymnastics
Tunceli Turkey   *area* –566
Tundra *see* Plains
Tungsten *see* Metals
Tungusic
  ethnic groups   *area* –174
  languages   494
  lingual groups   *area* –175
  see also other spec. subj.
Tunicata
  paleozoology   566
  zoology   596
Tunisia   *area* –61
Tunneling
  mining   622
  see also Tunnels
Tunnels
  architecture   725
  construction
    economics   338.4
    technology
      gen. wks.   624
      military   623.6
  govt. control
    gen. wks.   †350
    see also spec. levels of
      govt.
  transportation   388.1
  see also other spec.
    applications
Tupi *see* Amerindians

Ugro-Ostyak *see* Finno-Ugric
Uighur *see* Turkic
Ukraine   *area* –†477
Ukrainian
  ethnic groups   *area* –174
  language   491.79
  lingual groups   *area* –175
  see also other spec. subj.
Ukuleles *see* String instruments
Ulster Ireland   *area* –416
Ultramicrobes
  biology   576
  medicine
    animals
      gen. wks.   636.089
      see also spec. animals
    man   616.01
    see also spec. diseases
Ultrasonic
  vibrations *see* Ultrasonics
Ultrasonics
  engineering
    gen. wks.   †620.2
    see also spec. branches
  physics   534.5
  see also spec. applications
Ultraviolet *see* Paraphotic
    phenomena
Unarmed
  combat
    ethics   175
    gen. wks.   613.6
    mil. training *see* Training
      maneuvers
    sports
      management   658
      performance   796.8
Unconscious
  metaphysics   127
  psychology *see* Depth
    psychology
Unconventional
  warfare
    history *see hist. of spec.*
      countries
    services *see* Special
      services
Underconsumption
  economics
    gen. wks.   339.4
    see also spec. elements
  see also other spec. aspects

Undergraduate
  schools *see* Universities
Underground
  railways *see* Rapid transit
    railways
  waters *see* Ground waters
Underpasses *see* Bridges
Underprivileged
  classes *see* Social classes
Understanding *see* Perception
Undertaking
  customs *see* Funeral rites
  pub. health   614
Underwater
  operations
    engineering
      economics   338.4
      technology   627
    services   387.5
    see also Diving
  photography
    gen. wks.   778.7
    see also spec. applications
Underwear *see* Garments
Underweight
  people
    cookbooks   641.5
    hygiene   613.2
    see also Body contours
Unemployment
  insurance
    gen. wks.   368.4
    see also Financial
      institutions
  labor economics   331.1
  managerial aspects   †658.31
Unfunded
  debts *see* Public securities
Unguiculata
  paleozoology   569
  zoology   599.3
Ungulates *see* Hoofed
    mammals
Unicameral
  legislatures *see* Legislative
    bodies
Unicellular
  animals *see* Protozoa
  plants *see* Schizomycetes

Uniforms
  customs *see* Costume
  garments *see* Garments
  mil. sci.
    administration 355.6
    gen. wks. 355.8
    see also spec. mil.
      branches
Unincorporated
  companies
    economics 338.7
    management †658
    see also *s.s.–065*
Union
  Isls. *see* Tokelau
  of Soviet Socialist Republics
      see Soviet Union
Union
  catalogs
    books 017–019
    library functions †021.6
    see also *s.s.–021*
  rugby *see* Football
Union-management
  disputes
    conciliation practices 331.15
    gen. wks. 331.89
  relationships *see* Employer-
      employee
      relationships
Unions
  labor
    economics **331.88**
    management 658
  see also Organizations
Unit
  method *see* Project method
  operations
    gen. wks. 660.28
    see also spec. products
  packaging
    production *see*
      Operational
      management
  processes *see* Synthesis
Unitarian
  Church *see* Unitarianism
  Universalist Association *see*
      Unitarianism

Unitarianism
  religion 288
  see also Church buildings
Unitary
  states
    pol. sci. 321
    see also spec. areas
United
  Arab Republic *see* Egypt
  Kingdom *area* –42
  States of America *area* –73
United
  Brethren
    in Christ *see* Recent
      Christian sects
    Moravian *see* Moravian
      Church
  charities *see* Community
      welfare
  Church of Canada *see*
      Methodist churches
  Church of Christ *see*
      Congregationalism
  Confederate Veterans *see*
      Military societies
  Daughters of the
      Confederacy *see*
      Hereditary societies
  Free Church *see* Moravian
      Church
  Nations
    gen. wks. 341.13
    see also spec. services
  Society of True Believers in
      Christ's Second
      Appearing *see*
      Shakers
Uniterms *see* Subject headings
Unitized
  cargo *see* Transportation
      services
Unity
  metaphysics 111.8
  rhetoric *see* Rhetoric
Unity School of Christianity
      see Recent Christian
      sects
Universal
  algebra
    gen. wks. 512
    see also *s.s.–01*

Universal (continued)
bibliographies †011
history *see* World history
languages †401
Universalism *see* Economic
systems
Universalist
Church
religion 289.1
see also Church buildings
Universe *see* Cosmology
Universities
gen. wks. 378.1
govt. control
gen. wks. †350
*see also spec. levels of
govt.*
see also s.s.–071
University
buildings *see* College
buildings
libraries *see* College
libraries
songs *see* Student songs
Universology *see* Cosmology
Unlawful
assembly *see* Offenses
Unmarried
mothers
sociology †301.41
welfare services †362.8
Unsewered
structures
archeology †913.03
engineering
economics 338.4
technology 628
Unskilled
work
economics
labor 331.7
production 338.1–.4
see also spec. subj.
Untouchables *see* Social
classes
Upanishads
literature 891.2
religion 294.5
Upholstery
interior decoration
art 747
home economics 645

Upholstery (continued)
manufacture *see* Textiles
Upper
Volta *area* –66
Upper
atmosphere
meteorology
gen. wks. 551.5
*see also spec.
phenomena*
regional subj.
treatment *area* –16
Uppsala Sweden *area* –487
Uralic
ethnic groups *area* –174
languages 494
lingual groups *area* –175
see also other spec. subj.
Uranium *see* Metals
Uranography *see* Descriptive
astronomy
Urban
communities
geography *area* –173
planning *see* Planning
communities
see also spec. areas
land
economics
gen. wks. 333.7
see also Real-estate
living
psychology †155.9
sociology 301.3
parishes
govt. & admin. 254.2
see also spec. aspects
redevelopment *see* Slums
redevelopment
sanitation *see* Municipal
engineering
Urbanists *see* Religious
congregations
Urdu *see* Prakrits
Urfa Turkey *area* –565
Urns *see* Containers
Urodela *see* Amphibians
Ursidae
paleozoology 569
zoology 599.7
Ursulines *see* Religious
congregations

580

Vaulting *see* Track athletics
Veal *see* Red meats
Vectors (disease) *see* Disease
    carriers
Vedas
  literature   891.2
  religion   294
Vedic *see* Sanskrit
Vegetable
  fats *see* Fats
  juices *see* Soft drinks
  oils *see* Fixed oils
  waxes *see* Waxes
Vehicles
  architectural design   725
  construction
    economics   338.4
    technology
      gen. wks.   **629**
      military   623.7
  marketing   658.8
  see also Ships
Velocipedes *see* Cycles
    (vehicles)
Vending
  machines
    engineering *see* Automatic
      control
    marketing *see* Distribution
      channels
Veneering
  arch. decoration   729
  see also Woodcrafts
Veneers
  manufacture
    economics   338.4
    technology   674
  materials
    construction   691
    engineering   620.1
  see also spec. applications
Venezuela   *area* –87
Venison *see* Game food
Ventilating
  equipment
    ind. management   658.2
    manufacture *see spec.*
      items
Ventilation
  engineering
    gen. wks.   697.9

Ventilation
  engineering (continued)
    mines   622
    see also other spec.
      applications
  ind. management   658.2
  specific structures
    households   644
    libraries   022
    museums   069
    schools *see* School
      buildings
Ventriloquism *see* Magic arts
Vermes
  paleozoology   565
  zoology   595
Vermont   *area* –743
Versification *see* Prosody
Vertebrates
  paleozoology   566
  zoology   596
Vespidae *see* Hymenoptera
Vessels (aircraft) *see* Aircraft
    (vehicles)
Vessels (containers) *see*
    Containers
Vessels (ships) *see* Ships
Vest-Agder Norway   *area* –482
Vestfold Norway   *area* –482
Vestments
  art   **746**
  manufacture
    economics   338.4
    technology   687
  religion
    Christian   247
    gen. wks.   291.3
    see also other spec. rel.
Veterans'
  benefits *see* Postmilitary
    benefits
  Day *see* Holidays
Veterans of Foreign Wars *see*
    Military societies
Veterinary
  sciences
    gen. wks.   636.089
    see also spec. animals
  services
    mil. sci. *see* Special
      services

Vocal
  expressions
    ethics   177
    etiquette   395
    physiology *see* Physiology
    psychology
      animals   †156
      gen. wks.   †152.3
    rhetoric   808.5
  music *see* Songs
Vocation
  religious *see* Monastic life
Vocational
  education
    adults   †374
    young people   †373.2
    see also   *s.s.*–07
  guidance *see* Vocational
          interests
  interests
    education
      gen. wks.   371.42
      see also spec. levels
        of ed.
    psychology   †158.6
    see also Aptitudes
  schools *see* Vocational ed.
Voice
  gen. wks. *see* Vocal
      expressions
  music *see* Songs
  recording & reproducing
    see Electroacoustical
    devices
Volapük *see* Artificial
    languages
Volatile
  oils *see* Essential oils
Volcanoes
  geography
    gen. wks.   †910.02
    see also spec. places
  geology   551.2
  history
    gen. wks.   904
    see also spec. places
  see also Disasters
Volition *see* Will
Volleyball *see* Net (texture)
    games

Voluntarism
  philosophy   141
  see also spec. philosophers
Voluntary
  actions *see* Will
  revenues *see* Nontax
    revenues
Voodooism *see* Witchcraft
Voting
  laws   †340
  pol. sci.   324
Votyak *see* Finnic
Voyages *see* Travels
Vulcanism *see* Volcanoes
Vultures
  agricultural pests   632
  see also Falconiformes

W

Waffle
  irons *see* Household
    appliances
Wagers *see* Gambling
Wages
  administration
    business   †658.32
    government
      gen. wks.   †350
      see also spec. levels of
      govt.
    economics   331.2
Wagons *see* Wheeled
    supports
Wagtails (birds) *see*
    Passeriformes
Wake
  Isl.   *area* –96
Waldensian
  Church   284
  see also Heresies
Wales   *area* –429
Walking (activity) *see*
    Outdoor life
Walkouts
  labor *see* Union-management
    disputes
  sociology *see* Group
    behavior
Walks *see* Trafficways
Wallabies *see* Marsupials

Waste
  disposal
    engineering *see* Waste
      treatment
    govt. control   352
    pub. health   614
  salvage
    management   658.5
    see also spec. industries
  treatment
    engineering
      economics   338.4
      technology   628
  utilization
    economics   338.4
    technology
      gen. wks.   679
    see also spec. products
Wasteland
  economics
    gen. wks.   333.7
    see also Real-estate
  reclamation *see* Land
    reclamation
Watch-animals *see* Working
  animals
Watchcases
  art metalwork   739.3
  see also Horology
Watches *see* Timepieces
Water
  bodies
    economics *see* Water
      supply
    engineering *see* Hydraulic
      engineering
    geography
      gen. wks.   910.09
      physical   †910.02
    geology
      activities   551.3
      morphology   551.4
      resources   553
    landscape elements   714
    regional subj.
      treatment   *area* −166
    safety measures *see* Safety
      measures
  buffaloes
    culture   636.2
    see also Bovoidea

Water (continued)
  conservation
    agriculture
      economics
        policies   333.9
        production   338.2
      technology   631.7
    engineering *see* Water
      reclamation
  games
    customs   394
    sports   797.2
  gardens
    culture
      gen. wks.   635.96
      see also spec. plants
    landscaping   714
  pageants
    customs   394
    performance   797.2
  plants *see* Hydrophytes
  pollution *see* Water supply
  polo *see* Water games
  purification *see* Water supply
    engineering
  reclamation
    agriculture *see* Water
      conservation
    engineering
      economics   338.4
      technology   627
  safety *see* Safety measures
  sports *see* Aquatic sports
  storage
    flood control *see* Flood
      control
    gen. wks. *see* Water
      supply
  supply
    economics
      production   **338.2**
      resources   333.9
    engineering
      economics   338.4
      technology
        gen. wks.   628
        military   623.7
        see also other spec.
          branches
      see also Plumbing
    geology *see* Water bodies

Weather	
folklore	
hist. & criticism	398.3
legends	398.2
physical geology	†551.6
Weathering	
materials *see* Deterioration	
soils *see* Soil erosion	
Weatherings	
installation	695
manufacture *see spec.*	
materials	
Weather-satellites *see*	
Artificial satellites	
Weaver	
finches *see* Passeriformes	
Weaverbirds *see* Passeriformes	
Weaving	
crafts	746.1
industry	677
study & teaching	
elementary ed.	372.5
see also	*s.s.*–07
Wedding	
music	
gen. wks.	783.2
see also spec. mediums	
rites *see* Marriage rites	
Wedges *see* Simple machines	
Weed	
killers *see* Pesticides	
Weeds	
agricultural pests	632
botany	
gen. wks.	581.6
see also spec. plants	
Weeks (feast of) *see* Holy	
days	
Weight	
gaining programs *see*	
Underweight people	
lifting *see* Gymnastics	
losing programs *see*	
Overweight people	
Weights *see* Metrology	
Weimaraners *see* Gun dogs	
Weirs	
hydraulic eng.	627
see also Hydrodynamics	
Welding	
metals	
arts	739
shipbuilding *see* Hull	
construction	
technology	
gen. wks.	671.5
see also spec. metals	
see also spec. products	
Welfare	
administration	
private	658
public	
gen. wks.	†350
see also spec. levels of	
govt.	
social	
gen. wks.	†350
see also spec. levels of	
govt.	
buildings	
architecture	725
construction	
economics	338.4
technology	690.5
departments *see* Executive	
departments	
services	
personnel management	
business	658.38
government	
gen. wks.	†350
see also spec. levels	
of govt.	
public	**†363**
religion	
Christian	258–259
gen. wks.	291.7
see also other spec. rel.	
social	**361–362**
work	
private	361.7
public	361.6
see also Community welfare	
Welsh	
corgis *see* Working dogs	
language *see* Celtic	
Wendish	
ethnic groups	*area* –174
language	491.8
lingual groups	*area* –175
see also other spec. subj.	

Wigs
  manufacture
    economics   338.4
    technology   679
  marketing
    services   †380.1
    technology   658.8
  see also Hairdressing
Wigtown Scotland   *area* –414
Wild
  flower
    gardens
      gen. wks.   635.96
      see also spec. plants
  flowers *see* Flowering plants
Wildcats *see* Cats
Wildings *see* Exceptional
         children
Wildlife
  conservation
    economics
      policies   333.7
      production   338.3
    laws   †340
    practices   †639
  refuges *see* Wildlife reserves
  reserves
    area planning   719
    conservation practices   †639
    geography *see spec. areas*
    land economics   333.7
Will
  metaphysics   123
  psychology   †153.8
  religion
    Christian
      gen. wks.   233
      salvation   234
    gen. wks.   291.2
    see also other spec. rel.
Wills
  law *see* Succession law
Wiltshire Eng.   *area* –423
Wind
  engines
    engineering
      economics   338.4
      technology
        gen. wks.   621.4
        see also spec.
          branches
    see also spec. applications

Wind (continued)
  instruments (musical)
    manufacture
      economics   338.4
      technology   681
    music   788
Wind-driven
  craft *see* Sailing craft
Windmills *see* Wind engines
Windows
  architecture   721
  construction
    economics   338.4
    technology
      carpentry   694.6
      gen. wks.   690
  glazing
    economics   338.4
    technology   698.5
  see also spec. structures
Winds
  geography
    gen. wks.   †910.02
    see also spec. places
  geology
    activities   551.3
    climatology   †551.6
    meteorology   551.5
  see also Storms
Windstorms *see* Storms
Windward Isls. West
         Indies   *area* –729 8
Wine
  cookery   641.6
  drinking *see* Drinking
  making *see* Wines
Wines
  manufacture
    economics   338.4
    technology
      commercial   663
      domestic   641.8
  marketing
    technology   658.8
    see also Liquor traffic
  pub. health meas.   614
Winnetka
  system *see* Individualized
       instruction

Wooden
  primary products *see* Wood-
      using industries
  shoes *see* Footwear
Woodland
  gardens *see* Wild flower
      gardens
  reserves *see* Forest reserves
Woodpeckers *see* Piciformes
Woods (forests) *see* Forests
Woods (substance)
  materials
    construction   691
    engineering   620.1
  processing *see* Lumber
  see also spec. products
Wood-using
  industries
    economics   338.4
    technology   674
Woodwinds *see* Wind
     instruments (musical)
Woodwork
  crafts *see* Woodcrafts
  trim *see* Trims
Woodworking
  tools *see* Tools
Woody
  plants
    floriculture   **635.93**
    landscaping   715
    see also Spermatophyta
Woolens *see* Textiles
Worcester Eng.   *area* –424
Word
  games *see* Puzzles
Words
  linguistics *see* Etymology
  spec. subj.   *s.s.*–01
Work
  efficiency
    economics   331.8
  management
    private   658.38
    public
      gen. wks.   †350
      see also spec. levels
          of govt.
  psychology   158.7
  songs *see* Topical songs

Working
  animals
    culture
      gen. wks.   †636.08
      see also spec. animals
    see also Draft animals
  classes *see* Social classes
  dogs
    culture   636.7
    use *see spec. purposes*
    see also Canidae
Workmen's
  compensation insurance *see*
       Disability insurance
Workshops
  education *see* Extension
Work-study
  programs *see* Laboratory
      methods
World
  government *see*
     International
     relations
  history
    gen. wks.   **909**
    see also spec. subj.
  order
    pol. sci. *see* International
      relations
    religion
      Christian   †261.8
      gen. wks.   291
      see also other spec. rel.
  peace *see* Peace movements
  state
    pol. sci.   321
    see also World history
  trade *see* Trade (activity)
  see also Cosmology
World War I
  gen. wks.   940.3
  see also spec. countries
World War II
  gen. wks.   **940.53**
  see also spec. countries
Worms
  agricultural pests   632
  culture   †639
  see also Vermes

Young
  people (continued)
    organizations
      gen. wks. 369
      see also spec. activities
    psychology †155.5
    sociology
      gen. wks. 301.43
      welfare services 362.7
    see also Children
  Women's
    Christian Associations
      gen. wks. 267
      see also spec. services
    Hebrew Associations
      gen. wks. 296.6
      see also spec. services
Youth *see* Young people
Yozgat Turkey *area* –563
Yugoslav *see* Serbo-Croatian
Yugoslavia *area* –497
Yukian *see* Hokan-Siouan
Yukon (ter.) *area* –712
Yurak *see* Samoyedic

Z

Zacharias (O.T.) *see* Prophetic books
Zambia *see* Northern Rhodesia
Zanzibar *area* –678
Zapotec *see* Macro-Otomanguean
Zebras
  husbandry 636.1
  see also Equidae
Zebrula
  husbandry 636.1
  see also Equidae
Zebrule *see* Zebrula
Zebus
  culture 636.2
  see also Bovoidea
Zechariah (O.T.) *see* Prophetic books
Zen *see* Buddhism
Zephaniah (O.T.) *see* Prophetic books
Zeppelins *see* Lighter-than-air aircraft
Zetland Scotland *see* Shetland Isls.

Zinc *see* Metals
Zincographs *see* Prints
Zincography *see* Planographic processes
Zircon
  glyptics 736
  mineralogy 549.6
Zithers *see* String instruments
Zodiac
  astrology 133.5
  astronomy 523.2
  folklore 398.3
Zodiacal
  light
    astronomy 523.5
    meteorology 551.5
  signs *see* Zodiac
Zonguldak Turkey *area* –563
Zoning
  govt. control 352
  laws †340
Zoo
  animals
    culture
      gen. wks. 636.08
      see also spec. animals
    zoology 591
Zoogeography *see* Biogeography
Zoological
  gardens
    gen. wks. 590.74
    see also Recreational land
  sciences
    agriculture **636–638**
    paleozoology 562–569
    zoology **591**
    see also s.s.–01
Zoology *see* Zoological sciences
Zootechny *see* Livestock
Zoroastrianism
  culture groups
    geography 910.09
    history 909
    subj. treatment *area* –176
  philosophy 181
  religion 295
Zulu *see* Niger-Congo
Zululand *area* –68
Zwinglianism *see* Reformed churches